Introduction to
Acupuncture and Moxibustion

World Century Compendium to TCM

World Century Compendium to TCM – Vol. 6

Introduction to
Acupuncture
and Moxibustion

Ren Zhang
Shanghai Literature Institute of Traditional Chinese Medicine, China

translated by
Xue-min Wang

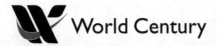
World Century

Published by

World Century Publishing Corporation
27 Warren Street
Suite 401-402
Hackensack, NJ 07601

Distributed by

World Scientific Publishing Co. Pte. Ltd.

5 Toh Tuck Link, Singapore 596224

USA office: 27 Warren Street, Suite 401-402, Hackensack, NJ 07601

UK office: 57 Shelton Street, Covent Garden, London WC2H 9HE

Library of Congress Cataloging-in-Publication Data
Zhang, Ren (Acupuncturist), author.
   Introduction to acupuncture and moxibustion / by Zhang Ren ; translated by Xuemin Wang.
      pages ; cm. -- (World Century compendium to TCM ; v. 6)
   Includes index.
   ISBN 978-1-938134-25-8 (softcover: alk. paper)
   I. Title.
   [DNLM: 1. Acupuncture Therapy. 2. Moxibustion. WB 369]
   RM184
   615.8'92--dc23
                                        2013018323

British Library Cataloguing-in-Publication Data
A catalogue record for this book is available from the British Library.

**World Century Compendium to TCM
A 7-Volume Set**

INTRODUCTION TO ACUPUNCTURE AND MOXIBUSTION
Volume 6
Copyright © 2013 by World Century Publishing Corporation

Published by arrangement with Shanghai Scientific & Technical Publishers.

Originally published in Chinese
Copyright © Shanghai Scientific & Technical Publishers, 2005
All Rights Reserved.

ISBN 978-1-938134-34-0 (Set)
ISBN 978-1-938134-25-8 (pbk)

Typeset by Stallion Press
Email: enquiries@stallionpress.com

Printed in Singapore

Foreword

The science of acupuncture and moxibustion is an indispensable part of traditional Chinese medicine and has made great contribution to the development and prosperity of the Chinese nation. For the thousands of years the Chinese people have appreciated it for its non-pharmaceutical treatment, simple application, wide range of use, good curative effect, and low cost.

As a part of Chinese science and culture, acupuncture and moxibustion have long been known in the world as a result of cultural exchange between China and other countries. However, a global interest in acupuncture and moxibustion and special enthusiasm for the subject have been growing in recent years. This edition will definitely satisfy those who are really interested in learning acupuncture and moxibustion therapy.

This book consists five parts: introduction to acupuncture and moxibustion, meridians and collaterals, acupoints, techniques of acupuncture and moxibustion, and clinical applications of acupuncture and moxibustion. It covers 167 acupoints, the characteristics and appropriate methods for more than 100 diseases.

As a valued scientific gift from the home of acupuncture and moxibustion, *The Gateway to Acupuncture and Moxibustion*, we hope, will be a good teacher and helpful friend to students and practitioners of acupuncture and moxibustion in the world.

Contents

CHAPTER 1

Old Yet Young Chinese Acupuncture and Moxibustion

The science of acupuncture and moxibustion is one of the most important contributions our ancestors have made to humankind. In a narrow sense, "acupuncture and moxibustion" refers to a medical therapy, and broadly speaking it is an integral science which consists of four subdisciplines: meridians and acupoints; acupuncture and moxibustion techniques; acupuncture and moxibustion therapy; experimental acupuncture and moxibustion.

LONG HISTORY

Acupuncture and moxibustion therapy is believed to have originated as early as in the New Stone Age. The ancient literature indicates that moxibustion was employed earlier than acupuncture. The earliest needle was made of *bian* stone and was used mainly for incising an abscess, draining pus and letting blood out for therapeutic purposes.

From the Warring States Period to the Qin Dynasty and to the Western Han Dynasty, with the introduction and application of iron instruments, *bian* stone needles were replaced by metal medical needles. This broadened the field of acupuncture practice, bringing about the development of acupuncture by leaps and bounds. The book *Huang Di Nei Jing (The Yellow Emperor's Inner Classic)* — in particular its second part, *Ling Shu (The Spiritual Pivot)* — passed on to the present day is a medical classic based on medical practice with acupuncture and moxibustion as the main therapeutic techniques, and it laid a theoretical foundation for Chinese acupuncture.

From the Eastern Han Dynasty to the Jin Dynasty and to the Northern and Southern Dynasties, another generation and great development of

1

acupuncture medicine occurred. For example, Huo Tuo in late Eastern Han selected only one or two points in acupuncture treatment and paid much notice to the propagation of the needling sensation. He was credited with the authorship of *Zhen Zhong Jiu Ci Jing* (*Canon of Moxibustion and Acupuncture Preserved in a Pillow;* lost). The outstanding doctor Zhang Zhong-jing presented 35 items about acupuncture and moxibustion in his book *Shang Han Lun* (*Treatise on Cold Damage*), putting forward his important viewpoints on prevention with acupuncture and moxibustion, acupuncture for yang syndromes and moxibustion for yin syndromes. Another famous doctor, Mi Huang-fu of the Wei and Jin Dynasties, compiled the book *Zhen Jiu Jia Yi Jing* (*Systematic Classic of Acupuncture and Moxibustion*). It is the earliest exclusive and systematized book on acupuncture and moxibustion, and has been one of the most influential works in the history of acupuncture and moxibustion.

During the Sui and Tang Dynasties, the science of acupuncture and moxibustion underwent great development. The famous physician Zhen Quan and his contemporary Sun Si-miao both had a good command of the knowledge of traditional Chinese medicine and made in-depth study of acupuncture and moxibustion. Sun Si-miao compiled *Bei Ji Qian Jin Yao Fang* (*Important Formulas Worth a Thousand Gold Pieces for Emergencies*) and *Qian Jin Yi Fang* (*Supplement to "Important Formulas Worth a Thousand Gold Pieces"*), in which a great deal of clinical experience on acupuncture treatment of various schools was included. He also designed and made *Ming Tang San Ren Tu* ("Charts of Three Views"), in which the 12 regular meridians and the 8 extra meridians were illustrated in various colors. They are the earliest multicolored charts of meridians and points but have been lost. In addition, Wang Tao wrote the book *Wai Tai Mi Yao* (*Arcane Essentials from the Imperial Library*), in which a host of moxibustion methods of various schools were recorded. Acupuncture and moxibustion in the Tang Dynasty had already become a special branch of medicine, and those specializing in this field were called "acupuncturists" and "moxibustionists." The Imperial Medical Bureau, responsible for medical education, was divided into four departments of medical specialties, and an acupuncture department was one of them.

In the Song, Jin and Yuan Dynasties, the science of acupuncture and moxibustion underwent great development and summarization. The famous acupuncturist Wang Wei-yi wrote in 1206 a monograph about acupoints, *Tong Ren Shu Xue Zhen Jiu Tu Jing (Illustrated Classic of Acupoints on the Bronze Figure)*, which was block-printed and published by the government. Under the support of the government, two bronze figures designed by him were manufactured, with the internal organs set inside and the meridians and points engraved on the surface for visual teaching and examination. The famous acupuncturist Wang Zhi-zhong of the Southern Song Dynasty wrote the book *Zhen Jiu Zi Sheng Jing (Classic of Nourishing Life with Acupuncture and Moxibustion)*, in which he laid stress on practical experience (including folk experience), exerting a great influence on the later generations. The famous doctor Hua Shou of the Yuan Dynasty did textual research on the pathways of meridians and collaterals, as well as their relationship with acupuncture points. He wrote the book *Shi Si Jing Fa Hui (An Elucidation on the Fourteen Channels)*, which further developed the theory of meridians and acupuncture points. In this period many other books were published, like *Xiao Er Ming Tang Jiu Jing (Canon of Acupuncture and Moxibustion for Children's Diseases)*, *Bei Ji Jiu Fa (Moxibustion Techniques for Emergencies)*, *Yong Ju Shen Mi Jiu Jing (The Secret of Moxibustion for Abscesses and Ulcers)* and *Zhen Jing Zhi Nan (Guide to the Classics of Acupuncture)*.

In the Ming Dynasty, acupuncture and moxibustion were worked up to a climax and many problems were studied more deeply and broadly. There were more famous doctors specializing in this field, such as Chen Hui of the early stage of the Ming Dynasty, Ling Yun of the middle stage and Yang Ji-zhou of the later stage. The main accomplishments in the Ming Dynasty were: (1) extensive collection and revision of the literature on acupuncture and moxibustion, e.g. *Zhen Jiu Da Quan (The Complete Compendium of Acupuncture and Moxibustion)* by Xu Feng, *Zhen Jiu Ju Ying (A Collection of Gems in Acupuncture and Moxibustion)* by Gao Wu, and *Zhen Jiu Da Cheng (The Great Compendium of Acupuncture and Moxibustion)* by Yang Ji-zhou; (2) studies on the manipulating methods of acupuncture; on the basis of single manipulation of acupuncture, more than 20 kinds of compound manipulation were developed; (3) development of warm moxibustion with moxa sticks from burning moxibustion with moxa cones; (4) sorting out the previous records of acupuncture sites located away form the 14 meridians and forming a new category of extra points.

From the establishment of the Qing Dynasty, doctors regarded herbal medication as superior to acupuncture, and therefore acupuncture and moxibustion gradually turned into a failure. Some relatively important books about acupuncture and moxibustion are *Zhen Jiu Ji Chen* (*The Integration of Acupuncture and Moxibustion*) by Liao Hong-run; *Yi Zong Jin Jian-Ci Jiu Xin Fa Yao Jue* (*The Golden Mirror of the Medical Tradition: Essential Teachings on Acupuncture and Moxibustion*), compiled by Wu Qian and his collaborators under an imperial order, and taking the practical form of rhymed verse with illustrations; and *Zhen Jiu Feng Yuan* (*The Source of Acupuncture and Moxibustion*) by Li Xue-chuan, which is the first book to systematically list the 361 points. In 1822, the authorities of the Qing Dynasty declared an order to abolish permanently the acupuncture–moxibustion department from the Imperial Medical College because "acupuncture and moxibustion are not suitable to be applied to the Emperor."

MODERN DEVELOPMENT

In modern times, the science of acupuncture and moxibustion got its chance to spread among the folks. Many acupuncturists made unrelenting efforts to protect and develop this great medical legacy by founding acupuncture associations, publishing books and journals on acupuncture, and launching correspondence courses to teach acupuncture. Among those acupuncturists, Cheng Dan-an made a particular contribution. In this period, besides inheriting the traditional acupuncture and moxibustion, they made efforts to explain the theory of acupuncture and moxibustion with modern science and technology. In 1899, Liu Zhong-heng wrote a book entitled *Zhong Xi Hui Can Tong Ren Tu Shuo* (*Illustration of the Bronze Figure with Chinese and Western Medicine*), paving the way for studying acupuncture through combination of traditional Chinese and Western medicine in the history of acupuncture. In 1934, *The Technique and Principles of Electroacupuncture and the Study of Electroacupuncture*, written by Tang Shi-cheng, started the use of electroacupuncture in China.

After the founding of New China, acupuncture and moxibustion were unprecedentedly popularized and promoted. Firstly, research and education institutes of acupuncture and moxibustion were set up all over the country. In 1951, the Experimental Institute of Acupuncture–Moxibustion Therapy, affiliated directly to the Ministry of Public Health, was set up. By 1992 there had been 8 research institutes on meridians in China, and 28 medical colleges out of 30 had founded departments of acupuncture and moxibustion. And, in 1986, the Beijing Institute of Acupuncture and Moxibustion was set up. Many institutes and colleges of Western medicine have put that science on the teaching curriculum and taken it as a scientific research item.

To apply modern scientific knowledge to the research work on the basis of exploring and inheriting the traditional acupuncture and moxibustion is the prominent characteristic of the present research on acupuncture and moxibustion. In the 1950s, the main work was to systematize the basic theory of acupuncture and moxibustion, to observe its clinical indications, and to make a systematic exposition of acupuncture and moxibustion with modern methods. From the late 1950s to the 1960s, the following were carried out: extensive summarization of the clinical effect on various disease entities, propagation of acupuncture anesthesia in clinical use, and experimental researches. From the 1970s up to now, investigations have been made into the mechanism of acupuncture anesthesia and acupuncture analgesia from the viewpoints of operative surgery, anesthesiology, neuro-anatomy, histochemistry and psychology, into the phenomena and nature of the meridians from the viewpoint of propagated acupuncture sensation and other angles, and into the relationship between acupuncture points and the needling sensation, between points and *zang–fu* organs. Now, the science of acupuncture and moxibustion is becoming a modern clinical medicine integrating prevention, treatments, rehabilitation and healthcare, from the previous single purpose of treatment.

In the sixth century, acupuncture and moxibustion were introduced to Japan and Korea, and in the 16th century they began to be introduced to Europe. Now, with the increasing influence of acupuncture and moxibustion, the propagation to the world has been speeded up. In the 1950s, China gave assistance to the former Soviet Union and other Eastern European countries in training acupuncturists. Since 1975, at the request of the WHO, the International Acupuncture Training Courses have been run in Beijing, Shanghai and Nanjing, and acupuncturists have been trained for many countries. Up to now, more than 140 countries have had acupuncturists, and in some countries teaching and scientific research on acupuncture and moxibustion have been carried out with good results.

QUESTIONS

(1) List the important books on acupuncture and moxibustion in past dynasties.
(2) What were the main accomplishments in the Ming Dynasty in acupuncture and moxibustion?

CHAPTER 2

Meridians and Collaterals

The theory of meridians and collaterals, an important part of acupuncture and moxibustion, is the core of the basic theory of acupuncture and moxibustion and a great achievement made by ancient doctors. The meridians and collaterals are pathways in which the *qi* and blood of the human body are circulated. The meridians run longitudinally and interiorly with the body, while the collaterals run transversely and superficially from the meridians. They are collectively termed *"jingluo"* ("meridians and collaterals") in traditional Chinese medicine. Records about *jingluo* were seen as early as in *Meridians and Vessels*, one of the silk scrolls in the Spring and Autumn Period and the Warring States Period. The theory of meridians and collaterals is of great significance in guiding the clinical practice of acupuncture and moxibustion, and is a research focus nowadays.

OVERVIEW OF THE SYSTEM OF MERIDIANS AND COLLATERALS

The system of meridians and collaterals is an integral system consisting of three parts: the main body, the inner part and the outer part. The main body has two categories: *jingmai* and *huomai*. *Jingmai* comprises the 12 meridians (or the 12 regular medians), the 12 divergent meridians and the 8 extra meridians. The 12 meridians are the major trunks of the system, including the 3 yin meridians of the hand (the meridian of hand–*taiyin*, the meridian of hand–*shaoyin* and the meridian of hand–*jueying*), the 3 yang meridians of the hand (the meridian of hand–*taiyang*, the meridian of hand–*shaoyang* and the meridian of hand–*yangming*), the 3 yin meridians of the foot (the meridian of foot–*taiyin*, the meridian of foot–*shaoyin* and the meridian of foot–*jueying*), and the 3 yang meridians of the foot (the meridian of foot–*taiyang*, the meridian of foot–*shaoyang* and the meridian of foot–*yangming*). The 12 divergent meridians are the main branches of the 12 regular medians in the chest, the abdomen and the head, and are the same as the 12 regular meridians which fit the hand and foot, including 3 yin and 3 yang divergent meridians. The 8 extra meridians, different from the 12 regular meridians, are called the extra meridians in short, including 8 meridians: the *ren, du, chong, dai, yangqiao, yinqiao, yangwei* and *yinwei* meridians, functioning to govern, connect and regulate all the other meridians and collaterals. *Luomai* refers to branches respectively from each of the 12 regular meridians in the 4 limbs, and from the *ren* meridian (the front of the trunk), the *du* meridian (the back), and a large one (the major collateral of the spleen) from the spleen — a total of 15 collaterals responsible for connection of the interior and the exterior, and circulation of *qi* and blood, which are termed the 15 collaterals. There are further branches of the 15 collaterals, known as minute collaterals, superficial collaterals and superficial venules.

The inner part of the system refers to the *zang–fu* organs, associated with the 12 meridians and collaterals, and their relationship is mainly demonstrated as "pertaining and connection." *Zang* organs pertain to yin, and *fu* organs to yang. And yin meridians pertain to *zang* organs and connect with *fu* organs, while yang meridians pertain to *fu* organs and connect with *zang* organs. For the 3 yin meridians of the hand, the meridian of hand–*taiyin* pertains to the lung, and so is termed the lung meridian of hand–*taiyin*; The meridian of hand–*shaoyin* to the heart is termed the heart meridian of hand–*shaoyin*; and the meridian of hand–*jueyin* to the pericardium is termed the pericardium meridian of hand–*jueyin*. And, accordingly, the rest are the small intestine meridian of hand–*taiyang*, the *sanjiao* meridian of hand–*shaoyang*, the large intestine meridian of hand–*yangming*, the spleen meridian of foot–*taiyin*, the kidney meridian of foot–*shaoyin*, the liver meridian of foot–*jueyin*, the bladder meridian of foot–*taiyang*, the stomach meridian of foot–*yangming*, and so on.

The outer part of the system includes 12 muscle regions and 12 cutaneous regions. The former have the same nomenclature as the 12 meridians, distributing on the surface of the body along the 12 meridians, which have their own characteristics: (1) distributing from the ends of the four limbs to the trunk or the head and face; (2) distributing in a strip shape, accumulating in the joint and spreading in the rich muscles; (3) having no direct connection with *zang–fu* organs. The latter refer to the corresponding areas of the 12 meridians distributing on the skin, and so diseases and disorders of the meridians or *zang–fu* organs will be reflected on the local skins.

The System of Meridians and Collaterals

Inner Part	Zang–fu Organs
Body part	*Jingmai* (meridians)
	12 regular meridians
	12 divergent meridians
	8 extra meridians
	Luomai (collaterals)
	15 collaterals
	Minute collaterals, superficial
	collaterals, superficial venules
Outer part	12 muscle regions
	12 cutaneous regions

FUNCTIONS OF THE MERIDIANS AND COLLATERALS

The network of the meridians and collaterals is closely connected with the tissues and organs of the body, and plays an important role in human physiology and pathology of ailments.

(1) Connecting the interior and the exterior and transfixing the superior and the inferior: the system of meridians and collaterals associates all the organs of the body by pertaining and connecting, and thus the interior and the exterior, the upper and the lower portions and the left and right sides of the body are kept in a close association, and a relative equilibrium of normal life activities is maintained.

(2) Transporting *qi* and blood and nourishing the whole body: *qi* and blood are the primary substances of the human body, while meridians and collaterals are passages for circulation of *qi* and blood.

(3) Transmissive function: the meridians and collaterals assume the responsibility of transmitting pathogens and needling sensations so as to regulate the organic body.

RESEARCH ON THE MERIDIANS
AND COLLATERALS

It has been more than 2000 years since the meridians and collaterals were found, but acupuncturists remain confused about some questions regarding whether they exist or not, and what they are if they exist. In order to clarify the issue of the existence of the meridians and collaterals and their natures, much work has been done since the 1950s, especially since the 1970s. The modern researches, generally, focus on the following three aspects:

(1) *Running pattern*: the routes by which the meridians and collaterals distribute on the body surface. One way is to study the transmitting routes of the needling sensation through points stimulation; another is to use physical or chemical methods to demonstrate the running routes, including detection of the electrical characteristics of the skin, temperature changes, cold illumination, sound information, radioactive nuclides, fluorescein, and so on.

(2) *Association pattern*: whether meridians and collaterals are the passages for associating the interior with the exterior. Pathological changes are reflected on the body surface, i.e. the interior is reflected on the exterior; stimulating the surface works to the organs, i.e. the exterior affects the interior. Research has been done on the associations of the tenderness spot (sensitive point) and the internal organs.

(3) *Morphology basis*: anatomy and histology of modern medicine. This is to study whether or not there exist special structures of meridians and collaterals.

A great deal of effort by many acupuncturists of the world has confirmed the existence of meridians and collaterals, but the nature of the system remains unclear. Great importance has been attached to the research on the meridians and collaterals in China, and there are reasons to believe that the eternal mystery will be unraveled in the near future.

QUESTIONS

(1) Describe the composition of the system of meridians and collaterals.
(2) What are the functions of the meridians and collaterals?

CHAPTER 3

Distribution of the 14 Meridians and Collaterals

In the system of meridians and collaterals, there are only the 12 regular meridians and 2 extra meridians which have acupoints with them and are the most commonly used in the clinic, while the others have no points themselves except for confluence ones.

OVERVIEW

Distribution on the Surface of the Body

It was mentioned in the previous chapter that meridians and collaterals are the passages for the association of the interior and the exterior, and so they interiorly associate with the organs and exteriorly with the acupoints, also called the passage with points, which is the major part of the meridians and collaterals. Generally, the meridian lines on ordinary schemas or molds of the meridians and collaterals all refer to the passages with acupoints. Therefore, getting familiar with the distribution of the meridians and collaterals is of great significance.

The *ren* and *du* meridians run along the median line of the body up to the mouth and down to the anus. The *ren* meridian runs from the perineum, then the abdomen and the chest to the lower lip, while the *du* meridian runs from the upper gums through the face, the head, the back and the waist to the sacrococcygeal region.

The 12 regular meridians distribute symmetrically on the left and the right side of the body. Distribution in the limbs is as follows: the yin meridians distribute along the inner side of the four limbs, and the yang meridians on the lateral side. According to yin and yang, the *taiyin* and *yangming* meridians distribute along the anterior side, the *jueyin* and *shaoyang* ones along the middle side, and the *shaoyin* and *taiyang* ones along the posterior side. Among these meridians, only the meridian of foot–*jueyin* turns and converges with other distributions. In the head and face, only the yang meridians distribute, among which the *yangming* meridians distribute mainly in the face, the foot–*taiyang* ones in the vertex, and the occiput–*shaoyang* ones on the lateral side of the face. Only hand–*taiyang*, different from foot–*taiyang*, mainly distributes in the lateral face. In the trunk, the *yangming* meridians distribute on the front, the *shaoyang* ones on the lateral side, and the *taiyang* ones on the back.

Circulation of the 12 Meridians

The 12 meridians form a cycle to guarantee the circulation of *qi* and blood.

They originate from the lung meridians of hand–*taiyin*; one meridian after another and returning to the lung meridian form a cycle, followed by the next cycle. The route is: the lung meridian of hand–*taiyin* → the large intestine meridian of hand–*yangming* → the stomach meridian of foot–*yangming* → the spleen meridian of foot–*taiyin* → the heart meridians of hand–*shaoyin* → the small intestine meridian of hand–*taiyang* → the bladder meridian of foot–*tainyang* → the kidney meridian of foot–*shaoyin* → the pericardium meridian of hand–*jueyin* → the *sanjiao* meridian of hand–*shaoyang* → the gallbladder meridian of foot–*shaoyang* → the liver meridian of foot–*jueyin* → the lung meridian of hand–*taiyin*.

There are two features in this route:

(1) The 12 meridians circulate first in the exterior and interior meridians of the hand, then the exterior and interior meridians of the foot, and lastly the exterior and interior meridians of the hand.

(2) The running direction is that the three yin meridians of the hand run from the chest to the hand; the three yang meridians run from the hand to the head; the three yang meridians of the foot run from the head to the foot; and the three yin meridians run from the foot to the abdomen. Such a cycle is formed.

The *du* and *ren* meridians associate with each other and closely with the 12 meridians, but are different from the 12 meridians in circulation. They govern, connect and regulate the *qi* and blood of all the meridians. The *du* meridian governs all the yang meridians, and it is therefore described as the sea of the yang meridians. The *ren* meridian meets all the yin meridians, and thus it is called the sea of the yin meridians.

The three yin meridians of the hand

The three yin meridians of the hand distribute along the inner side (flexor side) and the chest, *taiyin* close to the thumb, *shaoyin* to the little finger, and *jueyin* in the middle. The connections are: the lung meridian of hand–*taiyin* to the large intestine meridian of hand–*yangming*, the heart meridian of hand–*shaoyin* to the small intestine of hand–*taiyang*, and the pericardium meridian of hand–*jueyin* to the *sanjiao* meridian of hand–*shaoyang*, which are all exteriorly–interiorly related or *qi*–blood-circulated in pairs. The following, introduced in detail, are the routes of the 12 meridians.

The lung meridian of hand–taiyin

On the surface: Chest → inner side of upper arm → inner elbow → inner side of forearm → *cunkou* (RP site) → thenar eminence → end of thumb (Fig. 1).

Inside: It originates from the middle *jiao*, and runs downward to connect with the large intestine. Winding back, it goes along the upper orifice of the stomach, passes through the diaphragm and enters the lung.

The heart meridian of hand–shaoyin

On the surface: Armpit → posterior border of inside upper arm → posterior part inner elbow → posterior border of inside forearm → lenticular bone of hand → rear palm → distal end of little finger (Fig. 2.)

Inside: It originates from the heart. On emerging, it spreads over the "heart system" (i.e. the tissues connecting the heart with the other *zang–fu* organs). It passes through the diaphragm to connect with the small intestine.

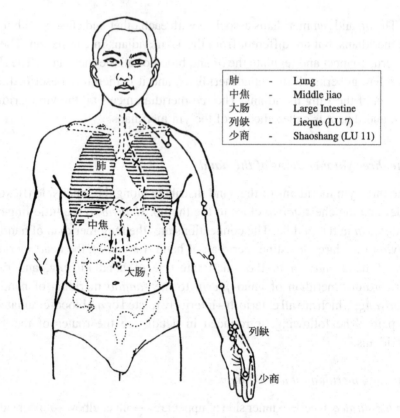

肺	-	Lung
中焦	-	Middle jiao
大肠	-	Large Intestine
列缺	-	Lieque (LU 7)
少商	-	Shaoshang (LU 11)

Fig. 1.   The lung meridian of hand–*taiyin*.

The pericardium meridian of hand–jueyin

On the surface: Flank (3 *cun* inferior to armpit) → armpit → inner side of upper arm → middle of inner elbow → forearm, running between two tendons (flexor cari radialis muscle tendon and cubitalis grailis) → palm center → end of middle finger along radialis (Fig. 3.)

Inside: It originates from the chest. On emerging, it enters the pericardium. Then it descends through the diaphragm to the abdomen, connecting successively with the upper, middle and lower *jiao*.

The three yang meridians of the hand

The three yang meridians of the hand distribute in the lateral side (extensor side) and the head and face, the hand–*yangming* meridians originating

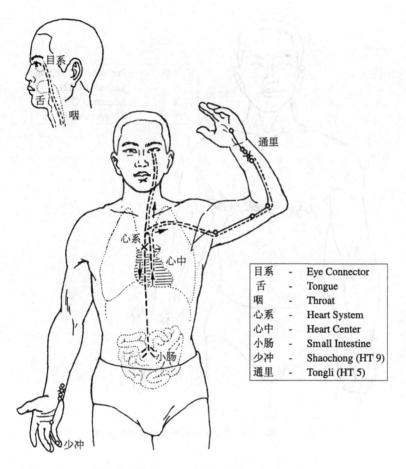

目系	-	Eye Connector
舌	-	Tongue
咽	-	Throat
心系	-	Heart System
心中	-	Heart Center
小肠	-	Small Intestine
少冲	-	Shaochong (HT 9)
通里	-	Tongli (HT 5)

Fig. 2. The heart meridian of hand–*shaoyin*.

fron the index finger, the hand–*taiyang* ones from the little finger, and the hand–*shaoyang* ones from the fourth finger. *Qi* and blood along the meridians run from hand to head, moving downward to connect with the three yang meridians of the foot. There are circulations of *qi* and blood between the three yang meridians of the hand and the three meridians of the foot, and the three yang meridians of the hand are exteriorly–interiorly related to the three yin meridians of the hand.

The large intestine meridian of hand–yangming

On the surface: End of index finger → margo radialis of index finger → interspace of first and second metacarpus → two tendons (extensor pol-

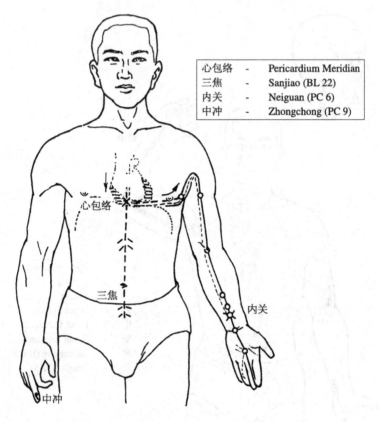

心包络	-	Pericardium Meridian
三焦	-	Sanjiao (BL 22)
内关	-	Neiguan (PC 6)
中冲	-	Zhongchong (PC 9)

Fig. 3.   The pericardium meridian of hand–*jueyin*.

licis longus muscle tendon and short extensor muscle of thumb) → radialis of forearm → lateral elbow → front part of outside of upper arm → front of acromial region → supraclavicular fossa → cheek → lower dental alveolus → beside mouth, joining at philtrum → left turning left and right turning right, up to the nose.

Inside: It starts from the supraclavicular fossa. On emerging, it descends to the supraclavicular fossa to connect with the lung. It then passes through the diaphragm and enters the large intestine. (See Fig. 4.)

The small intestine meridian of hand–taiyang

On the surface: End of lateral little finger → ulnaris of palm → wrist → capitulum ulnae → lower border of ulna → inner side of elbow (between

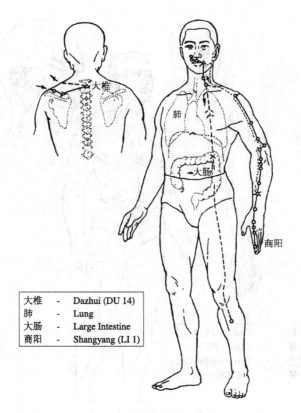

Fig. 4.　The large intestine meridian of hand–*yangming*.

大椎	-	Dazhui (DU 14)
肺	-	Lung
大肠	-	Large Intestine
商阳	-	Shangyang (LI 1)

internal epicondyle of humerus and decranon of ulna) → exterior–posterior side of upper arm → shoulder joint, meeting shoulder by circling round scapula → supraclavicular fossa → neck → cheek → external canthus → ear center.

Inside: It diverges from the supraclavicular fossa. On emerging, it connects with the heart. It then, along the esophagus, passes through the diaphragm and enters the small intestine. (See Fig. 5.)

The sanjiao meridian of hand–shaoyang

On the surface: End of ring finger → along dorsum of hand, emerging from the two bones on extensor side of forearm (ulna and radius) → apex of elbow → lateral side of upper arm → shoulder → supraclavicular

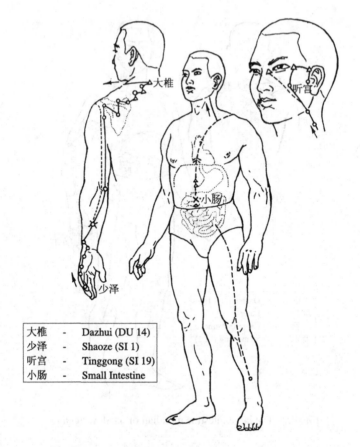

大椎	-	Dazhui (DU 14)
少泽	-	Shaoze (SI 1)
听宫	-	Tinggong (SI 19)
小肠	-	Small Intestine

Fig. 5. The small intestine meridian of hand–*taiyang*.

fossa → posterior vertex → back of ear → superior ear → winding over to cheek → inferior to eye. Another branch: back of ear → ear center → the front of ear → cheek → external canthus.

Inside: Winding over to the supraclavicular fossa, it spreads in the mediastinum to connect with the pericardium. It then descends through the diaphragm, and joins the upper, middle and lower *jiao*. (See Fig. 6.)

QUESTIONS

(1) What are the distribution characteristics of the 12 meridians?

(2) Demonstrate the running routes of the three yin meridians of the hand and the three yang meridians of the hand on the surface.

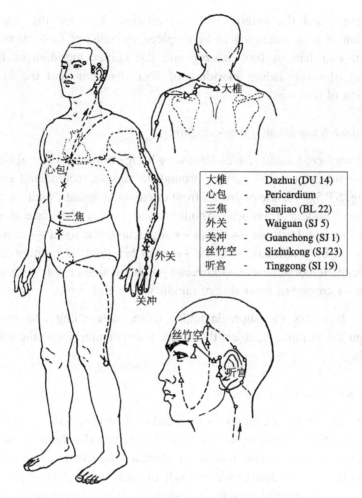

大椎	-	Dazhui (DU 14)
心包	-	Pericardium
三焦	-	Sanjiao (BL 22)
外关	-	Waiguan (SJ 5)
关冲	-	Guanchong (SJ 1)
丝竹空	-	Sizhukong (SJ 23)
听宫	-	Tinggong (SI 19)

Fig. 6.   The *sanjiao* meridian of hand–*shaoyang*.

The three yang meridians of the foot

The yang meridians of the foot distribute on the lateral side of the head, the trunk and the four limbs, the meridian of foot–*yangming* on the front reaching the second toe, that of foot–*taiyang* on the back reaching the little toe, and that of foot–*shaoyang* on the *lateral* reaching the fourth toe. *Qi* and blood circulate from the head to the foot, connecting the three yang meridians of the hand with the three yin meridians of the foot. Among the three yang meridians of the foot, there are the *qi* and blood circulation and the external–internal relations between the stomach meridian of foot–*yangming* and the spleen meridian of foot–*taiyin*, the bladder meridian of foot–*taiyang* and the kidney meridian of foot–*shaoyin*, the gallbladder meridian of foot–*shaoyang* and the kidney meridian of foot–*shaoyin*.

The stomach meridian of foot–yangming

On the surface: Lateral side of alanasi → bridge of nose → lateral side of nose → upper gums → curving around the tips → mentolabial groove (*daying*, ST 5) → angle of jaw → front of ear → aygomatic arch → along hairline → middle of forehead. Another branch: artery of the face (*daying*, ST 5) → carotid arteries → throat → supraclavicular fossa → center of breasts → by umbilicus → *qi jie* → front hip joint → prominence of quadriceps femoris muscle → kneecap → lateral side of tibia → dorsum of foot → crevice of inner side of middle toe → end of toe.

Inside: It enters the supraclavicular fossa, descending and passing through the diaphragm, enters the stomach and connects with the spleen. (See Fig. 7.)

The bladder meridian of foot–taiyang

On the surface: Inner canthus → forehead → joining at vertex → neck → inner aspect of scapula region → parallel to vertebral column → lumbar → gluteal region → popliteal fossa. Another branch: inner margin of scapula region → scapula → lateral side of back → hip joint → popliteal fossa → gastrocnemius muscle → posterior side of external malleulus → tuberosity of fifth metatarsal bone → lateral side of tip of little toe.

Inside: It enters the lumbar, connecting with the kidney, and joins the bladder (Fig. 8).

The gallbladder meridian of foot–shaoyang

On the surface: Outer canthus → corner of forehead → back of ear → side of neck → shoulder → supraclavicular fossa → armpit → along lateral side of chest, passing through hypochondrium → hip joint → lateral side

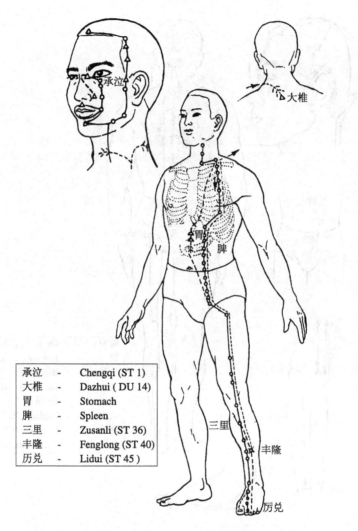

承泣 - Chengqi (ST 1)
大椎 - Dazhui (DU 14)
胃 - Stomach
脾 - Spleen
三里 - Zusanli (ST 36)
丰隆 - Fenglong (ST 40)
历兑 - Lidui (ST 45)

Fig. 7. The stomach meridian of foot–*yangming*.

of thigh → lateral side of knee → front of fibular head → inferior segment of fibula → anterior to external malleolus → lateral side of fourth toe along dorsum of foot. Another branch: back of ear → center of ear → front of ear → posterior side of outer canthus.

Inside: It enters the supraclavicular fossa through the diaphragm to connect with the liver and enters the gallbladder (Fig. 9).

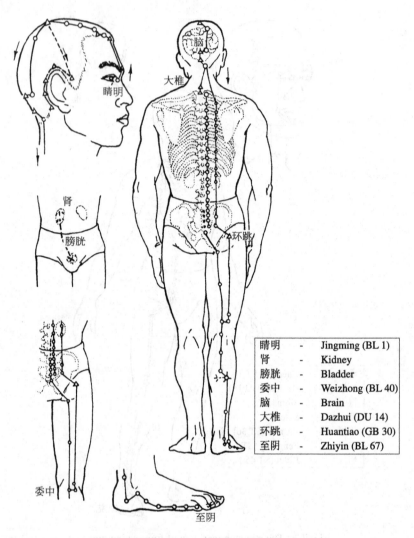

睛明	-	Jingming (BL 1)
肾	-	Kidney
膀胱	-	Bladder
委中	-	Weizhong (BL 40)
脑	-	Brain
大椎	-	Dazhui (DU 14)
环跳	-	Huantiao (GB 30)
至阴	-	Zhiyin (BL 67)

Fig. 8.   The bladder meridian of foot–*taiyang*.

The three meridians of the foot

The three meridians of the foot distribute on the inner side of the four limbs, the chest and the abdomen, the meridian of foot–*taiying* originating from the inner side of the big toe, that of foot–*shaoyin* from the little toe through the sole center, and that of foot–*jueyin* from the superior side of the big toe and passing between. Runing from the foot to the abdomen, the

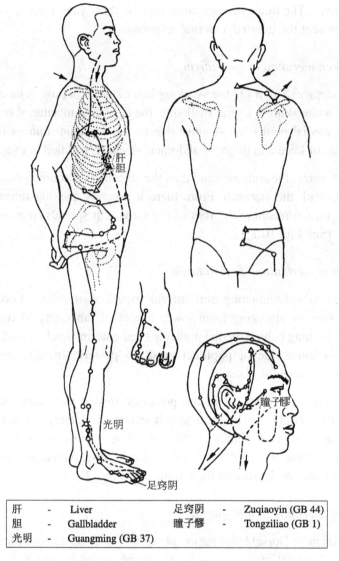

肝	-	Liver	足窍阴	-	Zuqiaoyin (GB 44)
胆	-	Gallbladder	瞳子髎	-	Tongziliao (GB 1)
光明	-	Guangming (GB 37)			

Fig. 9.   The gallbladder meridian of foot–*shaoyang*.

qi and blood connect the three yang meridians of the foot to the three yin meridians of the hand. *Qi* and blood circulate between the spleen meridian of foot–*taiyin* and the heart meridian of hand–*shaoyin*, the kidney meridian of foot–*shaoyin* and the pericardium meridian of hand–*jueyin*, and the liver meridian of foot–*jueyin* and the lung meridian of hand–*taiyin*. The three yin meridians and the three yang meridians of the foot represent the internal–external relations.

The spleen meridian of foot–taiyin

On the surface: Tip of big toe → along inner side of big toe at junction of red and white skin → lateral malleolus (head of first metatarsal bone) → front of medial malleolus → inner side of leg → along tibia → front of inner side of knee and thigh → abdomen → chest, paralled to esophagus.

Inside: It enters the abdomen and then the spleen, its pertaining organ, and connects with the stomach. From there it ascends, passing through the diaphragm. On reaching the root of the tongue, it spreads over its lower surface. (See Fig. 10.)

The kidney meridian of foot–shaoyin

On the surface: Originating from inferior aspect of small toe → obliquely toward sole → emerging from lower aspect of tuberosity of navicular bone → running behind medial malleolus and entering heel → medial side of leg → inner side of popliteal fossa → posterior–medial aspect of thigh → abdomen → chest.

Inside: It goes upward along the posterior–medial aspect of the thigh toward the vertebral column, where it enters the kidney, its pertaining organ, and connects with the bladder. Then it runs upward, passing through the liver and the diaphragm, enters the lung, runs along the throat and terminates at the root of the tongue. (See Fig. 11.)

The liver meridian of foot–jueyin

On the surface: Dorsal hairy region of big toe → along dorsum foot, 1 *cun* in front of medial malleolus → inner side of leg, at an area 8 *cun* above the medial malleolus, where it runs across and behind the spleen meridian of foot–*taiyin* → medial side of poples → pubic hair region, where it curves around the external genitalia → abdomen → lateral thorax.

Inside: It enters the abdomen, and then runs upward and curves around the stomach to enter the liver, its pertaining organ, and connects with the gallbladder. Then it ascends along the posterior aspect of the throat to the nasopharynx

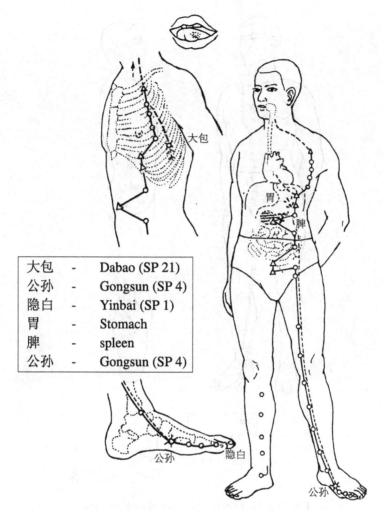

Fig. 10. The spleen meridian of foot–*taiyin*.

and connects with the eye system. Running further upward, it emerges from the forehead and meets the *du* meridian at the vertex. (See Fig. 12.)

The eight extra meridians

The eight extra meridians were named in *Nan Jing* (*The Classic of Difficult Issues*) but actually recorded in *Nei Jing* (*The Inner Classic*). They are different from the 12 regular meridians because none of them

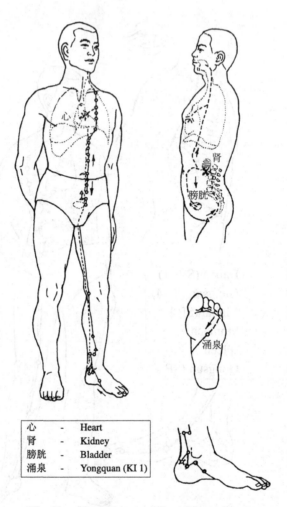

心	-	Heart
肾	-	Kidney
膀胱	-	Bladder
涌泉	-	Yongquan (KI 1)

Fig. 11.   The kidney meridian of foot–*shaoyin.*

pertains to the *zang* oragans and communicates with the *fu* organs or pertains to the *fu* organs and communicates with the *zang* organs. And they are not exteriorly–interiorly related, among which only the *du* and the *ren* meridians have their own acupoints. Strengthening the association among the meridians, they assume the responsibility to control, join, store and regulate the *qi* and blood of each meridian. Here, only the *du* and *ren* meridians are introduced; the other six (the *mai, dai, qinqiao, yangqiao, yinwei* and *yangwei* meridians) are omitted.

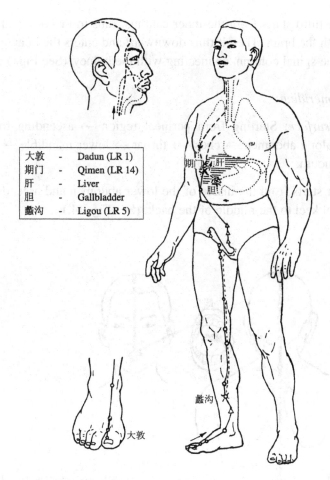

大敦	-	Dadun (LR 1)
期门	-	Qimen (LR 14)
肝	-	Liver
胆	-	Gallbladder
蠡沟	-	Ligou (LR 5)

Fig. 12. The liver meridian of foot–*jueyin*.

The du meridian

On the surface: Emerging from perineum → ascending along spinal column → back of neck → vertex → along forehead to columnella of nose → upper gums of teeth.

Inside: There are three branches. The first, together with the *chong* and *ren* meridians, originates from the inside of the lower abdomen, passes through the spine, and enters the kidney, its pertaining organ; the second ascends from the abdomen, passing through the favea umbilicalis, then the throat, curving around the lips, and reaches the middle part below the eyes; the third starts from the inner canthus, runs to the vertex and connects with the brain. Then it runs downward and enters the bilateral muscles to the spinal column, connecting with the kidney. (See Fig. 13.)

The ren meridian

On the surface: Starting from perineal region → ascending to pubic hair → along abdomen → chest → throat → lower mandible → lateral side of mouth.

Inside: It starts from the inside of the lower abdomen and ascends along the dorsal keel to the middle of the back. (See Fig. 14.)

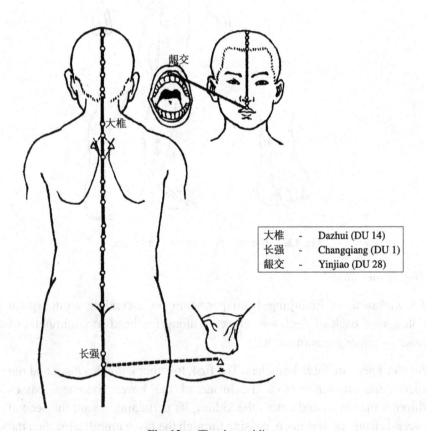

大椎	-	Dazhui (DU 14)
长强	-	Changqiang (DU 1)
龈交	-	Yinjiao (DU 28)

Fig. 13.   The *du* meridian.

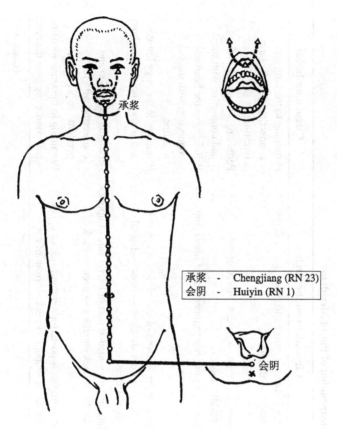

承浆 - Chengjiang (RN 23)
会阴 - Huiyin (RN 1)

Fig. 14. The *ren* meridian.

Distribution of the 14 Meridians

Fourteen Meridians		Circulation on the Surface	Circulation Inside
Three yin meridians of the hand	Lung meridian of hand–*taiyin*	Lateral chest → anterior to inner side of upper limbs → thumb	Pertaining to the lung and connecting with the large intestine
	Pericardium meridian of hand–*jueyin*	Lateral of breast → medial side of upper limbs → middle finger	Pertaining to the pericardium and connecting with *sanjiao*
	Heart meridian of hand–*shaoyin*	Armpit → posterior to inner side of upper limbs → little finger	Pertaining to the heart and connecting with the small intestine
Three yang meridians of the hand	Large intestine meridian of hand–*yangming*	Index finger → front of lateral side of upper limbs → front shoulder → neck → lateral side of nose	Pertaining to the large intestine and connecting with the lung
	Sanjiao meridian of hand–*shaoyang*	Ring finger → medial part of lateral side of upper limbs → back shoulder → neck → back of ear → brow tip	Pertaining to *sanjiao* and connecting with the pericardium
	Small intestine meridian of hand–*taiyang*	Little finger → posterior to lateral side of upper limbs → scapula → neck → front of ear	Pertaining to the small intestine and connecting with the heart

(Continued)

(Continued)

Fourteen Meridians		Circulation on the Surface	Circulation Inside
Three yang meridians of the foot	Stomach meridian of foot–*yangming*	Below eye → around face → front neck → second lateral line of chest and abdomen → anterior to lateral side of lower limbs → second toe	Pertaining to the stomach and connecting with the spleen
	Gallbladder meridian of foot–*shaoyang*	Outer canthus → temple → lateral side of neck → lateral side of lumbar → middle part of lateral of lower limbs → fourth toe	Pertaining to the gallbladder and connecting with the liver
	Bladder meridian of foot–*taiyang*	Inner canthus → first line lateral side of vertex → back of neck → first and second lateral lines of back and lumbar → sacrum → posterior part of lateral side of lower limbs → little toe	Pertaining to the bladder and connecting with the kidney
Three yin meridians of the foot	Spleen meridian of foot–*taiyin*	Inner side of big toe → front and middle parts of inner side of lower limbs → third lateral line of chest and abdomen	Pertaining to the spleen and connecting with the stomach
	Liver meridian of foot–*jueyin*	Outer side of big toe → front and middle parts of inner side of lower limbs → pudendum → flank	Pertaining to the liver and connecting with the gallbladder
	Kidney meridian of foot–*shaoyin*	Inferior part of little toe → sore → posterior part of inner side of lower limbs → first lateral line of chest and abdomen	Pertaining to the kidney and connecting with the bladder
Ren and *du* meridians	*Ren* meridian	Perineum → middle line of chest and abdomen → neck → lower lip	Originating from the inside of the lower abdomen
	Du meridian	Tip of coccyx → spinal column → middle line of vertex → column of nose → upper gums	Originating from the inside of the lower abdomen, pertaining to the kidney and connecting with the brain

QUESTIONS

(1) Describe the running routes of the three yang meridians of the foot and the three yin meridians of the foot on the body surface.

(2) What are the characteristics of the *ren* and *du* meridians in distribution?

CHAPTER 4

Introduction to Acupoints

Acupoints are the specific sites through which the *qi* of the *zang–fu* organs and meridians is transported to the body surface. The Chinese characters "腧穴" for an acupoint mean respectively "transportation" and "hole." In the medical literature of the past dynasties, acupoints, the sites where acupuncture and moxibustion treatment is applied, have other terms, such as *"qi* point" and "aperture." Acupoints are not only the pathways for the circulation of *qi* and blood, but also the loci of response to diseases. In acupuncture and moxibustion treatment, proper techniques are applied on the acupoints to regulate the functional activities of the body, and strengthen body resistance so as to prevent or treat diseases. Medical practitioners of past ages have left plentiful recordings describing the locations and indications of acupoints, formulating a systematical theory.

CLASSIFICATION OF ACUPOINTS

Generally speaking, acupoints fall into the following three categories in terms of their evolution.

Acupoints of the 14 Meridians

Also known as "regular points," acupoints of the 14 meridians are distributed along the 12 regular meridians and the *du* and *ren* meridians, amounting to 361. They are the most commonly used points and form the main part of all acupoints.

Extraordinary Points

These are of two kinds. One refers to the extraordinary points (or extra points for short), recorded in ancient acupuncture literature. These points are scattered over the body, or their curative effects have not been confirmed, so they are not added to the regular points of the 14 meridians. But, actually, some regular points were developed from the extraordinary points. Examples are *gaohuang* (BL 43) and *fengshi* (GB 31), which were extra points in *Bei Ji Qian Jin Fang* (*Important Formulas Worth a Thousand Gold Pieces for Emergencies*) in the Tang Dynasty; tu were added to the regular points in later acupuncture literature. The other kind refers to new points which have been summarized by many acupuncturists in China and foreign countries in modern times. The extraordinary points consist of extra points and the new points. There are more than 1500 extra points in some literature, among which 48 points are the standard points accepted in the world.

Ashi Points

In addition to regular points and extra points, tender spots can be used as acupoints in the clinic. These are termed *ashi* points, and were seen first in the Tang Dynasty; they are also known as reflexing points or unfixed points.

Acupoints of the three categories are closely related. During the development of acupoints, *ashi* points may become extra points that also may be changed into regular points. Besides, in treatment, they complement each other. For example, the treatment of acute lumbar sprain will involve three categories of points.

NOMENCLATURE OF ACUPOINTS

Acupoints of the 14 meridians and the extra points have definite locations and names. In early ages, they did not have names or had some confusing names. Clinically, they require unified and standardized names. Each point is named with profound significance. Most of them are named according to their locations or functions. The nomenclature of acupoints will be introduced in detail in the following chapters.

FUNCTION OF ACUPOINTS

Acupoints are the spots along the meridians, and they belong to meridians and collaterals. Generally, they have the followings functions:

To reflect diseases: Acupoints are able to reflect symptoms if the body is diseased, mainly manifested by disorders of feelings, colors and appearance, such as tenderness, soreness, sclerosis, prominence, depression or hyperemia. For example, in cases with cholelithiasis, the patient will feel obvious pain when pressing *tianzong* (SI 11); patients with gastroptosis will feel a trab-shaped object in *zusanli* (ST 36) or nodes in *zhongwan* (RN 12). Modern acupuncturists do further study on the relation of the acupoints and *zang–fu* organs and certain diseases by means of acupoint temperature determination, electricity determination and optics determination.

To receive stimulation: The stimulation of the body by acupuncture is achieved through acupoints, for acupoints, are able to receive stimulation and transmit the needling sensation to regulate the deficiency and excess, and balance yin and yang. Puncturing the acupoints will induce a sensation of soreness, distension, heaviness or numbness, which is a response to the stimulation. Much observation and research supports the view that acupuncture on some points will regulate the systemic functions of endocrine, immune, digestion, cadiovascular, discharge and reproduction, as well as neurological function.

METHODS OF LOCATING ACUPOINTS

Location of acupoints, whether accurate or not, will affect the therapeutic results. Precise location of acupoints therefore is of great significance. At present, four methods of acupoint location are commonly used in clinics.

Bone Proportional Measurements

In this method, which was first seen in *Ling Shu* (*The Spiritual Pivot*), the joints are taken as the main landmarks to measure the length and width of various portions of the human body. Keep in mind the following commonly used standards for proportional measurement:

(1) *Head*: It is converted to 12 *cun* from the anterior hairline to the posterior hairline; 9 *cun* between the two mastoid processes.
(2) *Chest, back, lumbar and abdomen*: 6 *cun* between the medial borders of the scapulas; 3 *cun* between the two sacroiliac joints; 8 *cun* between the two nipples or between the midpoints of the two collarbones; 8 *cun* from the sternocostal angle to the center of the umbilicus; 5 *cun* between the center of the umbilicus and the upper border of the symphysis pubis.
(3) *Four limbs*: 9 *cun* between the end of the axillary fold and the transverse cubital crease; 12 *cun* between the transverse cubital crease and the transverse wrist crease; 15 *cun* between the transverse gluteal crease and the transverse crease of the poples; 16 *cun* between the center of the patella and the tip of the lateral malleolus.

Surface Anatomical Landmarks

This is a method to determine the location of points on the basis of anatomical landmarks on the body surface, which are divided into fixed and moving landmarks. The fixed landmarks *include* the five sense organs, hair, nails, nipples, umbilicus, and prominence and depression of the bones. Examples are *yintang* (EX-HN3) between the two eyebrows, *suliao* (DU 25) on the tip of the nose, and *tanzhong* (RN 17) between the two nipples. The moving landmarks are the clefts, depressions, wrinkles or prominences appearing on the joints, muscles, tendons and skin during motion. For example, when the elbow is flexed and the cubital crease appears, *quchi* (LI 11) can be located; *jiache* (ST 6) is located in the prominence of the masseter muscle.

Finger Measurement

This is a method to locate the points by measuring the distance with either the length or the width of the patient's finger(s). The following three methods are commonly used in the clinic:

(1) *Middle finger measurement*: When the middle finger is flexed, the distance between the radial ends of the two interphalangeal creases of the patient's middle finger is taken as 1 *cun*. This method is employed for measuring the horizontal distance to locate the points on the limbs or the back.
(2) *Thumb measurement*: The width of the interphalangeal joint of the patient's thumb is taken as 1 *cun*. This method is employed to locate the points at an interval of 1 *cun*.
(3) *Four-finger measurement*: The width of the four fingers (index, middle, ring and little) close together at the level of the dorsal skin crease of the proximal interphalangeal joint of the middle finger is taken as 3 *cun*. This method is used to locate the points on the lower limbs, the lower abdomen or the back.

Simple Measurement

This is a simple method to locate the points developed from clinical practice. For example, *laogong* (PC 8) is located on the first transverse crease, where the tip of the middle finger is pressing when a hollow fist is made; *fengshi* (GB 31) is where the tip of the middle finger touches when the patient stands erect with the hands at laxation.

QUESTIONS

(1) What are the three classifications of acupoints?
(2) What functions do acupoints have?
(3) Describe the four methods of locating acupoints.

CHAPTER 5

Specific Points

Specific points are those of the 14 meridians that have special properties and are grouped under special names, including 5 *shu* points, *yuan*–primary points, *luo*–connecting points, *xi*–cleft points, 8 confluent points and lower *he*–sea points which are on the limbs below the elbow and the knee, front–*mu* points and back–*shu* points on the chest and the back, 8 influential points on the trunk, and crossing points on the whole body.

FIVE *SHU* POINTS

Each of the 12 regular meridians has, below the elbow and the knee, 5 specific points, namely *jing*–well, *ying*–spring, *shu*–stream, *jing*–river and *he*–sea, which are known as the 5 *shu* points in general. The names of the 5 *shu* points image the flow of meridian *qi* as the flow of water. The *jing*–well point is situated in the place where the meridian *qi* starts to bubble. The *ying*–spring point is where the meridian *qi* starts to gush. The *shu*–stream point is where the meridian *qi* flourishes. The *jing*–river point is where the meridian *qi* is pouring abundantly. Finally, the *he*–sea point signifies the confluence of rivers in the sea, where the meridian *qi* is the most flourishing.

The five *shu* points have their own characteristics in the treatment of diseases: the *jing*–well point is often used for loss of consciousness, owing to its enlightening and awakening function; the *ying*–spring point for heat diseases, because it is able to clear and disperse the evil heat; the *shu*–stream point for paroxysmal diseases or swelling and pain of joints; the *jing*–river point for asthma, cough and throat disorders; and the *he*–sea point for enterogastric diseases.

LOWER *HE*–SEA POINTS

The *he*–sea point mentioned above is the last of the five *shu* points located near the elbow and knee joints. In addition, each of the six *fu* organs has another *he*–sea point in the three yang meridians of the foot, known as the lower *he*–sea point. The lower *he*–sea points of the stomach, large intestine, small intestine, *sanjiao*, baldder and gallbladder are *zusanli* (ST 36), *shangjuxu* (ST 37), *xiajuxu* (ST 39), *weiyang* (BL 39), *weizhong* (BL 40) and *yanglingquan* (GB 34). The lower *he*–sea points are mostly employed to treat disorders of the six *fu* organs in the clinic, such as *shangjuxu* (ST 37) for diseases of the large intestine, *xiajuxu* (ST 39) for abdominal pain and *weiyang* (BL 39) for urinary retention.

YUAN–PRIMARY POINTS

Each of the 12 regular meridians has a *yuan*–primary point, which is located on the limbs. The Chinese character "原" (*yuan*) means the primary *qi* in this context. The *yuan*–primary points are where the primordial *qi* passes by and retains, and they consist of 12 points. In treatment, the *yuan*–primary points are able to dispel exogenous, reinforce deficiency and strengthen the body. Whatever diseases occur to *zang–fu* organs, corresponding *yuan*–primary points are applied, such as *taiyuan* (LU 9) for cough and shortness of breath, and *taibai* (SP 3) for borborygmus and enterorrhea.

LUO–CONNECTING POINTS

Each of the 12 regular meridians has, below the knee, a *luo*–connecting point to link its exteriorly–interiorly related meridian. Other *luo*–connecting points are *jiuwei* (RN 15) below the ensiform process of the sternum, *changqiang* (DU 1) at the sacrococcygeal region, and *dabao* (SP 21) in the lateral chest. In total there are 15 *luo*–connecting points.

A *luo*–connecting point is used to treat disorders involving the two exteriorly–interiorly related meridians and those in the area supplied by the two meridians. For example, *lieque* (LU 7) is applicable to both cough, shortness of breath and toothache, diseases on the vertex. According to

TCM, the disease occurs to meridians in the early stage while it enters collaterals if it lasts for a long time. Many chronic diseases induced by internal injuries can therefore be treated by *luo*–connecting points.

XI–CLEFT POINTS

"郄" (*xi*) means a space where *qi* and blood deeply converge. Each of the 12 regular meridians and the 4 extra meridians (*yinqiao, yangqiao, yinwei* and *yangwei*) has a *xi*–cleft point on the limbs, amounting to 16, including *jiaoxin* (KI 8) in the *yinqiao* meridian, *fuyang* (BL 59) in the *yangqiao* meridian, *zhubin* (KI 9) in the *yinwei* meridian and *yangjiao* (GB 35) in the *yangwei* meridian.

In the clinic, the *xi*–cleft point is used to treat acute disorders in the area supplied by its pertaining meridian and those of its pertaining *zang* or *fu* organ. Ancient literature supports the view that the *xi*–cleft points of yin meridians are applicable to blood troubles such as blood vomiting, rhinorrhagia, hemoptysis and acute functional uterine bleeding; the *xi*–cleft points of yang meridians are applicable to acute pains. Nowadays, they are used to help in diagnosis by pressing the *xi*–cleft point.

BACK–*SHU* AND FRONT–*MU* POINTS

Back–*shu* points are specific points on the back where the *qi* of the respective *zang–fu* organs is infused. Front–*mu* points are those points on the chest and abdomen where the *qi* of the respective *zang–fu* organs is infused and converged. In total there are 12 back–*shu* and 12 front–*mu* points. The names of the 24 points, except *jueyinshu* for the pericardium, come from their respective *zang–fu* organs, such as *feishu* (BL 13), *xinshu* (BL 15), *pishu* (BL 20), *weishu* (BL 21) and *sanjiaoshu* (BL 22).

In treatment, the back–*shu* and front–*mu* points are applicable to the diseases supplied by their respective *zang–fu* organs. It was believed in ancient times that the back–*shu* points were used mainly for yin syndromes, and the front–*mu* points contrariwise. Now, if a *zang* or *fu* organ is diseased, the corresponding point will have manifestations on it, such as changes in the skin color, a depression, a prominence, a node, a trab-like object, a hemisphere-like object when pressing, or tenderness. Some studies have been done on the back–*shu* and front–*mu* points by acupoint temperature and infrared imaging techniques.

EIGHT INFLUENTIAL POINTS

The eight influential points are important points where the *qi* of *zang*, *fu*, *qi*, blood, tendon, vessel, bone and marrow gathers, respectively. They are *zhangmen* (LR 13), *zhongwan* (RN 12), *tanzhong* (RN 17), *geshu* (BL 17), *yanglingquan* (GB 34), *taiyuan* (LU 9), *dazhu* (BL 11) and *juegu* (GB 39). They indicate respectively diseases of *zang*, *fu*, *qi*, blood, tendon, vessel, bone and marrow, such as *zhangmen* (LR 13) for abdominal distension, hypochondriac pain and abdominal mass; *zhongwan* (RN 12) for stomach-ache, borborygmus, vomiting and icterus; *yanglingquan* (GB 34) for paralysis, numbness and spasm; and *geshu* (BL 17) for blood troubles of various kinds.

EIGHT CONFLUENT POINTS

The eight confluent points are the points on the limbs where the regular meridians communicate with the eight extra meridians. They are *gongsun* (SP 4), *neiguan* (PC 6), *zulinqi* (GB 41), *waiguan* (SJ 5), *houxi* (SI 3), *shenmai* (BL 62), *lieque* (LU 7) and *zhaohai* (KI 6), among which *gong-sun* (SP 4) communicates with the *chong* meridian and *neiguan* (PC 6) with the *yinwei* meridian, meeting at the stomach, heart and chest; *houxi* (SI 3) with the *du* meridian and *shenmai* (BL 62) with the yangqiao merid-ian, meeting at the inner canthus, scapular region; *lieque* (LU 7) with the *ren* meridian and *zhaohai* (KI 6) with the *yinqiao* meridian, meeting at the throat, lung, chest and diaphragm.

In the clinic, the eight confluent points are used to treat a variety of disorders of the corresponding eight extra meridians, as well as diseases of regular meridians. For example, *gongsun* (SP 4) is applicable to both diseases of the spleen meridian and the *chong* meridian, and *neiguan* (PC 6) to both diseases of the pericardium meridian and the *yinwei* meridian. Especially, the eight points are divided into four pairs to enhance the curative effect. That is to say, *gongsun* (SP 4) and *neiguan* (PC 6) as a pair are applicable to diseases of the chest, heart, liver, spleen and stomach; *lieque* (LU 7) and *zhaohai* (KI 6) to diseases of the chest, throat, lung, diaphragm, liver and kidney; *houxi* (SI 3) and *shenmai* (BL 62) to diseases of the inner canthus, neck, scapula, back and lower back; and *waiguan* (SJ 5) and *zulinqi* (GB 41) to diseases of the outer canthus, back of the ear, cheek, neck, shoulder and lateral thorax.

In addition to the specific acupoints introduced above, there are crossing points at the intersections of two or more meridians.

QUESTIONS

(1) What do specific points include?
(2) Describe the characteristics of five *shu* points and the *yuan*–primary points.
(3) What are the differences between the eight confluent points and the eight influential points?

CHAPTER 6

Commonly Used Acupoints

According to statistics from 5700 pieces of clinical literature since the 1980s, among 361 regular points, about 120 are used at the highest frequency, 120 higher and 121 lower. Here, 150 regular points and 17 extra points are collected and introduced.

ACUPOINTS OF THE LUNG MERIDIAN OF HAND–TAIYIN[1]

(1) *Zhongfu* (LU 1, Front–*Mu* Point)

Definition

"*Zhong*" refers to the energy of the middle energizer among the triple energizers; "*fu*" means "collection." The lung meridian of hand–*taiyin* starts from the middle energizer. This point is the first point of the lung meridian, which is the collection place of all energy from the middle energizer, and so it is called *zhongfu*.

Location

(i) The patient is in the supine position, at the laterosuperior aspect of the anterior wall of the chest, 6 *cun* (finger measurement; the same below) lateral to the anterior midline, at the level of the first intercostal space.

(ii) Lateral to the junction of the straight line of the nipple and the third rib. It is easy to perform: restrict it to males.

---

[1]Figure 15.

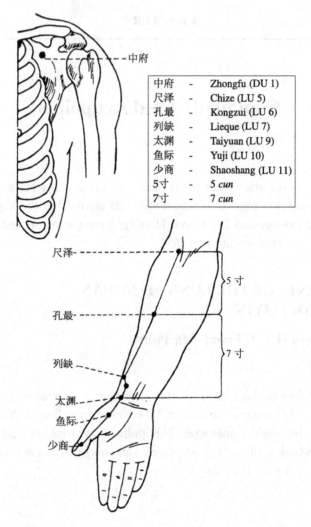

中府	-	Zhongfu (DU 1)
尺泽	-	Chize (LU 5)
孔最	-	Kongzui (LU 6)
列缺	-	Lieque (LU 7)
太渊	-	Taiyuan (LU 9)
鱼际	-	Yuji (LU 10)
少商	-	Shaoshang (LU 11)
5寸	-	5 *cun*
7寸	-	7 *cun*

Fig. 15. Acupoints of the lung meridian of hand–*taiyin*.

Method

Puncture obliquely downward with a 1-*cun*-long filiform needle, 0.5–0.8 *cun*, with the tip touching the rib margin, and a sensation of local soreness and distension. Revolving moxibustion with a moxa stick for 5–10 min is applicable.

Indications

Cough, asthma, chest pain.

Caution

Do not puncture too deeply toward the medial side, in case the lung gets hurt. It is safe to follow the structures mentioned above. Beginners are advised to use moxibustion or cupping therapies.

(2) *Chize* (LU 5, *He*–Sea Point)

Definition

"*Chi*" refers to the forearm; "ze" means "lowland in shallow water." It is named after its site.

Location

On the cubital crease, in the depression of the radial side of the tendon of the biceps muscle of the arm. This point is located with the elbow slightly flexed.

Method

Puncture perpendicularly 0.5–1 *cun* to induce the sensation of soreness and distension, or an electrified sensation radiating to the forearm. Warm moxibustion for 5–15 min.

Indications

Cough, asthma, tonsillitis, spasmodic pain of the elbow and arm.

Caution

Direct scarring moxibustion is not suitable.

(3) *Kongzui* (LU 6, *Xi*–Cleft Point)

Definition

"*Kong*" refers to poles; "*zui*" means "collecting." It is a cleft point, where *qi* and blood assemble.

Location

On the radial side of the palmar surface of the forearm, and on the line connecting *taiyuan* and *chize*, 7 *cun* above the wrist furrow.

Method

Puncture perpendicularly 1–1.5 *cun* to induce the sensation of soreness and distension in local area, or sometimes radiating to the forearm. Moxibustion with 3–7 moxa cones, or a moxa stick for 5–15 min.

Indications

Hemoptysis, cough, asthma, tonsillitis.

Caution

Tapping with a dermal needle is applicable with medium stimulation, effective for hemoptysis.

(4) *Lieque* (LU 7, *Luo*–Connecting Point)

Definition

"*Lie*" means "decomposition"; "*que*," "breaking." It is so named as it is the *luo*-connecting point hand-*taiyin* meridian where it enters hand-*yangming*, and it is located between the brachioradialis tendon and the long adductor muscle of the thumb, like a crevice. Besides, *lieque* in ancient times refers to lightning which is like a crevice in shape.

Location

(i)   On the radial side of the forearm, proximal to the processus styloideus of the radius, 1.5 *cun* proximal to the wrist furrow, between the brachioradial muscle and the tendon of the long adductor muscle of the thumb.

(ii) When the index fingers and thumbs of both hands are crossed with the wrist joint extended and the index finger of one hand placed on the processus styloideus of the radius of the other, the acupoint is in the depression on the dorsum on the wrist right under the tip of the index finger.

Method

Puncture 0.5–1 *cun* obliquely toward the elbow or horizontally toward the wrist with a local sensation of soreness and distension, or a sensation radiating to the elbow joint.

Indications

Cough, asthma, headache.

Caution

Avoid artery and direct scarring moxibustion.

(5) *Taiyuan* (LU 9, *Yuan*–Source Point)

Definition

"*Tai*" means "big"; "*yuan*," "depth of water." It is so named as it is a source point and one of the eight confluent points, where the blood and *qi* are thriving, great and deep at the *cunkou* artery.

Location

At the radial end of the crease of the wrist, when the pulsation of the radial artery is palpable.

Method

Puncture perpendicularly 0.3–0.5 *cun*, with soreness and distension in the local area.

Indications

Cough, asthma, sore throat, hemoptysis.

Caution

Avoid radial artery and direct moxibustion.

(6) *Yuji* (LU 10, *Ying*–Spring Point)

Definition

"*Yu*" means "thumb prominence like fish maw"; "*Ji*," "margin." It is named for being at the margin of the thumb prominence.

Location

In the depression proximal to the first metacarpophalangeal joint, on the radial side of the midpoint of the first metacarpal bone, and at the dorso-ventral boundary of the hand.

Method

Puncture perpendicularly 0.5 *cun* or slightly toward the palm 0.5–1 *cun*, with a sensation of soreness and distension.

Indications

Asthma, cough, dry pharynx, sore throat, infantile diarrhea.

Caution

Avoid direct moxibustion.

(7) *Shaoshang* (LU 11, *Jing*–Well Point)

Definition

"*Shao*" means "small"; "*shang*" refers to one of the five notes (*gong, shang, jiao, wei, yu*). According to *Nei Jing* (*The Inner Classic*), the sound of the lung is *shang*, so the point gets its name as it is a *jing*–well point and meridian *qi* is small at the beginning.

Location

On the radial side of the distal segment of the thumb, about 0.1 *cun* from the corner of the fingernail.

Methods

(i) Puncture obliquely upward 0.1–0.2 *cun*, with pain in the local area.
(ii) Prick for blood with a three-edged needle or a thick filiform needle.

Warm moxibustion is applicable, with a moxa stick, for 1–3 min.

Indications

Fever, swelling and pain in the throat, cough, asthma.

Summary

Location emphasis: Bone border, tendon border. Bone border for *kongzui* (LU 6) on the radial side of the palmar surface; tendon border for *chize* (LU 5) on the radial side of the biceps brachii tendon on the elbow transverse striation.

Major indications: Cough, asthma, throat disease.

QUESTIONS

(1) Describe how to locate the seven points above.
(2) What are the differences and similarities between the indications of the seven points?

ACUPOINTS OF THE HEART MERIDIAN OF HAND–SHAOYIN[2]

(1) *Jiquan* (HT 1)

Definition

"*Ji*" means "the end," and here it refers to deep depression; "*quan*" refers to the source of water. The heart meridian of hand–*shaoyin* starts from the heart and comes to the surface from the point in the axillary fossa like spring flows.

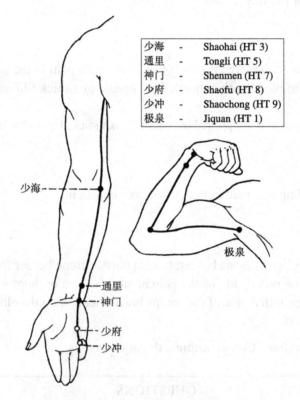

少海	-	Shaohai (HT 3)
通里	-	Tongli (HT 5)
神门	-	Shenmen (HT 7)
少府	-	Shaofu (HT 8)
少冲	-	Shaochong (HT 9)
极泉	-	Jiquan (HT 1)

Fig. 16. Acupoints of the heart meridian of hand–*shaoyin*.

[2]Figure 16.

Location

At the apex of the axillary fossa, where the pulsation of the axillary artery is palpable.

Method

With the upper arm extending, puncture perpendicularly 0.5–1.5 *cun*, with a sensation of soreness and distension in the local area or electric numbness radiating to the fingertip.

Indications

Periarthritis of the shoulder, hemiplegia by stroke, heartache.

Caution

Avoid the axillary artery. In order to make the needling sensation radiate to the fingertip, the needle should be inserted anterior to the artery. Be sure not to beat or jab after the electric numbness appears, for fear of injuring nerves. The point is unsuitable for moxibustion.

(2) *Shaohai* (HT 3, *He*–Sea Point)

Definition

"*Shao*" refers to the meridian of hand–*shaoyin*; "*hai*," the sea where rivers join.

Location

When the elbow is flexed, at the midpoint of the line connecting the ulnar end of the transverse cubital crease and the medial epicondyle of the humerus.

Method

Puncture perpendicularly or obliquely downward 0.5–1.5 *cun*, with local soreness and distension or electric numbness radiating to the forearm.

Indications

Pain in the cardiac region, schizophrenia, lymphadenitis, numbness and pain in the forearms.

Caution

Unsuitable for direct moxibustion.

(3) *Tongli* (HT 4, *Luo*–Connecting Point)

Definition

"*Tong*" means "access"; "*li*," "*inside*." It is a *luo*-connecting point where collaterals leave the meridian of hand-*taiyang*, whose branches return to the heart along this meridian.

Location

On the palmar side of the forearm, 1 *cun* proximal to the transverse crease of the wrist, at the radial border of the tendon of the m. flexor carpi ulnaris.

Method

Puncture perpendicularly 0.3–0.5 *cun*, which local soreness and distension, or numbness transmitting up and down along the ulnaris. Warm moxibustion is applicable.

Indications

Arrhythmia, pain in the cardiac region, neurasthenia, hysteria.

Caution

Unsuitable for direct moxibustion.

(4) *Shenmen* (HT 7, *Yuan*–Source Point)

Definition

"*Shen*" means "spirits, deities, heart–storing spirits"; "*men*," "door." It is a *yuan*-source point where spirits and deities come and go.

Location

On the wrist, at the ulnar end of the crease of the wrist, in the depression of the radial side of the tendon of the ulnar flexor muscle of the wrist.

Method

Puncture perpendicularly or slightly deviating to the ulnaris 0.3–0.5 *cun*, which local soreness or distension, or electric numbness radiating to the fingertips.

Indications

Insomnia, forgetfulness, dementia, palpitations, hysteria, schizophrenia.

Caution

Unsuitable for direction. Change the direction of the needle when electric numbness arises instead of grinding repeatedly.

(5) *Shaofu* (HT 8, *Ying*–Spring Point)

Definition

"*Shao*" refers to the meridian of hand–*shaoyin*; "*fu*," the place where *shen* and *qi* exist.

Location

(i) On the palm, between the fourth and fifth metacarpal bones, at the same level as *laogong* (PC 8);

(ii)   At the part of the palm touching the tip of the little finger when a fist is made.

Method

Puncture perpendicularly 0.3–0.5 *cun*, with distending pain in the local area.

Indications

Arrhythmia, pain in the cardiac region, spasm of the little finger.

Caution

Direct moxibustion is forbidden.

(6) *Shaochong* (HT 9, *Jing*–River Point)

Definition

"*Shao*" refers to the meridian of hand–*shaoyin*; "*chong*," the main route. It belongs to hand–*shaoyin* and the joint of hand–*shaoyin* and hand–*taiyang*, the main route of channel *qi* communication.

Location

On the radial side of the distal segment of the little finger, about 0.1 *cun* posterior to the corner of the nail.

Method

Puncture 0.1–0.2 *cun*, or prick for blood with a three-edged needle. Warm moxibustion for 5–10 min is applicable.

Indications

Palpitation, pain in the cardiac region, fainting, laryngitis.

Caution

Applicable to emergencies with pricking blood therapy; for others, with a shallow puncture.

Summary

Location emphasis: Stria end, tendon border, fingertip. Stripe head — *shaohai* (HT 2) is located at the end of the ulnar loop of flexed-elbow transverse striation; tendon border — *shenmen* (HT 7) and *tongli* (HT 5), 1 *cun* apart, is located lateral to the radialis of the ulnaris flexor tendon; finger tip — *shaofu* (HT 8) is located at the part of the palm touching the tip of the little finger when a fist is made.

Major indications: Heart and chest diseases.

ACUPOINTS OF THE PERICARDIUM MERIDIAN OF HAND–JUEYIN[3]

(1) *Quze* (PC 3, *He*–Sea Point)

Definition

"*Qu*" means "flexing," referring to the bend of the elbow; "*ze*," refers to a place where water joins in, which indicates that it is shallower and larger than chi ("pool") in *quchi*.

Location

At the midpoint of the cubital crease, on the lunar side of the tendon of the biceps muscle of the arm.

Method

Puncture perpendicularly 0.5–0.8 *cun*, with local soreness and distension, or electric numbness radiating to the finger, or prick with a three-edged needle for bloodletting. Warm moxibustion for 5–10 min is applicable.

---

[3]Figure 17.

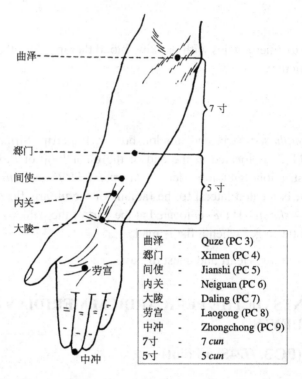

曲泽	-	Quze (PC 3)
郄门	-	Ximen (PC 4)
间使	-	Jianshi (PC 5)
内关	-	Neiguan (PC 6)
大陵	-	Daling (PC 7)
劳宫	-	Laogong (PC 8)
中冲	-	Zhongchong (PC 9)
7寸	-	7 *cun*
5寸	-	5 *cun*

Fig. 17. Acupoints of the pericardium meridian of hand–*jueyin*.

Indications

Pain in the cardiac region, palpitation, acute gastroenteritis, pain and numbness in the brachium, heatstroke.

Caution

Unsuitable for direct moxibustion. Avoid the artery while puncturing. Pricking is applicable to emergencies like acute gastroenteritis or heatstroke.

(2) *Ximen* (PC 4, *Xi*–Cleft Point)

Definition

"*Xi*," means "cleft"; "*men*," refers to a door, where *shen* ("spirit") and *qi* come and go.

Location

On the palmar side of the forearm, 5 *cun* proximal to the transverse crease of the wrist, at the line connecting *quze* with *daling*, between the tendons of the m. palmaris longus and the m. flexor carpi radialis.

Method

Puncture perpendicularly 0.8–1.2 *cun*, which local soreness and distension, or electric numbness radiating to the finger.

Indications

Coronary artery angina pectoris, arrhythmia, mania.

QUESTIONS

(1) Try to determine the selection method for *shaohai* (HT 3), *tongli* (HT 4) and *ximen* (PC 4).
(2) Which points can the pricking method be applicable to in this chapter?
(3) Which points indicate heart diseases?

---

(3) *Jianshi* (PC 9, *Jing*–River Point)

Definition

"*Jian*" refers to the cleft between two tendons; "*shi*" means "official". It belongs to the pericardium meridian, which is the official of the heart — the emperor.

Location

On the palmar side of the forearm, and on the line connecting *quze* and *daling*, 3 *cun* proximal to the transverse crease of the wrist, between the tendons of the m. palmaris longus and the m. flexor carpi radialis.

Method

Puncture perpendicularly 0.8–1.2 *cun*, with local soreness, distension and numbness radiating to the finger.

Indications

Coronary artery angina pectoris, arrhythmia, schizophrenia, hysteria, malaria.

Caution

Puncturing obliquely upward is applicable to angina pectoris and arrhythmia, with repeated twirling, rotating, lifting and thrusting of the needle to strengthen the sensation into transmitting upward. The point is unsuitable for direct moxibustion.

(4) *Neiguan* (PC 6, *Luo*–Connecting Point, One of the Eight Confluent Points)

Definition

"*Nei*" means "inside," for it is at the flexure surface of the forearm, opposite to *waiguan*; "*guan*" means "important pass." It is so named because the point is applicable to treating diseases of viscera.

Location

On the palmar side of the forearm, and on the line connecting *quze* and *daling*, 2 *cun* proximal to the transverse crease of the wrist, between the tendons of the m. palmaris longus and the m. flexor carpi radialis.

Methods

(i) Puncture perpendicularly 0.8–1.5 *cun*, penetrating to contralateral *waiguan* (SJ 5), with local soreness, distension, and numbness radiating to the fingertip.

(ii) Puncture obliquely upward (to the elbow joint) 1.5–2 *cun*, with numbness and distension diffusing to the elbow, armpit and chest.

(iii) Puncture shallowly with the tip slightly deviating to the radialis to 1.5–2 *cun*, with electric numbness radiating to the fingertip.

Indications

Coronary artery angina pectoris, arrhythmia, myocardial infarction, vomitting, hypertension, shock, diaphragmatic spasm, stomachache, as well as pain, numbness and paralysis of the upper limbs.

Caution

In treatment of heart disease, diaphragmatic spasm and vomiting, the tips should be inserted obliquely upward to make the sensation transmit upward; in treating pain, numbness and paralysis of the upper limbs, a shallow puncture should be made to induce a shocking sensation, but try to avoid repeatedly grinding in case of injuring the median nerve due to excessively strong stimulation.

(5) *Daling* (PC 7, *Yuan*–Source Point)

Definition

"*Da*" means "tall and big"; "ling," "hills." It is located behind the eminence of carpal bones, which is like a tall hill.

Location

At the midpoint of the transverse crease of the wrist, between the tendons of the m. palmaris longus and the m. flexor carpi radialis.

Method

Puncture perpendicularly 0.3–0.5 *cun*, with a local sensation of distending pain radiating to fingertips. Or puncture obliquely downward a little into the carpal, canal, with the same sensation.

Indications

Pain in the cardiac region, schizophrenia, numbness and pain in fingers.

Caution

Insert the needle rapidly, not too deep in case of injuring nerves for its apparent pain while puncturing.

(6) *Laogong* (PC 8, *Ying*–Spring Point)

Definition

"*Lao*" means "labor"; "*gong*," "palace," here meaning that the palm is the place where the heart and spirit live in. It is located at the point which the fingertip points to when the fingers are flexed.

Location

At the center of the palm, between the second and third metacarpal bones, but close to the latter, and in the part touching the tip of the middle finger when a fist is made.

Method

Puncture perpendicularly 0.3–0.8 *cun*, with a local sensation of distending pain. Warm moxibustion for 5–10 min is applicable.

Indications

Apoplectic coma, infantile convulsions, apthous stomatitis, hysteria.

Caution

Inform the patient about the pain during puncturing, and insert the needle rapidly after puncturing. It is unsuitable for direct moxibustion.

(7) *Zhongchong* (PC 9, *Jing*–Well Point)

Definition

"*Zhong*" refers to the middle finger; "*chong*" is similar to the "*chong*" in "*shaochong*" (HT 9). It is located at the tip of the middle finger, so it is named *zhongchong*.

Location

At the center of the tip of the middle finger.

Method

Puncture perpendicularly 0.1–0.2 *cun*, or prick for bloodletting with a three-edged needle.

Indications

Apoplectic coma, infantile convulsions, heatstroke, syncope.

Caution

It is used for emergencies, with strong stimulation and short-time retention. Direct moxibustion is forbidden.

Summary

Location emphasis: Tendon border, intertendon, fingertip. "Tendon border" refers to the elbow where *quze* (PC 3) is located at the ulnaris of the biceps brachii tendon, above the elbow transverse striation; "intertendon" means that *ximen* (PC 4), *jianshi* (PC 5), *neiguan* (PC 6) and *daling* (PC 7) are located between the two tendons (cubitalis grailis muscle tendon and flexor carpi radialis muscle tendon); "fingertip" refers to the tip of the middle finger, where *zhongchong* (PC 9) is located, while *laogong* (PC 8) is located at the site it directs to.

ACUPOINTS OF THE LARGE INTESTINE MERIDIAN OF HAND–YANGMING[4]

(1) *Shangyang* (LI 1, *Jing*–Well Point)

Definition

"*Shang*" refers to one of the five notes, similar to *shaoshang* (LU 11); "*yang*," a point of yang meridians, lateral to *shaoshang* (LU 11).

Location

On the radial side of the distal segment of the index finger, about 0.1 *cun* from the corner of the nail.

Method

Puncture perpendicularly 0.1–0.2 *cun*, or prick for bloodletting.

Indications

Apoplectic coma, swelling and pain in the throat, toothache, syncope.

Caution

The same as *zhongchong* (PC 9).

(2) *Erjian* (LI 2, *Ying*–Spring Point)

Definition

"*Er*" means "two," here referring to the second point in this meridian; "*jian*" means "cleft." The point is located at the cleft depression, so it gets the name *erjian*.

Location

With a slight fist made, at the dorsoventral boundary, in the depression of the radial side of the index finger, distal to the second metacarpal phalangeal joint.

---

[4]Figure 18.

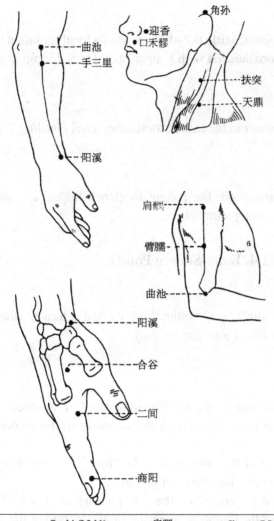

曲池	-	Quchi (LI 11)	肩髃	-	Jianyu (LI 15)
手三里	-	Shousanli (LI 13)	臂臑	-	Binao (LI 14)
阳溪	-	Yangxi (LI 5)	曲池	-	Quchi (LI 11)
迎香	-	Yjingxiang (LI 20)	阳溪	-	Yangxi (LI 5)
口禾髎	-	Kouheliao (LI 19)	合谷	-	Hegu (LI 4)
角孙	-	Jiaosun (SJ 20)	二间	-	Erjian (LI 2)
浮突	-	Futu (LI 18)	商阳	-	Shangyang (LI 1)
天鼎	-	Tianding (LI 17)			

Fig. 18. Acupoints of the large intestine meridian of hand–*yangming*.

Method

Puncture perpendicularly 0.2–0.3 *cun,* with a local sensation of distending pain. Warm moxibustion with a moxa stick for 5–15 min is applicable.

Indications

Swelling and pain in the throat, toothache, nasal bleeding.

Caution

While puncturing, ask the patient to clench his or her fist, with rapid insertion and strong stimulation.

(3) *Hegu* (LI 4, *Yuan*–Source Point)

Definition

"He" means "join"; *"gu,"* "valley." It is located at the site where the thumb and the index finger join like a valley.

Location:

   (i) On the dorsum of the hand between the first and second metacarpal bones, on the radial side of the midpoint of the second metacarpal bone;

  (ii) At the top of the eminence of the "tiger's mouth," when the thumb and the index finger are put together;

 (iii) Make the patient place the interphalangeal crease of the palmar surface of the thumb of one hand on the margin of the web between the thumb and the index finger of the other hand. The point is located just beneath the tip of the thumb when the thumb is at flexion.

Methods

   (i) Puncture perpendicularly 0.8–1.2 *cun,* with a local sensation of soreness and distension radiating to the fingertip.

(ii) Puncture 2–3 *cun* toward *laogong* (PC 8) or *houxi* (SI 3), with numbness and distension in the palm or radiating to the fingertips.

(iii) Puncture obliquely 1–1.5 *cun* along the periosteum of the second metacarpal bone, with numbness and distension radiating upward, sometimes to the elbow and shoulder joints.

Moxibustion with 3–5 moxa cones or warm moxibustion with moxa sticks for 10–15 min.

Indications

Cold, facial paralysis, hemiplegia by stroke, headache, toothache, tic douloureux, tonsillitis.

Caution

(i) The first point selection is the exact way, and the other two are easy, which may be referenced to each other.

(ii) While puncturing, hand half–clenched, avoid injuring the artery or major veins; while penetrating acupuncture is applied, be sure to avoid puncturing the arcus palmaris profundus. If branches of the cephalic vein in the dorsal fascia superficialis are pierced, local hematoma will appear; if the major artery is injured, hand muscle will contract to form abnormality due to too much bleeding. Improper point injection or excessive electrical stimulation will lead to hand muscle contraction, especially in infants.

QUESTIONS

(1) What are the characteristics in locating *jianshi* (PC 5), *neiguan* (PC 6) and *daling* (PC 7)?

(2) Compare the characteristics of the indications of the two meridian points introduced.

(3) What should be noted in locating and puncturing *hegu* (LI 4)?

(4) *Yangxi* (LI 5, *Jing*–River Point)

Definition

"*Yang*" refers to yang of yin–yang, because it is on the dorsum of the hand; "*xi*" means "stream in mountains," since it is at the depression between bones and muscles, like streams in mountains.

Location

At the radial end of the carpal transverse crease, in the depression between the tendons of the m. extensor pollicis brevis and longus when the thumb is tilted upward.

Method

Puncture perpendicularly 0.5–1 *cun*, with a local sensation of soreness and distension. Three to five cones of moxibustion are applicable, or warm moxibustion with moxa sticks for 10–15 min.

Indications

Headache, toothache, tenosynovitis, acute conjunctivitis.

(5) *Shousanli* (LI 10)

Definition

"*li*" means "*cun*," since the point is on the hand, 3 *cun* below elbow (condylus lateralis humeri).

Location

With the elbow flexed, on the radial side of the dorsal surface of the forearm and on the line connecting *yangxi* and *quchi*, 2 *cun* distal to *quchi*.

Method

Puncture perpendicularly 1.2–2 *cun*, with a local sensation of soreness and distension, sometimes radiating to the forearm and fingertips. Moxibustion with 3–7 cones is applicable, or warm moxibustion with moxa sticks for 10–15 min.

Indications

Hemiplegia by stroke, pain in the brachium, canker.

Caution

Besides local diseases (paralysis in the brachium, pain), it is applicable to abdominal diseases as adjuvant point.

(6) *Quchi* (LI 11, *He*–Sea Point)

Definition

"*Qu*" means "inflexion"; "*chi*," "pool." With the elbow flexed, a depression forms at the end of transverse striation like a shallow pool. "*Chi*" also means a place where *qi* and blood assemble like water flowing into a pool.

Location

(i) The elbow is flexed, at the midpoint of the line connecting *chize* (LU 5) and the condylus lateralis humeri;

(ii) The elbow is flexed, at the depression of the radial end of elbow transverse striation.

Methods

(i) Puncture perpendicularly 0.8–1.2 *cun* with the tip slightly oblique to the elbow joint, giving a local sensation of soreness and distension, or electric numbness radiating to the fingertips, when the patient flexes the elbow.

(ii) Puncture 2–2.5 *cun* penetrating to *shaohai* (HT 3), with a strong sensation of soreness and distension, sometimes radiating up to the shoulders or down to the fingers, when the patient flexes the elbow.

(iii) Puncture obliquely 1.5–2 *cun*, with the tip slightly toward the shoulder, giving a local sensation of soreness and distension radiating up to the shoulders.

Moxibustion with 5–7 cones is applicable, or moxibution with moxa sticks for 10–15 min.

Indications

Hemiplegia by stroke, high fever, urticaria, cold, hypertension, lateral epicondylitis, tonsillitis.

Caution

Choose a puncturing method according to different kinds of diseases: the first applicable to general diseases, the second to hemiplegia by stroke, and the third to periarthritis of the shoulder.

(7) *Binao* (LI 14)

Definition

"*Nao*" initially referred to the forelimbs of livestock; here it means the inside part of the upper arm. It is so named as it is located on the inside of the humerus.

Location

(i) On the lateral side of the arm, at the insertion of the deltoid muscle and on the line connecting *quchi* and *jianyu*, 7 *cun* above *quchi*.

(ii) The arm is raised to the level of the shoulders, at the depression above the inferior extremity of the deltoid muscle.

Methods

(i) Puncture perpendicularly 0.8–1.2 *cun,* with a local sensation of soreness and distension.

(ii) Puncture 1.2–1.5 *cun* penetrating to the anterior and posterior borders of the humerus, with a strong sensation of soreness and distension.

(iii) Puncture obliquely 1–1.2 *cun* upward to the deltoid muscle, with a local sensation of soreness and distension.

Moxibustion with 3–7 cones is applicable, or moxibution with moxa sticks for 10–15 min.

Indications

Periarthritis of the shoulder, hemiplegia by stroke, eye disease.

Caution

The two locating methods should be referenced to each other. Perpendicular insertion is applicable to paralysis of the upper extremities, and pain; penetrating insertion, to periarthritis of the shoulder; and oblique insertion, to eye diseases.

(8) *Jianyu* (LI 15)

Definition

"*Jian*" refers to the shouler; "*yu,*" acromion scapulae.

Location

On the shoulder superior to the deltoid muscle, in the depression anterior and inferior to the acromion when the arm is adducted or raised to the level of the shoulder.

Methods

(i) Puncture perpendicularly 1–1.5 *cun*, with a local sensation of soreness and distension.

(ii) Puncture 1.5–2.5 *cun* penetrating toward *jiquan* (HT 1) in the armpit, with a local sensation of soreness and distension.

(iii) Puncture obliquely toward *jianliao* (SJ 14) 1.5–2.0 *cun*, or retreat to subcutaneous and puncture obliquely toward the deltoid muscle and the anterior part of the shoulder, with soreness and distension diffusing to around the shoulder joint or to the upper limbs.

(iv) With the upper arm prostrating, puncture horizontally 2–3 *cun* toward the deltoid muscle, with a local sensation of soreness and distension.

Moxibustion with 3–7 cones is applicable, or moxibution with moxa sticks for 10–15 min.

Indications

Hemiplegia by stroke, periarthritis of the shoulder, hypertension, urticaria.

Caution

Different acupuncture methods are applicable to different diseases. The first is for beginners and for general diseases; the second and the third for periarthritis of the shoulder; the second and the fourth for hemiplegia by stroke.

(9) *Tianding* (LI 17)

Definition

"*Tian*" means "upper part or higher part"; "*ding*" refers to an ancient cooker with three legs. It is named thus because it is on the neck, in the middle of the head, cervical vertebrae and sternocleidomastoid.

Location

On the lateral side of the neck, at the posterior border of the sternocleidomastoid muscle beside the laryngeal protuberance, at the midpoint of the line connecting *futu* (LI 18) and *quepen* (ST 12).

Method

With the patient sitting with the head turning to the opposite side, puncture perpendicularly 0.3–0.8 *cun*, with a local sensation of soreness and distension reaching the back and the shoulder, sometimes with electric numbness radiating to the fingers. Warm moxibustion for 5–10 min is applicable.

Indications

Paralysis and numbness of the upper extremities, periarthritis of the shoulder, tonsillitis.

Caution

Avoid inserting too deep in case of pneumothorax. Experiences support the view that the tenderness spot may be found at this point in cases of hemiplegia by stroke or periarthritis of the shoulder. Then puncture the tenderness and induce a needling sensation radiating to the shoulders or fingers to achieve better efficacy.

(10) *Futu* (LI 18)

Definition

"*Fu*" means "help by arms"; "*tu*," "higher part." It is so named as it is located at the protrusion juncture of two tensions (the sternum end and clavicle end of the sternocleidomastoid).

Location

Ask the patient to sit upright and raise the head slightly, 3 *cun* lateral to the Adam's apple, at the midpoint between the sternal head and the clavicular head of the m. sternocleidomastoideus.

Method

Puncture obliquely downward 0.5–1 *cun* or perpendicularly 0.5–0.8 *cun*. Warm moxibustion is applicable.

Indications

Simple goiter, cough, asthma, swelling and pain in the throat.

Caution

Avoid inserting too deep or with high frequency of electroacupuncture, otherwise vagus reactions may occur, like slowing heartbeat, decreasing BP, nausea and vomiting, or a pale complexion.

(11) *Kouheliao* (LI 19)

Definition

"*He*" means "food"; "*liao*," "holes." It is near the mouth, which is for food intake, with a depression inside (a depression behind the foreteeth and the roots of tines). Since there are two points named *heliao*, it is called *kouheliao*.

Location

On the upper lip, directly below the lateral border of the nostril, on the level of *shuigou* (DU 26).

Method

 (i) Puncture perpendicularly 0.2–0.3 *cun*, with a local sensation of distending pain.
 (ii) Puncture 0.8–1.5 *cun* from *heliao* penetrating to the opposite one, with a sensation of distending pain.

Indications

Facial paralysis, rhinitis, chloasma.

Caution

The penetrating point is applicable to sequelae of facial paralysis. Direct moxibustion is forbidden.

QUESTIONS

(1) Describe the locations and indications of *quchi* (LI 11) and *jianyu* (LI 15).
(2) What should one be cautious about while puncturing *tianding* (LI 17) and *futu* (LI 18)?

---

(12) *Yingxiang* (LI 20)

Definition

"*Ying*" means "welcome"; "*xiang*" refers to flavors of various kinds. It is so named because the major indication of the point is the syndrome of anosmia.

Location

Lateral to the midpoint of the lateral border of the ala nasi in the nasolabial groove.

Methods

(i) Puncture perpendicularly 0.2–0.4 *cun* with a local sensation of distending pain.
(ii) Puncture 0.8–1 *cun* penetrating to *bitong* (EX-HN 8), with a local sensation of distending pain and lacrimation, the tip reaching the nose.
(iii) Puncture horizontally at an angle of 15°, then flatten the needle close to the skin and insert it toward the orbit 0.8–1.2 *cun*.

Indications

Rhinitis, nasal sinusitis, facial paralysis, ascariasis of the biliary tract.

Caution

Perpendicular puncture is applicable to acute rhinitis and facial paralysis in the acute stage, penetrating puncture to chronic rhinitis or nasal sinusitis, and horizontal puncture to ascariasis of the biliary tract and sequelae of facial paralysis.

Summary

Location emphasis: Intertendon, stria end, depression, ala nasi. "Intertendon" means that *yangxi* (LI 5) is located between the two wrist tendons (thumb long muscle tendon and short extensor tendon); "striae end" indicates that *quchi* (LI 11) is located at the depression of the radial end of elbow transverse striation while the elbow is flexed; "depression" refers to the depression below the acromion where *jianyu* (LI 15) is located when the arms are stretched out. "Ala nasi" means that *heliao* (LI 19) is located at the inferior border of the ala nasi, at the same level as *shougou* (DU 26) and *yingxiang* (LI 20), lateral to the midpoint of the lateral border of the ala nasi.

Major indications: Facial disease, local disease, skin disorder.

ACUPOINTS OF THE SMALL INTESTINE MERIDIAN OF HAND–*TAIYANG*[5]

(1) *Shaoze* (SI 1, *Jing*–Well Point)

Definition

"*Shao*" means "small," at the little finger aside *shaochong* (HT 9); "*ze*," "wetland or depression."

Location

On the ulnar side of the distal segment of the little finger, about 0.1 *cun* proximal to the corner of the nail.

Method

Puncture obliquely 0.1–0.2 *cun*, with a local sensation of distending pain, or prick with a three-edged needle for bloodletting. Warm moxibustion with moxa sticks for 5–15 min is applicable.

---

[5]Figure 19.

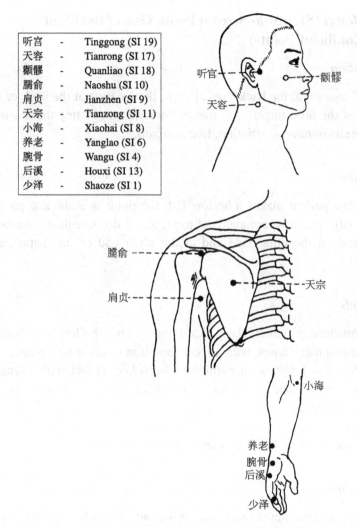

听宫	-	Tinggong (SI 19)
天容	-	Tianrong (SI 17)
颧髎	-	Quanliao (SI 18)
臑俞	-	Naoshu (SI 10)
肩贞	-	Jianzhen (SI 9)
天宗	-	Tianzong (SI 11)
小海	-	Xiaohai (SI 8)
养老	-	Yanglao (SI 6)
腕骨	-	Wangu (SI 4)
后溪	-	Houxi (SI 13)
少泽	-	Shaoze (SI 1)

Fig. 19. Acupoints of the small intestine meridian of hand–*taiyang*.

Indications

Lack of lactation after childbirth, apoplectic coma, mastitis.

Caution

Oblique acupuncture with retention and warm moxibustion are applicable to lack of lactation, and pricking needling to acute mastitis and apoplectic coma.

(2) *Houxi* (SI 3, *Shu*–Stream Point, One of the Eight Confluent Points)

Definition

"*Hou*" means "at the back," referring to the location at the back of basic joints of the little finger; "*xi*" means "stream," suggesting the location at the ulnaris transverse striation, like a stream.

Location

When the patient makes a hollow fist, the point is at the site proximal to the fifth meracarpophalangeal joint, at the dorsoventral boundary of the hand on the ulnar side and at the ulnar end of the distal palmar crease.

Methods

(i) Puncture perpendicularly 0.5–1 *cun* with a hollow fist along the lateral metacarpus, with a local sensation of distending pain.

(ii) Puncture 1.5–2 *cun* penetrating toward *hegu* (LI 4), with a sensation of soreness and distension on the whole palm, sometimes radiating to the finger.

Warm moxibustion for 5–10 min is applicable.

Indications

Malaria, mania, intercostal neuralgia, acute lumbar muscle sprain, poststroke syndrome.

Caution

Due to its severe pain, it is advised to insert swiftly. Penetrating puncture is applicable to induced poststroke syndrome like finger ankylosis.

(3) *Wangu* (SI 4, *Yuan*–Source Point)

Definition

Wangu, initially a name for the carpal bones, has the name because it is located near the carpal bones.

Location

On the ulnar border of the hand, in the depression between the proximal end of the fifth metacarpal bone and hamate bone, and at the dorsoventral boundary of the hand.

Method

Puncture perpendicularly 0.5–1 *cun*, with a local sensation of soreness and distension, sometimes radiating to the palm.

Indications

Swelling and pain in the wrist joints, diabetes, cholecystitis.

(4) *Yanglao* (SI 6, *Xi*–Cleft Point)

Definition

"*Yang*" means "to support"; "*lao*" means "the elderly," here referring to senile diseases. Ancient physicians thought that the point is effective in treating some senile conditions, like blurred vision.

Location

On the ulnar side of the posterior surface of the forearm, in the depression proximal to and on the radial side of the head of the ulna.

Method

Puncture perpendicularly 1–1.5 *cun*, with a sensation of soreness and numbness in the palm and wrist, sometimes radiating to the elbow or shoulder. Moxibustion with 3–5 cones is applicable, or warm moxibustion with moxa sticks for 10–15 min.

Indications

Stiff neck, hiccups, pain and numbness of the forearm, lumbar sprain, blurred vision.

Caution

(i) It hides itself in the bony suture, so it can be located only when the elbow is flexed with the palm turning to the chest.
(ii) Oblique acupuncture is applicable to acute stiff neck and lumbar sprain.

(5) *Xiaohai* (SI 8, *He*–Sea Point)

Definition

"*Xiao*," refers to the small intestine meridian; "*hai*" means "sea," a place with meridian *qi* aggregating.

Location

On the medial side of the elbow, in the depression between the olecranon of the ulna and the medial epicondyle of the humerus.

Methods

(i) Puncture perpendicularly 0.2–0.3 *cun*, with a local sensation of soreness and distension.
(ii) Puncture obliquely downward 0.5–1 *cun*, with a sensation of soreness and distension radiating to the forearm.

Warm moxibustion for 10–15 min is applicable.

Indications

Pain and numbness of the elbow and arm, schizophrenia, headache.

Caution

Oblique acupuncture is applicable to pain and numbness of the elbow and arm, and to patients who fail to respond to perpendicular acupuncture.

(6) *Jianzhen* (SI 9)

Definition

"*Jian*" means "shoulder"; "*zhen*," "right." Ancient people believed that the point is just at the end of the shoulder crevice on the back, which is the right position of the shoulder.

Location

Posterior–interior to the shoulder joint, 1 *cun* superior to the posterior end of the axillary fold when the upper limb is adducted.

Methods

 (i) Puncture perpendicularly 1.2–1.5 *cun*, with a local sensation of soreness and distension.
(ii) Puncture obliquely 1.2–2 *cun* at an angle of 70°, with a local sensation of soreness and distension, or soreness and numbness radiating to the fingertips.

Moxibustion with 3–5 cones is applicable, or warm moxibustion with moxa sticks for 10–15 min.

Indications

Periarthritis of the shoulder, hemiplegia by stroke, maschalephidrosis.

Caution

Oblique puncture is applicable to hemiplegia of the upper extremities, one of the poststroke syndromes. While puncturing the point, avoid inserting obliquely inward (toward the chest) too deep, in case of a pneumothorax.

(7) *Tianzong* (SI 11)

Definition

"*Tian*" means "upper part, high position"; "*zong*," "look up, adore." In ancient times the sun, moon and stars were called *tianzong* ("celestial watching"), while the point is at the highest site of the scapula, and so it gets the name *tianzong*.

Location

On the scapula, in the depression of the center of the subscapular fossa, and on the level of the fourth thoracic vertebra, or at the junction point of the upper third and middle third of the line connecting the lower border of the scapular spine and the interior angle of the scapula.

Method

(i) Puncture perpendicularly 0.8–1 *cun*, with a local sensation of soreness and distension.
(ii) Puncture obliquely 1–1.5 *cun* at an angle of 70°, with a sensation of soreness and numbness radiating to the shoulder.

Warm moxibustion for 10–20 min is applicable.

Indications

Acute mastitis, cyclomastopathy, periarthritis of the shoulder.

Caution

Oblique acupuncture is applicable to acute mastitis. And it is reported that obvious tenderness at *tianzong* (SI 11) can be regarded as the auxiliary diagnosis to biliary lithiasis.

QUESTIONS

(1) What are the characteristics of locating *houxi* (SI 3), *yanglao* (SI 6) and *xiaohai* (SI 8)?
(2) What are the characteristics of the indications of *yingxiang* (LI 20), *shaoze* (SI 1) and *tianzong* (SI 11)?

---

(8) *Tianrong* (SI 17)

Definition

"*Tian*" means "upper part"; "*rong*," "to house, to contain." It is on the neck, close to the throat, which contains things.

Location

On the lateral side of the neck, posterior to the mandibular angle, in the depression of the anterior border of the sternocleidomastoid muscle.

Methods

(i) *Routine acupuncture.* Puncture perpendicularly 0.3–0.5 *cun*, with a local sensation of soreness and distension.
(ii) *Special acupuncture.* The patient is in the supine position, with the shoulders padded up and the neck completely exposed. Feel the pulse with the left hand, and puncture between sternocleidomastoid and blood vessel, followed by inserting the needle slowly at an angle of 40° backward, inward and forward to 1–1.5 *cun*, with a sensation radiating to the forehead and shoulders.

Indications

Swelling and pain in the throat, central retinopathy, hemiplegia by stroke.

Caution

The first acupuncture is applicable to beginners, and the second mainly to eye disease and poststroke syndromes like hemiplegia, but be sure not to injure vessels. Direct moxibustion is not suitable.

(9) *Quanliao* (SI 18)

Definition

"*Quan*" refers to the jugal bone; "*liao*" means "holes." It is at the depression below the jugal bone.

Location

Ask the patient to sit upright with the eyes looking horizontally, on the face, directly below the outer canthus, in the depression on the lower border of the zygoma.

Method

Puncture perpendicularly 0.5–1 *cun*, with a local sensation of soreness and distension. Warm moxibustion for 10–15 min is applicable.

Indications

Trifacial neuralgia, facial paralysis, facial spasm, toothache, acupuncture anesthesia for craniocerebral operations and dental extraction.

(10) *Tinggong* (SI 19)

Definition

"*Ting*" means "hearing"; "*gong*" means "palace," here referring to the middle. It is so named because it is able to improve hearing and is located in the middle anterior to the ear.

Location

On the face, anterior to the tragus and posterior to the mandibular condyloid process, in the depression found when the mouth is open.

Method

With the mouth opening a little, puncture perpendicularly or obliquely downward 1.5–2 *cun*, with a local sensation of soreness and distension, or a sensation of soreness and distension in the ear and evagination of the tympanic membrane. Warm moxibustion for 10–20 min is applicable.

Indications

Deafness, otitis media, internal auditory vertigo.

Caution

While puncturing, open the mouth a little, otherwise it cannot reach the depth needed. And it requires skilled manipulation, rapid and correct because of its severe pain. The point is not suitable for direct moxibustion.

Summary

Location emphasis: Striae end, posterior to horns, depression. *Houxi* (SI 3) is located at the ulnar end of the distal palmar crease; *jianzhen* (SI 9) posterior–interior to the shoulder joint, 1 *cun* superior to the posterior end of the axillary fold. *Tianrong* (SI 17) is located posterior to the mandibular angle, in the depression of the anterior border of the sternocleidomastoid muscle. *Quanliao* (SI 18) is located at the depression of the inferior border of the jugal bone, directly below the outer canthus; *tinggong* (SI 19) is located anterior to the tragus and posterior to the mandibular condyloid process, in the depression found when the mouth is open.

Major indications: Diseases of the head and face, mastosis, local lesions.

ACUPOINTS OF THE *SANJIAO* MERIDIAN OF HAND–*SHAOYANG*[6]

(1) *Guanchong* (SJ 1)

Definition

"*Guan*" refers to an important pass. It is so named because the point is a well point of the *sanjiao* meridian of hand–*shaoyang*, where channel *qi* is generated, and it is located between *shaochong* (HT 9) and *zhongchong* (PC 9).

Location

On the ulnar side of the distal segment of the ring finger, about 0.1 *cun* posterior to the corner of the nail.

Method

A shallow puncture is performed to 0.1–0.2 *cun*, or pricking with a three-edged needle. Warm moxibustion for 5–10 min is applicable.

Indications

Apoplectic coma, heatstroke, swelling and pain in the throat, deafness.

Caution

Same as *zhongchong* (PC 9).

(2) *Zhongzhu* (SJ 3, *Shu*–Stream Point)

Definition

"*Zhong*" means "the middle"; "*zhu*," "small island." The point is the *shu*-stream point of the *sanjiao* meridian, which is like rivers flowing, where the meridian *qi* flows in and out, and so it is called *zhongzhu*.

---

[6]Figure 20.

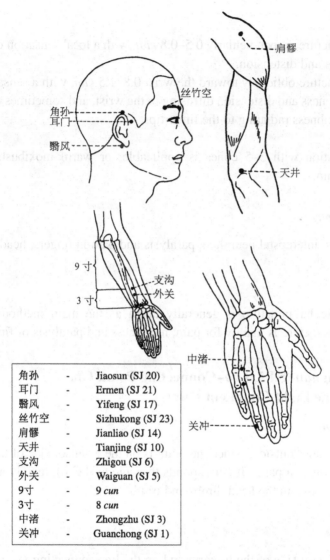

角孙	-	Jiaosun (SJ 20)
耳门	-	Ermen (SJ 21)
翳风	-	Yifeng (SJ 17)
丝竹空	-	Sizhukong (SJ 23)
肩髎	-	Jianliao (SJ 14)
天井	-	Tianjing (SJ 10)
支沟	-	Zhigou (SJ 6)
外关	-	Waiguan (SJ 5)
9寸	-	9 *cun*
3寸	-	8 *cun*
中渚	-	Zhongzhu (SJ 3)
关冲	-	Guanchong (SJ 1)

Fig. 20. Acupoints of the *sanjiao* meridian of hand–*shaoyang*.

Location

On the dorsum of the hand, proximal to the fourth metacarpophalangeal joint, in the depression between the fourth and fifth metacarpal bones.

Methods

(i) Puncture perpendicularly 0.5–0.8 *cun*, with a local sensation of sore-
     ness and distension.

(ii) Puncture obliquely toward the wrist 0.8–1.5 *cun*, with a sensation of
     soreness and distension diffusing to the wrist, and sometimes electric
     numbness radiating to the fingertips.

Moxibustion with 3–5 cones is applicable, or warm moxibustion for
10–15 min.

Indications

Deafness, intercostal neuralgia, paralysis and pain in fingers, headache.

Caution

Perpendicular puncture is generally taken as the main method, while
oblique puncture is mainly for pain, numbness and paralysis of fingers.

(3) Waiguan (SJ 5, Luo–Connecting Point, One of the Eight Confluent Points)

Definition

"*Wai*" means "outside," since the point is on the extensor side of the forearm; "*guan*", "a pass." It corresponds to *neiguan* (PC 6), mainly applicable to diseases in the head, limbs and trunk.

Location

On the dorsal side of the forearm and on the line connecting *yangchi* and
the tip of the olecranon, 2 *cun* proximal to the transverse crease of the
dorsal wrist, between the radius and the ulna.

Methods

(i) Puncture perpendicularly 0.8–1 *cun*, with a local sensation of
     soreness and distension.

(ii) Puncture 1.5–2 *cun* penetrating to *neiguan* (PC 6), with a strong sensation of soreness and distension, or electric numbness radiating to the fingertips.

(iii) Puncture obliquely 1.5–2 *cun* toward the elbow joint, with a local sensation of soreness and dissention radiating to the elbow and shoulder.

Moxibustion with 3–5 cones is applicable, or warm moxibustion for 10–15 min.

Indications

Cold, deafness, hypochondriac pain, parotitis, hemiplegia by stroke, pain and numbness in the elbow and wrist.

Caution

Perpendicular puncture is mainly applicable to local pain and numbness; penetrating puncture to *neiguan* (PC 6) for hemiplegia by stroke; oblique puncture to conditions in the head, face and trunk, such as deafness, cold and parotitis. It is worth noting that if electric numbness appears, withdraw the needle and insert it in another direction, instead of pounding aimlessly for fear of injuring the nerves.

(4) *Zhigou* (SJ 6, *Jing*–River Point)

Definition

"*Zhi*" refers to the four extremities, here meaning the forearms; "*gou*," means "ditch." It is so named as it is on the forearm, at a site depressed like a ditch.

Location

On the dorsal side of the forearm and on the line connecting *yangchi* and the tip of the olecranon, 3 *cun* proximal to the transverse crease of the dorsal wrist, between the radius and the ulna.

Method

Puncture perpendicularly 1–1.5 *cun*, with a local sensation of soreness and distension radiating to the elbow, and sometimes electric numbness radiating to the fingertips. Moxibustion with 3–5 cones is applicable, or warm moxibustion with moxa sticks for 10–15 min.

Indications

Intercostal neuralgia, contusions in the costal part, hemiplegia by stroke, habitual constipation.

(5) *Tianjing* (SJ 10, *He*–Sea Point)

Definition

"*Tian*" means "upper part"; "*jing*," "well, depression." It is so named as it is located on the olecranon, where the fossa olecrani is deep.

Location

On the lateral side of the upper arm, with the elbow flexed, at the depression about 1 *cun* proximal to the tip of the olecranon of the ulna.

Method

Puncture perpendicularly 0.5–0.8 *cun*, with a local sensation of soreness and distension. Moxibustion with 3–5 cones is applicable, or warm moxibustion with moxa sticks for 10–15 min.

Indications

Soreness in the elbow joint, lymphoid tuberculosis, urticaria, neurodermitis.

Caution

Lymphoid tuberculosis is treated with moxibustion, and other diseases with acupuncture.

QUESTIONS

(1) What is required in puncturing *tianrong* (SI 17) and *tinggong* (SI 19)?
(2) Describe how to locate *quanliao* (SI 18) and *zhongzhu* (SJ 3).

---

(6) *Jianliao* (SJ 14)

Definition

"*Jian*" means "shoulder;" "*liao*," "hole." It is so named as it is on the shoulder, which has depressions when lifted up.

Location

On the shoulder, posterior and inferior to the acromion, at the depression about 1 *cun* posterior to *jianyu* when the upper arm is horizontally adducted.

Methods

(i) Puncture perpendicularly 1–1.5 *cun* with a local sensation of soreness and distension.
(ii) Puncture 2–2.5 *cun* penetrating to *jiquan* (HT 1), with the arm adducted, a sensation of soreness and distension radiating to the whole articular cavity, and sometimes electric numbness induced to the fingertips.
(iii) Puncture obliquely 1.5 *cun*, with the tip toward the elbow, giving a sensation of soreness and distension diffusing to the shoulder. Moxibustion with 5–7 cones is applicable, or warm moxibustion with moxa sticks for 10–15 min.

Indications

Periarthritis of the shoulder, hemiplegia by stroke.

Caution

Perpendicular puncture is applicable to hemiplegia by stroke, and penetrating puncture and oblique puncture to periarthritis of the shoulder.
Beginners generally prefer perpendicular or oblique puncture.

(7) *Yifeng* (SJ 17)

Definition

"*Yi*" means "to cover"; "*feng*," "pathogenic wind." It is named *yifeng*
because it is effective in treating diseases induced by pathogenic wind,
and it is covered by auricular lobules.

Location

Posterior to the ear lobe, in the depression between the mastoid process
and the mandibular angle.

Methods

(i) Puncture perpendicularly 1–1.5 *cun* toward the contralateral eyeball,
     with a sensation of distending pain at the bottom of the external audi-
     tory canal.
(ii) Puncture obliquely 1.5–2 *cun*, with the tip anterior–inferior to the
     inside, giving a local sensation of soreness and distension, sometimes
     radiating to the throat.

Warm moxibustion with moxa sticks for 10–15 min is applicable.

Indications

Deafness, tinnitus, parotitis, facial paralysis.

Caution

Perpendicular puncture is mainly applicable to deafness and tinnitus;
oblique puncture, to facial paralysis and parotitis.

(8) *Jiaosun* (SJ 20)

Definition

"*Jiao*" refers to the superior angle of the ear; "*sun*," the minute collaterals. It is so named as it is located at the superior angle of the ear, where the lateral vein of the hand–*shaoyang* meridian passes.

Location

On the head, above the ear apex within the hairline.

Method

Puncture 0.5–1 *cun* downward along the skin or horizontally; or prick with a three-edged needle. Warm moxibustion with moxa sticks for 10–15 min is applicable, or rush-fire cauterization.

Indications

Parotitis, conjunctivitis, headache, deafness.

Caution

Parotitis and conjunctivitis are often treated with rush-fire cauterization, which will be introduced later in the book; other diseases, with acupuncture or moxibustion.

(9) *Ermen* (SJ 21)

Definition

"*Er*" means "earhole"; "*men*," "door." The point is located just in front of the earhole, like a door.

Location

On the face, anterior to the supratragic notch of the auricle, at the depression behind the posterior border of the condyloid process of the mandible.

Methods

(i) *Perpendicular puncture*: With the patient opening his or her mouth, find the depression and insert the needle rapidly to 0.8–1.5 *cun*, the tip being slightly posterior–inferior, with a sensation of distending pain radiating to the inner ear.

(ii) *Penetrating puncture*: With the tip downward, and the patient opening his or her mouth a little, insert the needle quickly, penetrating to *tinggong* (SI 19) and *tinghui* (GB 2), with a strong sensation of distending pain radiating to half of the face.

Warm moxibustion with moxa sticks for 10–15 min is applicable.

Indications

Deafness, tinnitus, otitis media, disorders of temporomandibular joint.

Caution

Puncturing *ermen* will cause pain, so it requires skilled operation and delicate manipulation, and a certain depth. Penetrating puncture is not suitable for infants and patients with a weak constitution or fearing acupuncture.

(10) *Sizhukong* (SJ 23)

Definition

"*Si*" means "finespun eyebrow"; "*zhu*," "bamboo leaves"; "*kong*," "holes." The point is located at the depression of the tip of the brow, like a bamboo leaf.

Location

On the face, in the depression at the lateral end of the eyebrow.

Methods

(i) Puncture perpendicularly 0.2–0.3 *cun*, with a local sensation of soreness and distension.
(ii) Puncture horizontally 0.5–1 *cun* backward or to the middle of the
eyebrow, with a local sensation of distension.

Indications

Headache, eye disease, facial paralysis.

Caution

Perpendicular puncture is applicable to eye disease, and horizontal puncture to others. Moxibustion was forbidden in ancient times.

Summary

Location emphasis: Interbone, olecranon, apex conchae auris. "Interbone"
refers to the two bones (ulna and radius) between which *waiguan* (SJ 5)
and *zhigou* (SJ 6) are located; *tianjing* (SJ 10) is located 1 *cun* above the
olecranon (the decranon of the ulna); *jiaosun* (SJ 20) is located at the apex
conchae auris when the auricle is folded.

Major indications: These meridian points are taken mainly for treating
diseases of the face, head and five organs, and local lesions.

ACUPOINTS OF THE STOMACH MERIDIAN OF FOOT-*YANGMING*[7]

(1) *Chengqi* (ST 1)

Definition

"*Cheng*" means "endure;" "*qi*," "tears." The point suggests that it can
endure when tears drop.

---

[7]Figure 21.

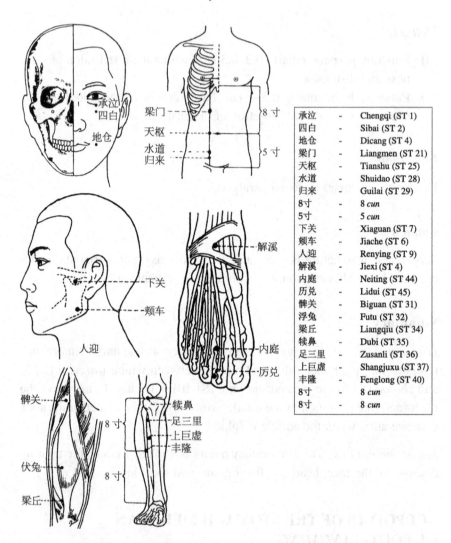

承泣	-	Chengqi (ST 1)
四白	-	Sibai (ST 2)
地仓	-	Dicang (ST 4)
梁门	-	Liangmen (ST 21)
天枢	-	Tianshu (ST 25)
水道	-	Shuidao (ST 28)
归来	-	Guilai (ST 29)
8寸	-	8 cun
5寸	-	5 cun
下关	-	Xiaguan (ST 7)
颊车	-	Jiache (ST 6)
人迎	-	Renying (ST 9)
解溪	-	Jiexi (ST 4)
内庭	-	Neiting (ST 44)
历兑	-	Lidui (ST 45)
髀关	-	Biguan (ST 31)
浮兔	-	Futu (ST 32)
梁丘	-	Liangqiu (ST 34)
犊鼻	-	Dubi (ST 35)
足三里	-	Zusanli (ST 36)
上巨虚	-	Shangjuxu (ST 37)
丰隆	-	Fenglong (ST 40)
8寸	-	8 cun
8寸	-	8 cun

Fig. 21.   Acupoints of the stomach meridian of foot–*yangming*.

Location

On the face, with the patient's eyes looking straight forward, directly below the pupil and between the eyeball and the infraorbital ridge.

Method

The patient closes the eyes. Use a fine filiform needle (No. 30–32) to pierce the skin rapidly, then insert the needle perpendicularly, close to the infraorbital border upward slightly to a depth of 1–1.5 *cun*; or insert the needle horizontally, to the angle of the eye. The sensation of soreness and distension may radiate to the whole eyeball, sometimes with lacrimation.

Indications

Conjunctivitis, central retinopathy, optic atrophy, chronic glaucoma.

Caution

Piercing the point may lead to hematoma, so it requires fine needles, rapid insertion and withdrawal. Avoid too much twirling, rotating, lifting and thrusting. Press the local skin with sterilized dry cotton balls after withdrawal. The point is unsuitable for moxibustion.

(2) *Sibai* (ST 2)

Definition

"*Si*" means "vast"; "*bai*," "bright and clear." The point is applicable to eye disease and effective in improving eyesight.

Location

On the face, with the patient's eyes looking straight forward, at the depression of the infraorbital foramen.

Methods

(i) Puncture perpendicularly 0.3–0.5 *cun*, with a local sensation of soreness and distension.
(ii) Puncture 1.5–2 *cun* toward *xiaguan* (ST 7) or *yingxiang* (LI 20), with a strong sensation of soreness and distension.

(iii) Puncture obliquely 0.3–0.5 *cun*, into the foramen infraorbitale from the lower part to *out upper*, with a sensation of electric numbness radiating to the upper lip.

Warm moxibustion with moxa sticks for 10–20 min is applicable.

Indications

Facial paralysis, trifacial neuralgia, conjunctivitis, rhinitis, keratitis.

Caution

Penetrating puncture is mainly applicable to obstinate facial paralysis; oblique puncture, to trifacial neuralgia. Beginners should take perpendicular acupuncture. The point is unsuitable for direct moxibustion.

(3) *Dicang* (ST 4)

Definition

"*Di*" means "lower part"; "*cang*," "granary." The point is located at the lower part of the face, near the mouth, where water and food are taken, and so it is name *dicang*.

Location

On the face, 0.4 *cun* lateral to the corner of the mouth, directly below the pupil.

Methods

(i) Puncture perpendicularly 0.2–0.3 *fen*.
(ii) Puncture 1.5–2 *cun* toward *jiache* (ST 6) or *yingxiang* (LI 20), with a sensation of soreness and distension in the local area or half of the face.

Warm moxibustion with moxa sticks for 3–5 min is applicable.

Indications

Facial paralysis, trifacial neuralgia, sialorrhea.

Caution

Penetrating puncture to *jiache* (ST 6) is applicable to obstinate facial paralysis; puncture to *yingxiang* (LI 20), to trifacial neuralgia.

QUESTIONS

(1) What should one be cautious about in puncturing *ermen* (SJ 21) and *chengqi* (ST 1)?
(2) Describe how to locate and puncture *jianliao* (SJ 14), *yifeng* (SJ 17), *sibai* (ST 2) and *sizhukong* (SJ 23).

---

(4) *Jiache* (ST 6)

Definition

"*Jia*" means "cheek;" "*che*," "maxillary joint." The mandible was called the mandibular joint, where the point is located.

Location

On the cheek, one fingerbreadth (middle finger) anterior and superior to the mandibular angle, in the depression where the masseter muscle is prominent.

Methods

(i) Puncture perpendicularly 0.5–0.8 *cun* with a local sensation of soreness and distension.
(ii) Puncture horizontally 2–2.5 *cun* toward *dicang* (ST 4) or *xiaguan* (ST 7), with a sensation of soreness and distension radiating to half of the face.

Warm moxibustion with moxa sticks for 5–10 min is applicable.

Indications

Facial paralysis, trifacial neuralgia, toothache, parotitis, disorders of the temporomandibular joint.

Caution

The second method is the main one for locating the point, with the first one as reference. Penetrating puncture is applicable to obstinate facial paralysis.

(5) *Xiaguan* (ST 7)

Definition

"*Xia*" means "lower part;" "*guan*," "maxillary joint," i.e. the anterior maxillary joint where the point is located, and so it is named *xiaoguan*, opposite to *shangguan*.

Location

On the face, anterior to the ear, in the depression between the zygomatic arch and the mandibular notch. It is where there is a hole with the mouth closed.

Methods

 (i) Puncture perpendicularly 1–1.5 *cun*, with the tip downward, giving a sensation of soreness and distension around.
 (ii) Puncture obliquely 0.8–1.5 *cun*, with the tip forward or backward.
(iii) Puncture 1.5–2.5 *cun*, penetrating toward *jiache* (ST 6) or *sibai* (ST 2).

Warm moxibustion with moxa sticks for 10–15 min is applicable.

Indications

Facial paralysis, trifacial neuralgia, toothache, deafness, disorders of the temporomandibular joint.

Caution

Common diseases are treated with perpendicular acupuncture. Oblique puncture is applicable to deafness; penetrating puncture, to obstinate facial paralysis.

(6) *RNying* (ST 9)

Definition

It is located at the carotid arterial pulse bilateral to the Adam's apple, called the *renying* pulse in ancient China, which was believed to welcome the *qi* of five *zang* viscera and six *fu* viscera to nourish the human body.

Location

On the neck, 1.5 *cun* lateral to the Adam's apple, at the anterior border of the m. sternocleidomastoideus, where the pulsation of the common carotid artery is palpable.

Method

Puncture perpendicularly 0.5–1 *cun* (avoiding the artery), with a local sensation of soreness and distension, sometimes radiating to the shoulder.

Indications

Hypertension, hypotension, acute or chronic laryngitis, tonsillitis, simple goiter.

Caution

During puncturing of the point, the patient should take the decubitus position instead of the sitting position. Do not puncture too deep, and stimulation should not be too strong. Avoid the artery. Generally, the point is unsuitable for moxibustion, and direct moxibustion is forbidden.

(7) *Liangmen* (ST 21)

Definition

"*Liang*" means "grains"; "*men*," "door." The point is located on the stomach, the place where food comes and goes.

Location

On the upper abdomen, 4 *cun* above the center of the umbilicus and 2 *cun* lateral to the anterior midline.

Method

With the patient in the supine position, puncture perpendicularly 1–1.5 *cun*, with a sensation of heaviness and distension in the upper abdomen. Three to five cones of moxa are applicable, or warm moxibustion with moxa sticks for 10–20 min.

Indications

Acute or chronic gastritis, peptic ulcer, vomiting.

Caution

Be sure not to puncture too deep. Generally, when the tip touches the peritoneum, the patient will complain of pain, and then stop the insertion.

(8) *Tianshu* (ST 25)

Definition

"*Shu*" means "hub." The point is located in the middle of the upper and the lower abdomen, transporting the *qi* of the middle and lower *jiao* like a traffic hub.

Location

On the middle abdomen, 2 *cun* lateral to the center of the umbilicus.

Method

Puncture perpendicularly 1–1.5 *cun*, with a local sensation of soreness and distension, sometimes radiating to the homolateral abdomen. Five-to-seven cones of moxa are applicable, or warm moxibustion with moxa sticks for 10–20 min.

Indications

Acute or chronic enteritis, bacillary dysentery, acute or chronic gastritis, appendicitis, constipation.

Caution

The same as for *liangmen* (ST 21).

(9) *Shuidao*

Definition

'*Shui*" means "stream," "current"; "*dao*," "pathway." The point works to induce diuresis and so is named *shuidao*.

Location

On the lower abdoman, 3 *cun* directly below the center of the umbilicus, 2 *cun* lateral to the middle of the abdomen.

Method

Puncture perpendicularly 1–1.5 *cun*, with a sensation of soreness and distension radiating to the homolateral lower abdomen. Five-to-seven cones of moxa are applicable, or warm moxibustion with moxa sticks for 10–15 min.

Indications

Nephritis, cystitis, urinary retention, enuresis, orchitis.

Caution

The same as for *liangmen* (ST 21).

(10) *Guilai* (ST 29)

Definition

Both "*gui*" and "*lai*" mean "recovery, restoration". The point is used to restore uterine prolapse to normal.

Location

On the lower abdomen, 4 *cun* directly below the center of the umbilicus, and 2 *cun* lateral to the midline of the abdomen, namely 1 *cun* directly below *shuidao*.

Methods

 (i) Puncture perpendicularly 1–1.5 *cun* with a local sensation of soreness and distension.
(ii) Puncture horizontally toward the pubic symphysis 5–2 *cun*, with a local sensation of soreness and distension sometimes radiating to lower abdomen and the external genitalia. Five-to-seven cones of moxa are applicable, or warm moxibustion with moxa sticks for 10–20 min.

Indications

Menoxenia, orchitis, uterine prolapse, infertility.

Caution

Horizontal acupuncture is applicable to orchitis and uterine prolapse.

(11) *Biguan* (ST 31)

Definition

"*Bi*" means "thigh"; "*guan*," "joint." The point is located at the thigh, close to the femur joint.

Location

(i) On the anterior side of the thigh and at the line connecting the anterior superior iliac spine and the superolateral corner of the patella, at the level of the perineum when the thigh is flexed, in the depression lateral to the sartorius muscle.

(ii) In the supine position, directly beneath the anterior superior iliac spine, on the transverse striation of the buttocks, opposite to *chengfu* (Bl 36).

Method

Puncture perpendicularly 1.5–2.5 *cun*, with a local sensation of soreness and distension, sometimes radiating to the knee. Three-to five cones of moxa are applicable, or warm moxibustion with moxa sticks for 10–15 min.

Indications

Hemiplegia by stroke, rheumatalgia, pain and numbness of the lower extremities.

Caution

In locating the point, the second one is easier while the first is exact, so the two should refer to each other.

QUESTIONS

(1) Descibe briefly the locations and acupuncture manipulations of *jiache* (ST 6), *xiaguan* (ST 7) and *renying* (ST 9).

(2) What are the indications of *liangmen* (ST 21), *tianshu* (ST 25), *shuidao* (ST 28) and *guilai* (ST 29)?

(12) *Futu* (ST 32)

Definition

"*Fu*" means "pronation"; "*tu*," "rabbit." The point is located at the eminence of the anterior side of the thigh; like a pronating rabbit.

Location

On the anterior side of the thigh and on the line connecting the anterior superior iliac spine and the superolateral corner of the pattela, 6 *cun* above this corner.

Method

Puncture perpendicularly 1.5–2.5 *cun*, with a sensation of soreness and distension radiating to the knee. Five-to-seven cones of moxa are applicable, or warm moxibustion with moxa sticks for 10–15 min.

Indications

Hemiplegia by stroke, paraplegia, lateral femoral cutaneous neuritis, gonarthritis.

(13) *Liangqiu* (ST 34)

Definition

"*Liang*" means "mountain ridge"; "*qiu*," "higher position." The point is located at the muscle eminence on the knee, like a hill.

Location

With the knee flexed, on the anterior side of the thigh and on the line connecting the anterior superior iliac spine and the superiolateral corner of the patella, 2 *cun* above this corner.

Method

Puncture perpendicularly 1–1.5 *cun*, with a sensation of soreness and distension radiating to the knee. Three-to-five cones of moxa are applicable, or warm moxibustion with moxa sticks for 10–15 min.

Indications

Gastritis, peptic ulcer disease, paralysis and pain of the lower extremities, mastitis, knee joint pain.

(14) *Dubi* (ST 35)

Definition

"*Du*" means "calf"; "*bi*," "nostril." The point is located in the depression lateral to the patella and its ligament on the knee, like the nostrils of a calf.

Location

With the knee flexed, on the knee, in the depression lateral to the patella and its ligament.

Methods

 (i) Puncture perpendicularly 1.5–2 *cun* from the back to the front, with a sensation of soreness and distension in the knee.
(ii) Puncture 2–2.5 *cun*, penetrating toward *neixiyan* (Ex-LE 4), with a local sensation of soreness and distension.

Warm needling is applicable with 1–2 moxa cones (1-*cun*-long cones pierced on the handle), or warm moxibustion for 15–20 min.

Indications

Gonarthrosis, hemiplegia by stroke.

Caution

During manipulation, the patient is to flex the knee at an angle of 90°. Perpendicular acupuncture is applicable to pain of the knee joint; penetrating puncture, to swelling of the knee joint.

(15) *Zusanli* (ST 36)

Definition

"*Zu*" means "foot"; "*li*," "cun." The point is located 3 *cun* below the knee, corresponding to *shousanli* (LI 10).

Location

On the anteriolateral side of the leg, 3 *cun* below *dubi*, one fingerbreadth lateral to the anterior crest of the tibia.

Methods

(i) Puncture perpendicularly 1–2 *cun*, slightly to the tibia, with a local sensation of soreness and distension, or electric numbness radiating to the dorsum of the foot.

(ii) Puncture obliquely 1.5–2.5 *cun*, with a sensation of soreness and distension, or electric numbness radiating downward to the dorsum of the foot, or upward to the knee. Five-to-ten cones of moxa are applicable, or warm moxibustion with moxa sticks for 10–20 min.

Indications

Acute or chronic gastritis, peptic ulcer disease, acute or chronic enteritis, dysentery, hypertension, neurasthenia, hyperlipidemia, hemiplegia by stroke, appendicitis, knee joint pain.

Caution

The second location method is simple and easy, and the first exact. Oblique acupuncture is mainly applicable to hemiplegia by stroke and lap diseases.

(16) *Shangjuxu* (ST 37, Lower Confluent Point of the Large Intestine Meridian)

Definition

"Shang" means "upper part;" *"juxu,"* "giant and empty," here referring to the big space between the tibiofibulas where the point is located and above *xiajuxu* (ST 39).

Location

On the anteriolateral side of the leg, 6 *cun* below *dubi*, one fingerbreadth (middle finger) from the anterior crest of the tibia.

Method

Puncture perpendicularly 1.5–2 *cun*, with a local sensation of soreness and distension, or electric numbness radiating to the foot. Three-to-seven cones of moxibustion are applicable, or warm moxibustion with moxa sticks for 10–20 min.

Indications

Appendicitis, acute or chronic enteritis, bacillary dysentery, parapysis and pain of the lower extremities.

(17) Fenglong (ST 40, Luo–Connecting Point)

Definition

 (i) *"Feng"* means "fullness"; *"long,"* "eminence." The point is located at a site with the full and ridgy muscle.
 (ii) *"Fenglong"* originally referred to the thunderclap, the name of thunder god, after which the point is named, like *lieque* (LU 7) after lightning.

Location

On the anteriolateral side of the leg, 8 *cun* proximal to the tip of the lateral malleolus, two fingerbreadths (middle finger) from the anterior crest of the tibia.

Method

Puncture perpendicularly 1.5–2.5 *cun*, the tip being slightly inward, with a sensation of soreness and distension radiating up to the knee or down to the external malleolus. Five-to-seven cones of moxa are applicable, or warm moxibustion with moxa sticks for 10–15 min.

Indications

Cough and excessive phlegm, bronchitis, hypertension, hyperlipemia, paraplegia.

(18) *Jiexi* (ST 41, *Jing*–River Point)

Definition

"*Jie*" refers to the interosseous raphe, the junction of bones; "*xi*" means "stream, depression." The point is located in the depression between the tendons of the ankle joint.

Location

At the central depression of the crease between the instep of the foot and the leg, between the tendons of the m. extensor digitorum longus and hallucis.

Methods

 (i) Puncture perpendicularly 0.3–0.5 *cun*, with a local sensation of soreness and distension.
(ii) Puncture 1–1.5 *cun*, penetrating toward both sides, with a sensation radiating to the whole ankle joint.

Five-to-seven cones of moxibustion are applicable, or warm moxibustion with moxa sticks for 10–15 min.

Indications

Pain and swelling in the ankle, headache, nephritis, thromboangiitis obliterans.

Caution

Generally, perpendicular acupuncture is used, and penetrating acupuncture is applicable to ankle diseases.

(19) *Neiting* (ST 44, *Ying*–Spring Point)

Definition

"*Nei*" means "enter"; "*ting*," "gate and yard." The point is located between toes, like a gate to a yard.

Location

At the dorsum of the foot, at the junction of the red and white skin proximal to the margin of the web between the second and third toes.

Methods

 (i) Puncture perpendicularly upward 0.3–0.5 *cun*, with a local sensation of distending pain.
(ii) Puncture obliquely 0.5–1 *cun*, with a local sensation of soreness and distension.

Warm moxibustion with moxa sticks for 10–15 min is applicable.

Indications

Toothache, trifacial neuralgia, acute or chronic enteritis, stomachache, numbness and pain of the foot.

Caution

Generally, oblique acupuncture is applicable except for local lesions, treated by perpendicular acupuncture.

(20) *Lidui* (ST 45)

Definition

"*Li*" "foot"; "*dui*," "pointed end." The point is located at the anterior end of the toe.

Location

On the lateral side of the distal segment of the second toe, 0.1 *cun* from the corner of the nail.

Method

Puncture horizontally upward 0.2–0.3 *cun*, or prick for bloodletting. Warm moxibustion with moxa sticks for 5–10 min is applicable.

Indications

Tonsillitis, neurasthenia, hysteria.

Summary

Location emphasis: The connecting line between the pupil and the angle of the lips, where *chengqi* (ST 1), *sibai* (ST 2) and *dicang* (ST 4) are located; the line lateral to the abdomen where abdominal acupoints are located 2 *cun* to the midline; the line between the anterior superior iliac spine and exterior margin of the patella, where *biguan* (ST 31) and *liangqiu* (ST 34) are located.

Major indications: Gastroenteropathy; diseases of the head and face.

QUESTIONS

(1) What are the differences and similarities in the indications of *zusanli* (ST 36), *shangjuxu* (ST 37) and *fenglong* (ST 40)?

(2) Desribe how to locate and puncture *dubi* (ST 35) and *jiexi* (ST 41).

ACUPOINTS OF THE BLADDER MERIDIAN OF FOOT–*TAIYANG*[8]

(1) *Jingming* (Bl 1)

Definition

"*Jing*" means "eyes"; "*ming*," "bright." The point is able to brighten the eyes.

Location

On the face, in the depression 0.1 *cun* superior to the inner canthus.

Method

 (i) *Shallow puncture*: Puncture perpendicularly 0.2–0.3 *cun*, with a local sensation of soreness and distension.

(ii) *Deep puncture*: Ask the patient to close his or her eyes, push the eyeball outward the left hand, take a fine filiform needle (Nos. 32–34) to insert rapidly and puncture slowly 1–1.5 *cun* along the orbital border, with a local sensation of soreness and distension radiating behind and around the eyeball.

Indications

Acute conjunctivitis, optic atrophy, central retinopathy, myopia, chronic simple glaucoma, mild cataract in the early stage.

---

[8]Figure 22.

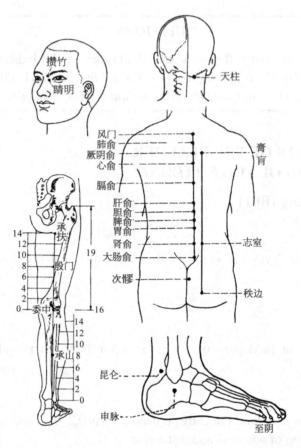

攒竹	-	Cuanzhu (Bl 2)	大肠俞	-	Dachangshu (Bl 25)
睛明	-	Jingming (Bl 1)	次髎	-	Ciliao (Bl 32)
天柱	-	Tianzhu (Bl 10)	承扶	-	Chengfu (Bl 36)
风门	-	Fengmen (Bl 12)	殷门	-	Yinmen (Bl 37)
肺俞	-	Feishu (Bl 13)	委中	-	Weizhong (Bl 40)
厥阴俞	-	Jueyinshu (Bl 14)	承山	-	Chengshan (Bl 57)
心俞	-	Xinshu (Bl 15)	膏肓	-	Gaohuang (Bl 43)
膈俞	-	Geshu (Bl 17)	志室	-	Zhishi (Bl 52)
肝俞	-	Ganshu (Bl 18)	秩边	-	Zhibian (Bl 54)
胆俞	-	Danshu (Bl 19)	昆仑	-	Kunlun (Bl 60)
脾俞	-	Pishu (Bl 20)	申脉	-	Shenmai (Bl 62)
胃俞	-	Weishu (Bl 21)	至阴	-	Zhiyin (Bl 67)
肾俞	-	Shenshu (Bl 23)			

Fig. 22.   Acupoints of the bladder meridian of foot–*taiyang*.

Caution

Beginners should take shallow puncture rather than deep puncture, for this will lead to ocular hematoma. While puncturing deeply, be sure to push the needle slowly and change the direction if there is any resistance till the sensation appears, the needle is retained without lifting or twirling, and do not insert it too deeply. Withdraw the needle slowly then press the local skin with disinfection dry cotton balls for 1–2 min. Do observe whether there is blood in the pinhole. Too much bleeding suggests injury of the vessel, which requires a cold compress to stop the bleeding, followed by a hot compress to disperse the blood stasis. Moxibustion is not suitable for the point.

(2) *Cuanzhu* (Bl 2)

Definition

"*Zan*" means "assemble, gather'; "*zhu*," "bamboo leaf," here referring to the eyebrow. The point is located on the inner side of the eyebrow, like bamboo leaves gathering together, when the patient frowns.

Location

On the face, in the depression at the medial end of the eyebrow, at the supraorbital notch.

Methods

(i) *Shallow acupuncture*: Puncture perpendicularly 0.2–0.3 *cun*, or puncture obliquely downward to *jingming* (Bl 1) 0.5–0.8 *cun*, with a sensation of soreness and distension in the local area or around the eye.

(ii) *Deep acupuncture*: A No. 30 filiform needle is inserted slowly along the foramen sive incisura supraorbitalis to 1–1.5 *cun*, with a sensation of soreness and distension in the orbit or the eyeball.

(iii) *Horizontal acupuncture*: Insert the needle 1.2–1.5 *cun*, with the tip to the middle of the eyebrow, giving a sensation of distending pain in the local area or around the eye.

Warm moxibustion with moxa sticks for 3–5 min is applicable.

Indications

Headache, acute conjunctivitis, facial paralysis, optic atrophy.

Caution

Shallow acupuncture is mainly applicable to headache and acute conjunctivitis; deep acupuncture to optic atrophy; and horizontal acupuncture to facial paralysis. Deep acupuncture always results in bleeding, so what one should be cautious about is the same as for puncturing *jingming* (Bl 1). Direct moxibustion is unsuitable for the point.

(3) *Tianzhu* (BL 10)

Definition

"*Tian*" means "head"; "*zhu*," "post, pillar." Nuchal muscle bulges like a pillar where the point is located.

Location

On the nape, 1.3 *cun* lateral to the posterior midline, at the depression at the lateral border of the m. trapezius.

Method

Puncture perpendicularly 0.5–1 *cun*, with a local sensation of soreness and distension radiating to the parietal region. Warm moxibustion with moxa sticks for 5–10 min is applicable.

Indications

Posterior headache, stiff neck, laryngopharyngitis, neurasthenia.

Caution

The point is unsuitable for deep acupuncture upward, in case of hurting by mistake the medulla oblongata. Generally, direction moxibustion is not applied.

(4) *Fengmen* (BL 12)

Definition

"*Feng*" refers to pathogenic wind; "men" means "door." The point was believed in ancient times to be the door for pathogenic wind coming and going.

Location

On the back, 1.5 *cun* lateral to the posterior midline, below the spinous process of the first thoracic vertebra.

Methods

(i)   *Oblique acupuncture*: At 1 *cm* outside the point, insert the needle toward the apinal column at an angle of 45° to a depth of 1–1.5 *cun*, with a local sensation of soreness and distension, sometimes radiating to the ribs.

(ii) *Horizontal acupuncture*: Puncture 1.5–2 *cun*, penetrating from up to down, with a local sensation of soreness and distension.

Moxibustion with 3–5 cones is applicable, or warm moxibustion with moxa sticks for 10–15 min.

Indications

Cold, bronchitis, pneumonia, pertussis, urticaria.

Caution

It is a little difficult for beginners to puncture perpendicularly, for too-deep acupuncture will injure the lung and induce a pneumothorax.

(5) *Feishu* (BL 13, Back–*Shu* Point of the Lung)

Definition

"*Fei*" refers to the lung; "*shu*," the back–*shu* point, i.e. the place for viscus *qi* transfusion where the point is located.

Location

On the back, 1.5 *cun* lateral to the posterior midline, below the spinous process of the third thoracic vertebra.

Method

The same as for *fengmen* (BL 12).

Indications

Bronchitis, asthma, pertussis, pneumonia.

Caution

The same as for *fengmen* (BL 12).

(6) *Jueyinshu* (BL 14, Back–*Shu* Point)

Definition

"*Yueyin*" refers to the pericardium of hand–*jueyin*, meaning that the point is corresponding to the pericardium, where *qi* and blood infuse.

Location

On the back, 1.5 *cun* lateral to the posterior midline, below the spinous process of the fourth thoracic vertebra.

Method

Puncture obliquely (toward thoracic vertebrae) 1.5–2 *cun* till the tip touches the basivertebral. The needling sensation may radiate to the brisket. Moxibustion with 3–7 cones is applicable, or warm moxibustion with moxa sticks for 10–15 min.

Indications

Coronary artery disease, arrhythmia, intercostal neuralgia, rheumatic heart disease.

Caution

Too-deep puncture at this point will injure the lung and, generally, oblique acupuncture is applied, especially for beginners.

(7) *Xinshu* (BL 15, Back–*Shu* Point)

Definition

"*Xin*" means "heart." The point is the place where heart *qi* is transported.

Location

On the back, 1.5 *cun* lateral to the posterior midline, below the spinous process of the fifth thoracic vertebra.

Method

The same as for *jueyinshu* (BL 14).

Indications

Coronary artery disease, arrhythmia, neurasthenia, schizophrenia, intercostal neuralgia.

Caution

The same as for *jueyinshu* (BL 14).

(8) *Gesu* (BL 17, Back–*Shu* Point, the Influential Point Relating to the blood)

Definition

"*Ge*" refers to the diaphragm, corresponding to the point.

Location

On the back, 1.5 *cun* lateral to the posterior midline, below the spinous process of the seventh thoracic vertebra.

Method

Puncture obliquely downward or beside the vertebral column 0.5–0.8 *cun*, with a local sensation of soreness and distension. Three-to-five cones of moxa are applicable, or warm moxibustion with moxa sticks for 10–15 min.

Indications

Hiccups (diaphragmatic spasm), nervous vomitting, hemoptysis.

Caution

The same as for *jueyinshu* (BL 14). Regional anatomy shows that the point is located in the thinnest muscle layer, and deep puncture should be avoided.

(9) *Ganshu* (BL 18, Back–*Shu* Point)

Definition

"*Gan*" refers to the liver. The point is the place where liver *qi* is transported.

Location

On the back, 1.5 *cun* lateral to the posterior midline, below the spinous process of the ninth thoracic vertebra.

Method

The same as for *geshu* (BL 17).

Indications

Acute or chronic hepatitis, cholecystitis, eye disease, neurasthenia.

Caution

Avoid too-deep puncture, in case of injuring the lung to induce a pneumothorax.

(10) *Danshu* (BL 19, Back–*Shu* Point)

Definition

"Dan" refers to the gallbladder. The point is a back–*shu* point of the gallbladder.

Location

On the back, 1.5 *cun* lateral to the posterior midline, below the spinous process of the tenth thoracic vertebra.

Method

The same as for *geshu* (BL 17).

Indications

Cholecystitis, hepatitis.

Caution

The same as for *ganshu* (BL 18).

QUESTIONS

(1) What should one be cautious about in puncturing *jingming* (BL 1) and *zanzhu* (BL 2)?

(2) What are the back–*shu* points? What should one be cautious about in puncturing the points of the back?

(11) *Pishu* (BL 20, Back–*Shu* Point)

Definition

"*Pi*" refers to the spleen. The point is the back–*shu* point of the spleen.

Location

On the back, 1.5 *cun* lateral to the posterior midline, below the spinous process of the 11th thoracic vertebra.

Method

Puncture perpendicularly 0.8–1 *cun*, slightly inclined to the vertebral body, with a local sensation of soreness, numbness and distension. Three-to-five cones of moxibustion are applicable, or warm moxibustion with moxa sticks for 10–20 min.

Indications

Gastritis, peptic ulcer disease, gastroptosis, uterine prolapse, anergy of limbs.

Caution

Too-deep puncture should be avoided, for fear of injuring the kidney or the liver.

(12) *Weishu* (BL 21, Back–*Shu* Point)

Definition

"*Wei*" refers to the stomach. The point is the back–*shu* point of the stomach.

Location

On the back, 1.5 *cun* lateral to the posterior midline, below the spinous process of the 12th thoracic vertebra.

Method

The same as for *pishu* (BL 20).

Indications

Stomachache, peptic ulcer disease, pancreatitis, gastritis.

Caution

The same as for *pishu* (BL 20).

(13) *Shenshu* (BL 23, Back–*Shu* Point)

Definition

"*Shen*" refers to the kidney. The point is the place where kidney *qi* is transported.

Location

On the back, 1.5 *cun* lateral to the posterior midline, below the spinous process of the second thoracic vertebra.

Method

Puncture perpendicularly 1.5–2 *cun*, slightly inlined to the vertebral body, with a sensation of soreness and distension in the lower back, or electric numbness radiating to the buttocks or the lower limbs. Three-to-five cones of moxibustion are applicable, or warm moxibustion with moxa sticks for 10–15 min.

Indications

Nephritis, kidney calculi, UTI (urinary tract infection), infantile enuresis, soft tissue injuries in the lower back, lumbago leg pain.

Caution

While puncturing, the tip should be directed to the vertebral body instead of deviating to the outside, for fear of injuring the kidney.

(14) *Dachangshu* (BL 25, Back–*Shu* Point)

Definition

"*Dachang*" refers to the large intestine. The point is the place where large intestine *qi* is transported.

Location

On the back, 1.5 *cun* lateral to the posterior midline, below the spinous process of the fourth thoracic vertebra.

Methods

(i) Puncture perpendiculary 1–2 *cun*, with a local sensation of soreness and distension.
(ii) Puncture obliquely 2–3 *cun*, with the tip outward a little, giving a sensation of electric numbness radiating to the lower limbs.

Moxibustion with 5–7 cones is applicable, or warm moxibustion with moxa sticks for 10–20 min.

Indications

Acute or chronic enteritis, enuresis, soft tissue injuries in the lower back, sciatica.

Caution

Perpendicular puncture is applicable to common diseases; oblique puncture, to sciatica.

(15) *Ciliao* (BL 32)

Definition

"*Ci*" means "second"; "*liao*," means "hole," here referring to the deuter-ostoma of the sacrum where the point is located.

Location

On the sacrum, at the second posterior sacral foramen, medial and inferior to the posterior superior iliac spine and the governor vessel.

Method

Puncture perpendicularly into the dorsal sacral foramina 1–2 *cun*, with a sensation of soreness and distension in the sacral region, or radiating to the abdomen or lower limbs. Three-to-five cones of moxibustion are applicable, or warm moxibustion with moxa sticks for 10–15 min.

Indications

Sciatica, amenorrhea, menalgia, urinary incontinence, paraplegia.

Caution

The crevice hole must be found exact; puncture it perpendicularly or slightly upward. Too-deep insertion should be avoided, for fear of injuring the rectum or bladder.

(16) *Chengfu* (BL 36)

Definition

"*Cheng*" means "bear, endure"; "*fu*," "support." The point is able to bear the upper body and to support the lower body.

Location

On the posterior side of the thigh and on the midpoint of the inferior transverse gluteal fold.

Method

Puncture perpendicularly 2–2.5 *cun*, with a local sensation of soreness and distension, or electric numbness radiating to the foot. Three-to-five cones of moxibustion are applicable, or warm moxibustion with moxa sticks for 10–15 min.

Indications

Sciatica, paraplegia.

(17) *Yinmen* (BL 37)

Definition

"*Yin*" means "profound, medianus"; "*men*" refers to the door where meridian *qi* comes and goes. The point is located at the thick muscles in the posterior middle of the thigh.

Location

On the posterior side of the thigh and on the line connecting *chengfu* and *weizhong*, 6 *cun* distal to *chengfu*.

Method

Puncture perpendicularly 2–2.5 *cun* with a local sensation of soreness and distension, or electric numbness radiating up to the buttocks, or down to the foot. Three-to-five cones of moxibustion are applicable, or warm moxibustion with moxa sticks for 10–15 min.

Indications

Lumbago, sciatica, paraplegia.

(18) *Weizhong* (BL 40, *He*–Sea Point)

Definition

"*Wei*" means "bending," here referring to the bending part of the knee; "*zhong*," "center." The points located at the center of the bending part of the knee.

Location

At the midpoint of the transverse popliteal fold, between the tendons of the biceps muscle of the thigh and the semitendinous muscle.

Method

Puncture perpendicularly 0.5–1 *cun*, with a local sensation of soreness and distension, or electric numbness radiating to the foot; Or prick with a three-edged needle for bloodletting. Warm moxibustion with moxa sticks for 5–7 min is applicable.

Indications

Acute lumbar muscle sprain, hemiplegia by stroke, sciatica, swelling and pain in the knee joint.

Caution

In order to transmit the needling sensation downward, ask the patient to lie on the back with leg-raising (if this cannot be done, seek help from others). Insert the needle to the middle of the point 0.5–0.8 *fen*. In most cases, the sensation of electric numbness will be induced and will radiate to the foot. But remember that 2–3-time stimulation is enough. The method is applicable to sciatica and hemiplegia by stroke; pricking with three-edged needles, to acute lumbar muscle sprain.

(19) *Gaohuang* (BL 43)

Definition

"*Gao*" refers to lipoids; "*huang*," membranes. It was thought in ancient times that *gao* was the inferior part of the heart while *huang* was located under the heart and above the diaphragm. The point is the place where *gaohuang qi* is transported.

Location

On the back, 3 *cun* lateral to the posterior midline, below the spinous process of the fourth thoracic vertebra.

Method

Puncture obliquely 0.5–1 *cun* from the anterior exterior to the dorsal part, with local sensation of soreness and distension, sometimes radiating to the scapular region. Moxibustion with 5–15 cones is applicable, or warm moxibustion with moxa sticks for 10–20 min.

Indications

Bronchitis, asthma, weakness due to chronic disease.

Caution

The point is generally given moxibustion. Acupuncture is applied to a depth of no more than 0.8 *cun* (regional anatomy shows that its maximum depth is 3.5 cm), otherwise it will injure the lung.

(20) *Zhishi* (BL 52)

Definition

"*Zhi*" means "will"; "*shi*," "house." According to TCM theory, the kidney stores will. The point is located bilateral to *shenshu* (BL 23), the place where kidney *qi* is infused.

Location

On the lower back, 3 *cun* lateral to the posterior midline, below the spinous process of the second thoracic vertebra.

Methods

(i) Puncture perpendicularly 0.5–0.8 *cun*, with a local sensation of soreness and distension.
(ii) Puncture obliquely toward *shenshu* (BL 23) 2–3 *cun*, with a local sensation of soreness and distension radiating to the buttocks or lower limbs.

Five-to-seven cones of moxibustion are applicable, or warm moxibustion with moxa sticks for 10–20 min.

Indications

Nephroptosia, lumbago, nephritis, prostatitis.

Caution

The maximum depth in this point is 1 *cun*. Oblique puncture is applicable to lower back pain.

QUESTIONS

(1) Describe the locations of *pishu* (BL 20), *gaohuang* (BL 43) and *ciliao* (BL 32).
(2) What are the differences and similarities between the indications and the acupuncture methods of *yinmen* (BL 37) and *weizhong* (BL 40)?

---

(21) *Zhibian* (BL 54)

Definition

"*Zhi*" means "order, sequence"; "*bian*," "border." The point is located at the lowest along the back of the bladder meridian.

Location

On the buttock and on the level of the fourth posterior sacral foramen, 3 *cun* lateral to the median sacral crest.

Methods

(i) Puncture perpendicularly 2–3 *cun* with a local sensation of soreness and distension, or electric numbness radiating to the foot.

(ii) Puncture obliquely at an angle of 45° 2.5–4 *cun* with a sensation radiating to the abdomen and the perineal region.

Five-to-seven cones of moxa are applicable, or warm moxibustion with moxa sticks for 10–20 min.

Indications

Sciatica, paraplegia, impotence, functional ejaculation failure.

Caution

Perpendicular puncture is applicable to sciatica and paraplegia; oblique puncture, to diseases of the genital system.

(22) *Chengshan* (BL 57)

Definition

"*Cheng*" means "continue"; "*shan*," "valley." The lower end of the gastrocnemius muscle in the leg is like a valley, with a depression in it where the point is located.

Location

On the posterior midline of the leg, between *weizhong* and *kunlun*, in the pointed depression formed below the gastrocnemius muscle belly when the leg is stretched or the heel is lifted.

Method

Puncture perpendicularly 1–1.5 *cun*, with a local sensation of soreness and distension. Warm moxibustion with moxa sticks for 10–15 min is applicable.

Indications

Sciatica, sural spasm, piles.

Caution

Puncturing *chengshan* (BL 57) should avoid lifting and thrusting or twirling and rotating with a large amplitude, otherwise discomfort will occur.

(23) *Kunlun* (BL 60, *Jing*–River Point)

Definition

"*Kunlun*" originally meant "high mountains"; here it refers to the external ankle protruding high like a mountain, beside which the point is located.

Location

Posterior to the lateral malleolus, at the depression between the tendon of the m. calcaneus and the tip of the external malleolus.

Methods

(i) Puncture perpendicularly 0.5–1 *cun*, with a local sensation of soreness and distension radiating to the little toe.
(ii) Puncture obliquely, with the tip upward, 1–2 *cun*, giving a local sensation of soreness and distension radiating to the heel and/or the toe.

Three-to-five cones of moxibustion are applicable, or warm moxibustion with moxa sticks for 5–15 min.

Indications

Headache, acute lumbar muscle sprain, paraplegia, thyromegaly, abnormal fetal position, sciatica.

Caution

Perpendicular puncture is applicable to common diseases; oblique puncture, to thyromegaly.

(24) *Shenmai* (BL 62, One of the Eight Confluent Points)

Definition

"*Shen*" means "extend, stretch"; "*mai*," the yang heel channel where the points pass.

Location

On the lateral side of the foot, in the depression directly below the external malleolus.

Methods

 (i) Puncture perpendicularly 0.3–0.5 *cun*, with a local sensation of soreness and distension.
(ii) Puncture obliquely 0.5–0.8 *cun*, with the tip downward, giving a local sensation of soreness and distension.

Three-to-five cones of moxibustion are applicable, or warm moxibustion with moxa sticks for 10–15 min.

Indications

Internal auditory vertigo, mania, an ankle sprain, headache.

Caution

Oblique puncture is applicable to an ankle sprain.

(25) *Zhiyin* (BL 67, *Jing*–Well Point)

Definition

"*Zhi*" means "arrive"; "*yin*" refers to the kidney meridian of foot–*shaoyin*, where the bladder meridian of foot–*taiyang* and of foot–*shaoyin* make contact.

Location

On the lateral side of the distal segment of the small toe, about 0.1 *cun* posterior to the corner of the nail.

Method

Puncture obliquely upward 0.1–0.2 *cun*, or prick for bloodletting, with pain in the local area. Warm moxibustion with moxa sticks for 10–30 min is applicable.

Indications

Abnormal fetal position, prolonged labor, headache.

Caution

Moxibustion is applicable to abnormal fetal position.

Summary

Location emphasis: Vertebral column, buttock striation, ham striation, interval between muscles, ankle. Back-*shu* points of the first lateral line are located 1.5 *cun* lateral to the middle of vertebrae, and points of the second lateral line are located 3 *cun* lateral to it; *chengfu* (BL 36) in the middle of buttock striation; *weizhong* (BL 40) in the middle of ham striation; *chengshan* (BL 57) at the divergence of the two ends of the gastrocnemius muscle; *kunlun* (Bl 60) in the depression between the ankle and the achilles tendon.

Major indications: Diseases of *zang–fu* viscera, diseases of the head and face, local disease.

ACUPOINTS OF THE GALLBLADDER MERIDIAN OF FOOT–*SHAOYANG*[9]

(1) *Tongziliao* (GB 1)

Definition

"*Tongzi*" means "eye"; "*liao*," "hole." The point is located beside the eye.

Location

On the face, 0.5 *cun* lateral to the outer canthus, at the depression on the lateral border of the orbit.

Method

Puncture horizontally toward the temple (backward) to 0.8–1 *cun*, with a local sensation of soreness and distension, sometimes radiating to the ear canal. Warm moxibustion with moxa sticks for 5–10 min is applicable.

Indications

Headache, central retinitis, optic atrophy, facial paralysis.

Caution

Unsuitable for direct moxibustion.

(2) *Tinghui* (GB 2)

Definition

"*Ting*" refers to the sense of hearing; "*hui*" means "convergence". "The point may converge the sense of hearing.

Location

On the face, anterior to the intertragic notch, at the depression posterior to the condyloid process of the mandible when the mouth is open.

---

[9]Figure 23.

阳白	-	Yangbai (GB 14)
瞳子髎	-	Tongziliao (GB 1)
听会	-	Tinghui (GB 2)
风池	-	Fengchi (GB 20)
肩井	-	Jianjing (GB 21)
居髎	-	Juliao (GB 29)
环跳	-	Huantiao (GB 30)
风市	-	Fengshi (GB 31)
阳陵泉	-	Yanglingquan (GB 34)
光明	-	Guangming (GB 37)
悬钟	-	Xuanzhong (GB 39)
丘墟	-	Qiuxu (GB 40)
足临泣	-	Zulinqi (GB 41)
足窍阴	-	Zuqiaoyin (GB 44)

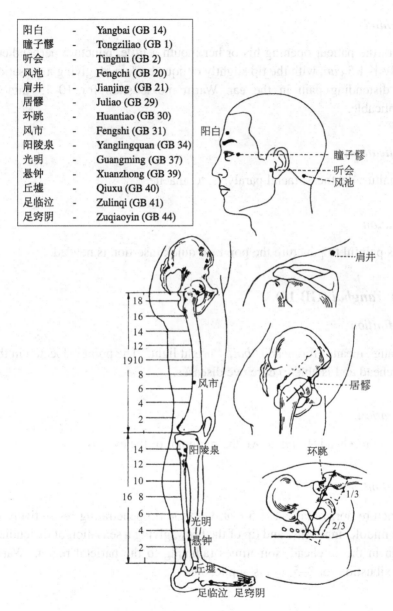

Fig. 23. Acupoints of the gallbladder meridian of foot–*shaoyang*.

Method

With the patient opening his or her mouth a little, puncture perpendicularly 1–1.5 *cun*, with the tip slightly oblique backward, giving a sensation of distending pain in the ear. Warm moxibustion for 10–15 min is applicable.

Indications

Tinnitus, deafness, facial paralysis, toothache.

Caution

It is painful to puncture the point, so quick insertion is needed.

(3) *Yangbai* (GB 14)

Definition

"Yang" means "forehead" "*bai*," "bright light." The point is located in the forehead and is able to cure eye diseases.

Location

At the forehead, 1 *cun* above the midpoint of the eyebrow.

Method

Puncture horizontally 1–1.5 *cun*, with the tip penetrating respectively to the middle, inner side and tip of the brow, giving a sensation of distending pain in the forehead, sometimes radiating to the parietal region. Warm moxibustion for 3–5 min is applicable.

Indications

Frontal headache, paralysis, ptosis, eye disease.

Caution

Generally, horizontal puncture to the middle of eyebrow is applied to the point, and penetrating needling to the inner side or tip is available for facial paralysis.

(4) *Fengchi* (GB 20)

Definition

"*Feng*" refers to pathogenic wind; "*chi*," means "pool," here referring to a depression. The point is located in the depression of the lateral neck, which is a place pathogenic wind will easily attack.

Location

In the posterior aspect of the neck, below the occipital bone, on the level of *fengfu*, at the depression between the upper ends of the m. sternocleido-mastoid and m. trapezius.

Methods

(i) Puncture perpendicularly to the nasal tip 0.5–1.2 *cun*, with a local sensation of soreness and distension radiating to the calvaria, temporalis part, forehead or orbit.

(ii) Puncture penetrating to contralateral *fengchi* (GB 20), with a local sensation of soreness and distension radiating to the nuchal region.

Warm moxibustion for 10–15 min is applicable.

Indications

Cold, headache, eye disease, hypertension, mania, painful spasm of the nape.

Caution

Being one of the dangerous points, the point is inserted no deeper than 1.2 *cun*. Avoid deep puncture to the contralateral tragus or its anterior border, for fear of piercing the cranial cavity. Among the acupuncture techniques, perpendicular puncture is the most common one and penetrating puncture is more applicable to headache or painful spasm of the nape.

QUESTIONS

(1)   What should one be cautious about in puncturing *fengchi* (GB 20) and *chengshan* (BL 57)?
(2)   Recall the locations and indications of the points learned about.

---

(5) *Jianjing* (GB 21)

Definition

"*Jian*" means "shoulder"; "*jing*," "depression." The point is located in the depression of the shoulder.

Location

On the shoulder, directly above the nipple, at the midpoint of the line connecting *dazhui* and the acomion.

Method

Puncture perpendicularly or obliquely backward a bit 0.5–1 *cun*, with a local sensation of soreness and distension radiating to the shoulder and back. Three-to-seven cones of moxibustion are applicable, or warm moxibustion for 10–15 min.

Indications

Shoulder pain, hemiplegia by stroke, mastitis, drowsiness.

Caution

Being one of the dangerous points, *jianjing* (GB 21) is punctured no deeper than 1 *cun*, especially for emaciated old men. Inserting to the anterior interna should be avoided.

(6) *Juliao* (GB 29)

Definition

"*Ju*" means "squat down"; "*liao*," air space. The point refers to the depression in the thigh when the person is squatting down.

Location

On the hip at the midpoint of the line connecting the anteriosuperior iliac spine and the prominence of the great trochanter.

Methods

(i)   Puncture perpendicularly 1–2 *cun*, with a local sensation of soreness and distension.
(ii) Puncture obliquely 2–3 *cun*, with the tip toward the hip joint, giving a sensation of soreness and distension radiating to the hip joint.

Five-to-seven cones of moxibustion are applicable, or warm moxibustion for 10–15 min.

Indications

Pain and swelling in coxa, acute lumbar muscle sprain, paraplegia, lumbago leg pain.

Caution

Perpendicular puncture is always taken as the main method, and oblique puncture is applicable to pain and swelling in coxa.

(7) *Huantiao* (GB 30)

Definition

"*Huan*" means "round," here referring to the buttocks; "*tiao*," "jump." The point is located on the buttock and is able to cure diseases of lower limb movement.

Location

On the lateral side of the thigh, when the patient is in the lateral recumbent position with the thigh flexed, at the junction of the lateral one-third and medial two-thirds of the line connecting the highest point of the greater trochanter and the hiatus of the sacrum.

Methods

 (i) Puncture perpendicularly 2–3 *cun*, with the tip slightly leaning to the perineum, giving a local sensation of soreness and distension or electric numbness radiating to the foot.
(ii) Puncture obliquely 1.5–2.5 *cun*, with the tip probing near the hip joint, giving a sensation radiating to the hip joint.

Seven-to-ten cones of moxibustion are applicable, or warm moxibustion for 10–20 min.

Indications

Sciatica, paraplegia, soft tissue injury in the gluteal region.

Caution

Perpendicular puncture is mainly applicable to sciatica and paraplegia; oblique puncture, to soft tissue injury in the gluteal region.

(8) *Fengshi* (GB 31)

Definition

"*Feng*" refers to disease affected by pathogenic wind; "*shi*" means "market, assemble." The point is able to cure different diseases affected by pathogenic wind.

Location

At the midline of the lateral aspect of the thigh, 7 *cun* proximal to the transverse popliteal crease; or, when the patient is standing upright with the hands hanging by the sides of the body, the point is where the tip of the middle finger reaches.

Method

Puncture perpendicularly 1.5–2 *cun*, with a local sensation of soreness and distension, sometimes radiating downward. Five-to-seven cones of moxa are applicable, or warm moxibustion for 10–15 min.

Indications

Paraplegia, sciatica, lateral femoral cutaneous neuritis, urticaria.

(9) *Yanglingquan* (GB 34, *He*–Sea Point)

Definition

"*Yang*" refers to the facies lateralis cruris; "*ling*" means "protrusion," here referring to the capitulum fibulae; "*quan*," "depression." The point is located at the facies lateralis cruris, in the depression of the capitulum fibulae.

Location

On the lateral side of the leg, at the depression inferior and anterior to the head of the fibula.

Method

Puncture perpendicularly 1.5–2 *cun*, with insertion obliquely downward to the posterior border of the tibia, giving a sensation of soreness and distension radiating downward. Four-to-seven cones of moxibustion are applicable, or warm moxibustion for 10–15 min.

Indications

Cholecystitis, Barbados distemper, biliary ascariasis, paraplegia, sciatica, intercostal neuralgia.

(10) *Zuguangming* (GB 37, *Luo*–Connecting Point)

Definition

The point is able to cure eye diseases and improve the eyesight. There are two points both named *guangming*, and this point is located in the foot, so it is called *zuguangming* (GB 37).

Location

On the lateral side of the leg, 5 *cun* proximal to the tip of the external malleolus, at the anterior border of the fibula.

Method

Puncture perpendicularly 1–1.5 *cun*, with the tip slightly upward, giving a sensation of soreness and distension, sometimes radiating to the knee or lateral to the dorsum of the foot. Three-to-five cones of moxibustion are applicable, or warm moxibustion for 10–15 min.

Indications

Optic atrophy, chronic simple glaucoma, early cataract, headache, paraplegia and pain of the lower extremities.

(11) *Xuanzhong* (GB 39, Influential Point Dominating the Marrow)

Definition

"*Xuan*" means "hang up"; "*zhong*," "heel." The point is located above the heel while the heel hangs below, so it is named *xuanzhong*.

Location

On the lateral side of the leg, 3 *cun* proximal to the tip of the external malleolus, at the anterior border of the fibula.

Methods

 (i) Puncture perpendicularly 0.8–1 *cun*, with a local sensation of soreness and distension.
 (ii) Puncture 1.5–2 *cun*, penetrating to *sanyinjiao* (SP 6), with a sensation of soreness and distension radiating to the sole.

Three-to-five cones of moxa are applicable, or warm moxibustion for 10–15 min.

Indications

Hemiplegia by stroke, sciatica, stiff neck, headache.

Caution

Generally, perpendicular puncture is applied while penetrating acupuncture is applicable to hemiplegia by stroke.

(12) *Qiuxu* (GB 40, *Yuan*–Source Point)

Definition

"*Qiu*" means "high place"; "*xu*," "larger and higher," here referring to the external malleulus. The point is beside it and so is named *qiuxu*.

Location

At the depression inferoanterior to the lateral malleolus, lateral to the tendon of the long extensor muscle of the toes.

Method

Puncture perpendicularly aiming at the inferior border of the medial malleolus 1–1.5 *cun* with a local sensation of soreness and distension. One-to-three cones of moxibustion are applicable, or warm moxibustion for 5–10 min.

Indications

An ankle joint sprain, thoraxicohypochondriac pain, cholecystitis.

QUESTIONS

(1) Describe the characteristics of locating *juliao* (GB 29), *huantiao* (GB 30), *Yanglingquan* (GB 34) and *qiuxu* (GB 40).

(2) What should be paid attention to in puncturing *jianjing* (GB 21)?

---

(13) *Zulinqi* (GB 41, *Shu*–Stream Point, One of the Eight Confluent Points)

Definition

"*Lin*" means "from up to down"; "*qi*" tears which are believed to be the liquid of the liver in TCM. The point is located above the foot and indicates eye diseases, so it is named *linqi*. In order to be distinguished from the other *linqi* (GB 15), of the head, it is named *zulinqi* (GB 41).

Location

On the lateral side of the instep of the foot, posterior to the fourth metatarsophalangeal joint, in the depression lateral to the tendon of the extensor muscle of the little toe.

Method

Puncture perpendicularly 0.5–0.7 *cun*, with a local sensation of soreness and distension, sometimes radiating to the fourth digit of the foot. One-to-three cones of moxibustion are applicable, or warm moxibustion for 5–10 min.

Indications

Headache, hemiplegia by stroke, conjunctivitis, mastitis.

(14) *Zuqiaoyin* (GB 44, *Jing*–Well Point)

Definition

"*Qiao*" means "a pass;" "*yin*" refers to the meridian of foot–*jueyin*. The point is the last of the meridians of *zu–shaoyang*, conjoint with the meridian of foot-*jueyin*. In order to be distinguished from the other *qiaoyin* (GB 11), of the head, it is named *zuqiaoyin* (GB 44).

Location

On the lateral side of the distal segment of the fourth toe, 0.1 *cun* from the corner of the toenail.

Method

Puncture obliquely 0.2–0.3 *cun*, with the tip upward and a sensation of pain; or prick with a three-edged needle for bloodletting. Warm moxibustion for 5–10 min is applicable.

Indications

Migraine, conjunctivitis, fever.

Caution

Pricking with a three-edged needle is mainly applicable to conjunctivitis; oblique puncture, to common diseases.

Summary

Location emphasis: Outer canthus, under the tragus, greater trochanter of the femur, anterior and posterior borders of the fibula. *Tongziliao* (GB 1) is located at the outer canthus; *tinghui* (GB 2) under the canthus; *juliao* (GB 29) at the middle of the connecting line of the greater trochanter of the femur and the anterior superior iliac spine; *huantiao* (GB 30) at the one-third of the line connecting with the sacral hiatus; *yanglingquan* (GB 34) and *zuguangming* (GB 37) at the anterior border of the fibula; *xuanzhong* (GB 39) at the posterior border.

Major indications: Diseases of the head and face, diseases of the gallbladder, local diseases.

ACUPOINTS OF THE SPLEEN MERIDIAN OF FOOT–*TAIYIN*[10]

(1) *Yinbai* (SP 1, *Jing*–Well Point)

Definition

"*Yin*" means "to hide;" "*bai*," means "white," here referring to the border between the red and the white flesh. The point is located on the inside of distal phalanx of the big toe, as if hiding in the border between the red and the white flesh.

Location

On the medial side of the distal segment of the big toe, 0.1 *cun* posterior to the corner of the nail of the big toe.

Method

Puncture obliquely 0.1–0.2 *cun*, with the tip upward and a sensation of pain; or prick with a three-edged needle for bloodletting. Warm moxibustion for 5–7 min is applicable.

---

[10]Figure 24.

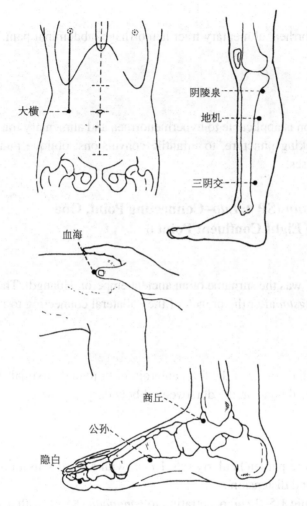

大横	-	Daheng (SP 15)	血海	-	Xuehai (SP 10)
阴陵泉	-	Yinlingquan (SP 9)	商丘	-	Shangqiu (SP 5)
地机	-	Diji (SP 8)	公孙	-	Gongsun (SP 4)
三阴交	-	Sanyinjiao (SP 6)	隐白	-	Yinbai (SP 1)

Fig. 24. Acupoints of the spleen meridian of foot–*taiyin*.

Indications

Hypermenorrhea, alimentary tract hemorrhage, abdominal pain, infantile convulsion.

Caution

Moxibustion is applicable to hypermenorrhea and alimentary tract hemorrhage; pricking puncture, to infantile convulsions; oblique puncture, to other diseases.

(2) *Gongsun* (SP 4, *Luo*–Connecting Point, One of the Eight Confluent Points)

Definition

"*Gongsun*" was the surname of an ancient emperor, Huangdi. The point is named *gongsun* after the branch of the collateral connecting to it.

Location

On the medial border of the foot, anteroinferior to the proximal end of the fist metatarsal bone, at the dorsoventral boundary.

Methods

 (i) Puncture perpendicularly 0.5–1 *cun*, with a local sensation of soreness and distension.
(ii) Puncture 1.5–2 *cun* penetrating to *yongquan* (KI 1), with a sensation radiating to the sole.

Warm moxibustion for 10–15 min is applicable.

Indications

Stomachache, vomiting, acute or chronic enteritis, menalgia, agitation and insomnia.

Caution

When one is treating gastrointestinal affections, the point is often combined with *neiguan* (PC 6). Generally, perpendicular acupuncture is applied and penetrating acupuncture is applicable to agitation and insomnia.

(3) *Shangqiu* (SP 5, *Jing*–River Point)

Definition

Shang was one of the five notes in ancient times and *jin* in five phases; "*qiu*" means earth hill. The point is a *Jing*–river point, attributing to *jin* in five phases, and it is located under the medial malleolus, protruding like a hill.

Location

At the depression anteroinferior to the medial malleolus, at the midpoint of the line connecting the tip of the medial malleolus with the tubercle of the scaphoid bone.

Methods

 (i) Puncture perpendicularly 0.3–0.5 *cun*, with a local sensation of soreness and distension.
 (ii) Puncture toward *jiexi* (ST 41) 1–1.5 *cun*, with a sensation of soreness and distension in the ankle joint.

Three or four cones of moxibustion are applicable, or warm moxibustion for 10–15 min.

Indications

Swelling and pain of the ankle, gastroenteritis, dyspepsia.

Caution

Penetrating acupuncture is applicable to swelling and pain of the ankle, and should be performed by experienced practitioners. Perpendicular puncture is applicable to other diseases.

(4) *Sanyinjiao* (SP 6)

Definition

"*Sanyin*" refers to the three yin meridians in the foot (the meridians of the liver, spleen and kidney); "*jiao*" means "intersection." The point is at the intersection of the three yin meridians.

Location

On the medial side of the leg, 3 *cun* proximal to the tip of the meidal malleolus, posterior to the medial border of the tibia.

Methods

  (i) Puncture perpendicularly 0.5–1.5 *cun*, with a local sensation of soreness and distension.
 (ii) Puncture toward *xuanzhong* (GB 39) 1.5–2 *cun*, with an obvious sensation of soreness and distension, or electric numbness radiating to the foot.
(iii) Puncture obliquely 1.5–2.5 *cun*, with a sensation radiating up to the knee.

Three to seven cones of moxa are applicable, or warm moxibustion for 10–15 min.

Indications

Acute or chronic nephritis, acute or chronic enteritis, metrorrhagia, urinary retention, enuresis, impotence, insomnia, hypertension, prolonged labor, hemiplegia by stroke.

Caution

The point is unsuitable for pregnant women. Perpendicular puncture is applicable to common diseases; penetrating puncture, to hemiplegia by stroke; oblique puncture, to diseases of the urogenital system.

(5) *Diji* (SP 8, *Xi*–Cleft Point)

Definition

"*Di*" means "earth, soil," here referring to the spleen meridian as the spleen belongs to *tu* in five phases; "*ji*," "key place." The point is the *xi*-cleft point, where *qi* and blood aggregate.

Location

On the medial side of the leg, 3 *cun* distal to *yinlingquan*, at the line connecting *yinlingquan* and *sanyinjiao*.

Method

Puncture perpendicularly 1.2–1.5 *cun*, with a local sensation of soreness and distension, sometimes radiating to the leg. Three-to-five cones of moxa are applicable, or warm moxibustion for 10–15 min.

Indications

Menalgia, menoxenia, functional uterine bleeding, abdominal pain and distension.

(6) *Yinlingquan* (SP 9, *He*–Sea Point)

Definition

"Yin" refers to the inner side of the leg; "*ling*" means "protruding hill," here referring to the condylus medialis tibiae; "*quan*," "depression." The point is located in the depression of the condylus medialis tibiae on the inner side of the leg, so it is named *yinglingquan*; corresponding to *yanglingquan* (GB 34).

Location

On the medial side of the leg, in the depression posterior and inferior to the medial condyle of the tibia.

Methods

(i) Puncture perpendicularly along the posterior border of the tibia 1–1.5 *cun*, with a local sensation of soreness and distension radiating downward.

(ii) Puncture obliquely with the tip upward, giving a sensation of soreness and distension, sometimes radiating to the knee.

Three-to-five cones of moxa are applicable, or warm moxibustion for 10–15 min.

Indications

Edema, urinary retention, enteritis, nephritis, swelling and pain of the knee and leg.

Caution

The point is good at inducing diuresis and, generally, perpendicular acupuncture is applied. Oblique puncture is applicable to urinary retention, as well as swelling and pain of the knee and leg.

QUESTIONS

(1) What are the differences between the indications of *zuqiaoyin* (GB 44) and *yinbai* (SP 1)?

(2) What are the differences and similarities between the acupuncture methods and indications of *gongsun* (SP 4), *sanyinjiao* (SP 6), *diji* (SP 8) and *yinlingquan* (SP 9)?

---

(7) Xuehai (SP 10)

Definition

"*Xue*" means "blood"; "*hai*," "sea." TCM believes that spleen controls blood, and the point is the place where the spleen blood gathers like a vast sea.

Location

(i) When the knee is flexed, on the medial side of the thigh, 2 *cun* proximal to the superinternal border of the patella, on the bulge of the medial portion of the m. quadriceps femoris of the thigh.

(ii) The operator puts his or her left hand over the patient's right patella with the center of the palm just on the upper border of the patella, and the second-to-fifth fingers directed upward and the thumb at an angle of 45° with the index finger; the spot beneath the tip of the thumb is the location.

Method

Puncture perpendicularly 0.8–1.5 *cun*, with a local sensation of soreness and distension sometimes radiating to the coxa. Three-to-five cones of moxibustion are applicable, or warm moxibustion for 10–15 min.

Indications

Menoxenia, functional uterine bleeding, urticaria, pruritus of skin.

Caution

The second method of location is easy and convenient but should refer to the first.

(8) *Daheng* (SP 15)

Definition

"*Heng*" means "sidelong." The point is horizontally opposite the umbilicus center at a longer distance than *tianshu* (ST 25), so it is named *daheng*.

Location

On the middle abdomen, 4 *cun* lateral to the center of the umbilicus.

Methods

(i) Puncture perpendicularly 1–1.5 *cun*, with a sensation of distension and heaviness in the local area.

(ii) Puncture horizontally 2–2.5 *cun*, with the tip toward the umbilicus center, giving a sensation radiating to the homolateral abdomen.

Three-to-five cones of moxibustion are applicable, or warm moxibustion for 10–15 min.

Indications

Ascariasis in the biliary tract and intestinal tract, diarrhea, constipation.

Caution

The point is effective in treating ascariasis with the manipulation of horizontal acupuncture. Perpendicular puncture is applicable to common diseases.

Summary

Location emphasis: Posterior border of the tibia where *yinlingquan* (SP 9), *diji* (SP 8) and *sanyinjiao* (SP 6) are located, swelling part of muscles where *xuehai* (SP 10) is located in the medial vastus muscle, and lateral to the umbilicus where daheng (SP 15) is located 4 *cun* away.

ACUPOINTS OF THE KIDNEY MERIDIAN OF FOOT–*SHAOYIN*[11]

(1) *Yongquan* (KI 1, *Jing*–Well Point)

Definition

"Yong" means "bubbling up or rushing forth of water"; "*quan*," "spring water." The point is the well point, which means that channel *qi* rushes forth from the sole.

---

[11] Figure 25.

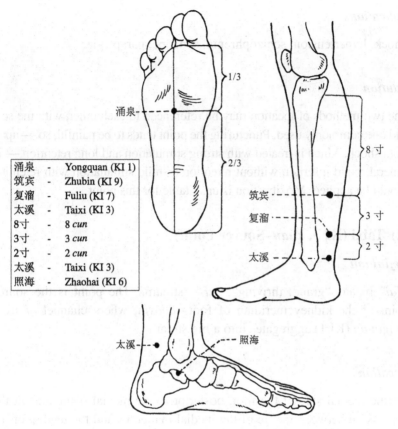

Fig. 25. Acupoints of the kidney meridian of foot–*shaoyin*.

Location

(i) On the sole, in the depression appearing on its anterior part when the foot is in plantar flexion, approximately at the junction of the anterior third and posterior two-thirds of the line connecting the base of the second and third toes and the heel.

(ii) When the foot flexed, on the depression of the forepart of the foot.

Method

Puncture perpendicularly 0.5–0.8 *cun*, with a local sensation of distending pain, sometimes radiating to the ankle. Warm moxibustion for 5–10 min is applicable.

Indications

Shock, hypertension, schizophrenia, syncope, paraplegia.

Caution

The two methods of location may be referenced to each other, with the second one commonly used. Puncturing the point tends to be painful, so — apart from shock, which is treated with strong stimulation and long retention — in general, rapid insertion without retention or mild stimulation with retention should be applied. Moxibustion is unsuitable for this point.

(2) Taixi (KI 3, *Yuan*–Source Point)

Definition

"*Tai*" means "grand, thriving"; "*xi*," "stream." The point is the source point of the kidney meridian of foot–*shaoyin*, where channel *qi* from *yongquan* (KI 1) aggregates into a big stream.

Location

On the medial side of the foot, posterior to the medial malleolus, at the depression between the tip of the medial malleolus and the tendon of the m. calcaneus.

Methods

(i) Puncture perpendicularly 0.5–0.8 *cun*, with a local sensation of soreness and distension.

(ii) Puncture 0.8–1 *cun*, with the tip penetrating to *kunlun* (BL 60), giving a sensation of soreness and distension radiating to the heel.

(iii) Puncture obliquely toward the medial malleolus, with a sensation of electric numbness radiating to the sole.

Three-to-five cones of moxa are applicable, or warm moxibustion for 5–10 min.

Indications

Chronic pharyngolaryngitis, pedialgia, dizziness, insomnia, toothache.

Caution

Oblique acupuncture is applicable to heel pain, the other two methods, to common diseases.

(3) *Zhaohai* (KI 6, One of the Eight Confluent Points)

Definition

"*Zhao*" means "apparent"; "*hai*," "sea." The point has obvious channel *qi*, like a vast sea.

Location

On the medial side of the foot, in the depression of the lower border of the medial malleolus.

Methods

 (i) Puncture perpendicularly 0.5–0.8 *cun*, with a local sensation of soreness and distension.
(ii) Puncture obliquely 0.8–1 *cun*, with the tip downward, giving a sensation of soreness and numbness radiating to the ankle or inside of the foot.

Three to five cones of moxa are applicable, or warm moxibustion for 10–15 min.

Indications

Pharyngolaryngitis, insomnia, hypertension, mania, heel pain.

Caution

Oblique acupuncture is applicable to heel pain and hypertension.

(4) *Fuliu* (KI 7, *Jing*–River Point)

Definition

"*Fu*" means "repeat, return"; "*liu*," "flow." Channel *qi* of the kidney meridian of foot–*shaoyin* flows from *yongquan* (KI 1) to *taixi* (KI 3), moves around to *zhaohai* (KI 6), and then flows from *taixi* (KI 3) to this point, which is thus named *fuliu* (KI 7).

Location

On the medial side of the leg, 2 *cun* above *taixi*, anterior to the tendon calcaneus.

Method

Puncture perpendicularly 1–1.5 *cun*, with a local sensation of soreness and distension, or electric numbness radiating to the sole. Three-to-seven cones of moxibustion are applicable, or warm moxibustion for 10–15 min.

Indications

Orchitis, functional uterine bleeding, hyperhidrosis, paraplegia.

(5) *Zhubin* (KI 9, *Xi*–Cleft Point of the *Yinwei* Channel)

Definition

"*Zhu*" originally referred to the pestle for building walls, which is solid and substantial; here it seems to refer to the gastrocnemius muscle beside which the point is located, which means "*bin*", or "the guest."

Location

On the medial side of the leg, 5 *cun* proximal to *taixi*, at the line connecting *taixi* and *yinggu*, medial and inferior to the gastrocnemius muscle belly.

Method

Puncture perpendicularly 1–1.5 *cun*, with a local sensation of soreness and distension, sometimes radiating up to the thigh or down to the sole. Three-to-five cones of moxa are applicable, or warm moxibustion for 10–15 min.

Indications

Nephritis, UTI, pelvic inflammation, sural spasm.

Summary

Location emphasis: Depression, medial malleolus, Achilles tendon. *Yongquan* (KI 1) is located on the depression of the sole when the foot is flexed; *taichi* (KI 3) on the posterior border of the medial malleolus and *zhaohai* (KI 6) on the inferior border; *fuliu* (KI 7) and *zhubin* (KI 9) on the anterior border of the inside Achilles tendon.

Major indications: Diseases of the genitourinary system, diseases of the mental and nervous systems, local diseases.

ACUPOINTS OF THE LIVER MERIDIAN OF FOOT–*JUEYIN*[12]

(1) *Dadun* (LR 1, *Jing*–Well Point)

Definition

"*Da*" means "big"; "*dun*," "thick." The point is located on the lateral to the big toe, which is big and thick.

Location

At the lateral aspect of the dorsum of the terminal phalanx of the big toe, 0.1 *cun* from the corner of the nail.

---

[12] Figure 26.

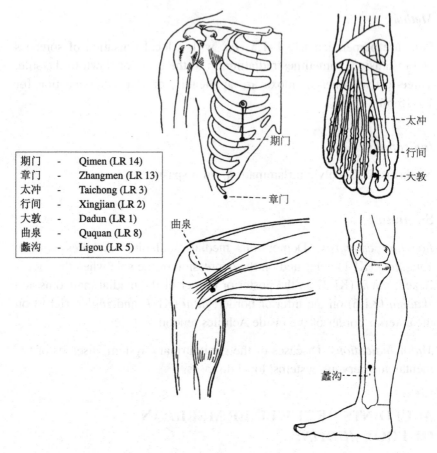

期门	-	Qimen (LR 14)
章门	-	Zhangmen (LR 13)
太冲	-	Taichong (LR 3)
行间	-	Xingjian (LR 2)
大敦	-	Dadun (LR 1)
曲泉	-	Ququan (LR 8)
蠡沟	-	Ligou (LR 5)

Fig. 26. Acupoints of the liver meridian of foot-*jueyin*.

Method

Puncture obliquely upward 0.2–0.3 *cun*, or prick with a three-edged needle for bloodletting, with a pain sensation in the local area. Warm moxibustion for 5–10 min is applicable.

Indications

Functional ejaculation failure, functional uterine bleeding, prolonged labor, syncope.

Caution

Puncturing the point needs rapid manipulation, because of its severe pain. Moxibustion is applicable to functional ejaculation failure; acupuncture, to syncope.

QUESTIONS

(1) Describe the location and indications of the *jing*-well points of the kidney and liver meridians.
(2) Describe the accupuncture methods and indications of *xuehai* (SP 10) and *daheng* (SP 15).
(3) Describe briefly the location methods of *zhaohai* (KI 6), *fuliu* (KI 7) and *zhubin* (KI 9).

---

(2) *Xingjian* (LR 2, *Ying*–Spring Point)

Definition

"*Xing*" means "go through"; "*jian*," "middle." Channel *qi* of the liver meridian of foot–*jueyin* goes through the point between toes.

Location

On the instep of the foot, between the first and second toes, at the junction of the red and white skin proximal to the margin of the web.

Method

Puncture obliquely upward 0.5–1 *cun*, with a local sensation of distending pain radiating to the dorsum of the foot. Warm moxibustion for 5–10 min is applicable.

Indications

Hypertension, chronic simple glaucoma, hypermenorrhea, infantile convulsions.

(3) *Taichong* (LR 3, *Yuan*–Source Point)

Definition

"*Tai*" means "grand"; "*chong*," "abundant." The point is the *yuan*–source point, which is abundant in *qi* and blood, and so is named *taichong*.

Location

At the dorsum of the foot, at the depression of the posterior end of the first interosseous metatarsal space.

Methods

 (i) Puncture perpendicularly 0.5–1 *cun*, with a local sensation of soreness and distension.
 (ii) Puncture toward *yongquan* (KI 1) 1.2–1.5 *cun*, with a local sensation of soreness and distension, or electric numbness radiating to the sole.

Three to five cones of moxibustion are applicable, or warm moxibustion for 10–15 min.

Indications

Headache, dizziness, functional uterine bleeding, hypertension, neurasthenia, hepatitis, mastitis.

Caution

Generally, perpendicular acupuncture is used, and penetrating acupuncture is applicable to hypertension and neurasthenia.

(4) *Ligou* (LR 5, *Luo*–Connecting Point)

Definition

"*Li*" means "ladle"; "*gou*," "ditch." The calf, where the point is located, is like a ladle in shape, and the inside tibia is like a ditch.

Location

On the medial side of the leg, 5 *cun* proximal to the tip of the medial aspect of the tibia.

Methods

(i) Puncture perpendicularly 0.5–1 *cun* along the posterior border of the tibia, with a local sensation of soreness and distension.

(ii) Puncture obliquely upward 1.5–2 *cun* along the posterior border of the tibia with the manipulation of lifting, thrusting, twirling and rotating, giving a sensation of soreness and distension radiating to the knee, and even to the genitalia.

Two or three cones of moxa are applicable, or warm moxibustion for 10–15 min.

Indications

Menoxenia, orchitis, hepatitis, eczema.

Caution

Oblique acupuncture is applicable to diseases of the genitalia; perpendicular puncture, to common diseases.

(5) *Zhangmen* (LR 13, Front–*Mu* Point of the Spleen, Influential Point Dominating the *Zang* Organs)

Definition

"*Zhang*" means "magnificent"; "*men*," "door." The point, both a *mu*-point of the spleen and an influential point dominating the *zang* organs, is a site where the *qi* and blood of the five *zang* organs magnificently meet.

Location

Right below the free end of the 11th rib, on the lateral side of the chest.

Methods

(i) Puncture obliquely toward short ribs (free end) 0.5–1 *cun*, with a local sensation of soreness, distension and heaviness.
(ii) Puncture horizontally anterior–inferior 1–1.5 *cun*, with a sensation of distension and heaviness in the lateral region of the abdomen.

Three cones of moxa are applicable, or warm moxibustion for 10–20 min.

Indications

Barbados distemper, hypochondriac pain, icterus, dyspepsia.

Caution

Accidents often occur to the point. Autopsy shows that the insertion should not be deeper than 0.5 *cun*. Generally, oblique acupuncture is applied toward the short ribs, with the tip touching the rib, which is applicable to common diseases. Horizontal acupuncture, at an angle of 15°, is for hypochondriac pain.

(6) *Qimen* (LR 14, Front–*Mu* Point of the Liver)

Definition

"*Qi*" means "cycle"; "*men*," "door." The *qi* and blood of the 12 meridians flow in a cycle from *yunmen* (LU 2) to this point, so it is named *qimen*.

Location

On the chest, when the patient lies supine, directly below the nipple, at the sixth intercostal space, 4 *cun* lateral to the anterior midline.

Method

Puncture obliquely to the upper or lower costal margin about 0.5 *cun*, with a sensation of distending pain, sometimes radiating to the posterior wall of the abdomen. Three to five cones of moxibustion are applicable, or warm moxibustion for 10–15 min.

Indications

Intercostal neuralgia, mastitis, cyclomastopathy, cholecystitis, hepatitis.

Caution

Accidents often occur to the point and the insertion should not be deeper than 0.5 *cun*. Generally, oblique acupuncture is applied till the tip touches the margin of the rib. With electric stimulation, the tip should be inserted horizontally along the intercostal space subcutaeously.

Summary

Location emphasis: Metatarsophalangeal joint, tibia, ribs. *Xingjian* (LR 2) is located anterior to the metatarsophalangeal joint, *taichong* (LR 3) posterior; *ligou* (LR 5) is located on the medialis tibiae; *zhangmen* (LR 13) on the end of the 11th rib and *qimen* (LR 14) on the 6th intercostal space.

ACUPOINTS OF THE DU MERIDIAN[13]

(1) *Changqiang* (DU 1, *Luo*–Connecting Point)

Definition

"*Chang*" means "higher position, commander"; "*qiang*," "strong." The point is the first of the *du* meridians, commanding all the yang meridians with strong *qi* and blood.

Location

Below the tip of the coccyx, at the midpoint of the line connecting the tip of the coccyx and the anus.

---

[13]Figure 27.

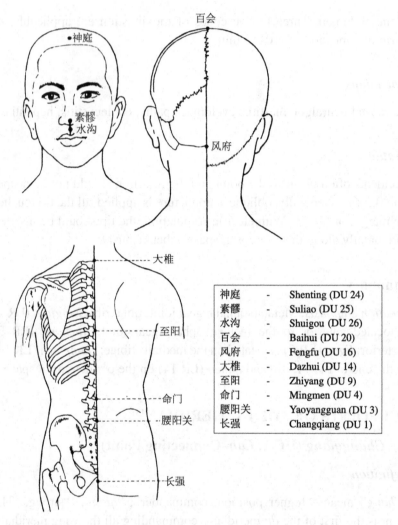

Fig. 27. Acupoints of the *Du* meridian (governor vessel).

神庭	-	Shenting (DU 24)
素髎	-	Suliao (DU 25)
水沟	-	Shuigou (DU 26)
百会	-	Baihui (DU 20)
风府	-	Fengfu (DU 16)
大椎	-	Dazhui (DU 14)
至阳	-	Zhiyang (DU 9)
命门	-	Mingmen (DU 4)
腰阳关	-	Yaoyangguan (DU 3)
长强	-	Changqiang (DU 1)

Method

With the patient in the genucubital position, puncture obliquely at an angle of 45° close to the tip of the coccyx to a depth of 1 *cun*, with a local sensation of soreness and distension radiating to the anus. Warm moxibustion for 10–15 min is applicable.

Indications

Mania, proctoptosis, hemorrhoids, prostatitis.

Caution

Puncture close to the anterior border of the coccyx and try to avoid injuring the front rectum. Direct moxibustion is unsuitable here.

(2) *Yaoyangguan* (DU 3)

Definition

"*Yang*" refers to yang *qi*; "*guan*" means "key place." The point is the key place for yang *qi* going through. As there is another *yangguan* (GB 33) in the knee, it is named *yaoyangguan* (DU 3).

Location

On the lower back and on the posterior midline, at the depression below the spinous process of the fourth lumbar vertebra, paralled to the iliac crest.

Method

Three-to-five cones of moxibustion are applicable, or warm moxibustion for 10–15 min.

Indications

Lumbago leg pain, paraplegia, impotence, pelvic inflammation.

Caution

Do not puncture perpendicularly too deep. If electric numbness appears, lift the tip a little. Horizontal puncture is mainly applicable to beginners.

(3) *Mingmen* (DU 4)

Definition

"*Ming*" means "life"; "*men*," "door." The point is located in the middle of left and right *shenshu* (BL 23), while kidney *qi* is the root of the body, and so it is named *mingmen*.

Location

On the lower back and on the posterior midline, at the depression below the spinous process of the second lumbar vertebra.

Methods

 (i) Puncture perpendicularly 1–1.5 *cun*, with a local sensation of distension and heaviness, or electric numbness radiating to the lower limbs when one is puncturing deep.
(ii) Puncture horizontally 1.5–2 *cun* from the processus spinosus, with a local sensation of distension and heaviness.

Five-to-seven cones of moxibustion are applicable, or warm moxibustion for 10–20 min.

Indications

Acute lumbar muscle sprain, paraplegia, infertility, enuresis, pelvic inflammation.

Caution

The same as for *yaoyangguan* (DU 3).

QUESTIONS

 (i) What should be paid attention to when one is puncturing *zhangmen* (LR 13) and *qimen* (LR 14)?
(ii) Since *changqiang* (DU 1), *mingmen* (DU 4) and *yaoyangguan* (DU 3) are all points of *du* meridians, what are the differences in indications?

(4) Zhiyang (DU 9)

Definition

"*Zhi*" means "extremity"; "*yang*" refers to yang *qi*. It is believed in TCM that the back is yang while the *du* meridian governs yang, and the part above the diaphragm is yang within yang. The point is just above the diaphragm, so it is named *zhiyang*.

Location

On the lower back and on the posterior midline, at the depression below the spinous process of the seventh thoracic vertebra, parallel to the inferior angle of the scapula.

Methods

(i) Puncture perpendicularly 0.5–1 *cun*, with a local sensation of distension and heaviness, or electric numbness radiating to the lower back.

(ii) Puncture horizontally 1–2 *cun*, from the processus apinosus downward along the skin, with a local sensation of distension and heaviness.

Three-to-five cones of moxibustion are applicable, or warm moxibustion for 10–15 min.

Indications

Hepatitis, cholecystitis, coronary angina pectoris, malaria, ascariasis of the biliary tract.

Caution

The same as for *yaoyangguan* (DU 3).

(5) *Dazhui* (DU 14)

Definition

"*Da*" means "big;" "*zhui*," "vertebra." The point is below the seventh cervical vertebra, the highest part of the protruding processus spinosus, and so is named *dazhui*.

Location

On the lower back and on the posterior midline, at the depression below the spinous process of the seventh cervical vertebra.

Methods

 (i) Puncture perpendicularly, slightly downward, 1–1.2 *cun*, with a local sensation of distension and heaviness radiating downward or to the shoulders, or strong electric numbness induced by deeper insertion.
(ii) Puncture horizontally 1.5–2 *cun*, from the processus apinosus downward along the skin, with a local sensation of distension and heaviness.

Three-to-seven cones of moxibustion are applicable, or warm moxibustion for 10–15 min.

Indications

Fever, cold, malaria, schizophrenia, mania, bronchitis, asthma, heatstroke.

Caution

Accidents may occur to the point, so avoid deep insertion. Electric numbness suggests deep insertion; withdraw the needle rapidly.

(6) *Fengfu* (DU 16)

Definition

"*Feng*" refers to pathogenic wind; "*fu*" means "the place to meet." The point is the place where pathogenic winds meet.

Location

On the nape, at the depression between the m. trapezius of the two sides, directly below the external occipital protuberance, or at the midline of the back of the head, 1 *cun* above the posterior hairline.

Method

With the patient sitting on a desk, the head slightly forward and the neck muscle relaxed, puncture perpendicularly toward the lower mandible 0.8–1 *cun*, with a local sensation of soreness and distension. Warm moxibustion for 5–10 min is applicable.

Indications

Headache, cold, internal aural vertigo, pseudobulbar paralysis.

Caution

The point is one of those to which accidents will occur. 1.5-*cun*-deep insertion may injure the medulla oblongata, so for this point one should avoid deep insertion or repeatedly lifting and thrusting, twirling and rotating. If the patient feels the soreness and distension radiating up and down, this shows that the tip has reached the dura mater of the spinal cord; then withdraw the needle rapidly, for fear of serious consequencs. It the patient complains of headache or dizziness after the acupuncture, it should be thought over whether subarachnoid hemorrhage has occurred and the patient should be turned to other departments for examination and observation.

(7) *Baihui* (DU 20)

Definition

"*Bai*" means "a lot"; "*hui*," "meet." The point is located on the calvaria, where all meridians and channels meet.

Location

On the head, 5 *cun* directly above the midpoint of the anterior hairline, at the midpoint of the line connecting the apexes of both ears; or, at the cross point of the line connecting the apexes of the two auricles and the midline of the head.

Method

Puncture horizontally forward–backward or left–right 0.5–1.5 *cun*, with a local sensation of distending pain. Three to ten cones of moxibustion are applicable, or warm moxibustion for 5–15 min.

Indications

Headache, hypertension, internal aural vertigo, shock, athletic syndrome, prolapse of the rectum, neurasthenia.

Caution

The point should not be taken for infants with patent fontanelles. Bleeding often happens to the point, so remember to press the hole with sterilized dry cotton balls after withdrawal.

(8) *Shangxing* (DU 23)

Definition

"*Shang*" means "upper part"; "*xing*," "stars," here referring to the bright light. The point is located on the upper part of the head and works to cure eye diseases.

Location

One *cun* directly above the midpoint of the anterior hairline, at the midline of the head.

Method

Puncture horizontally backward 0.5–1 *cun* along the scalp, with a local sensation of distending pain. Warm moxibustion for 5–10 min is applicable.

Indications

Headache, rhinitis, eye disease.

(9) *Suliao* (DU 25)

Definition

"*Su*" means "white." It is believed in TCM that the lung opens at the nose and governs the color white. "*Liao*" means "hole." The point is located at the nasal tip, so it is named *suliao*.

Location

On the face, at the center of the nose apex.

Method

To puncture obliquely up words by 0.3–0.5 *cun*, or to prick it with a three-edged needle to caused bleeding. Moxibustion is applicable.

Indications

Shock, bradycardia, rhinitis, hiccups.

Caution

Puncture obliquely 0.3–0.5 *cun*, with the tip inserted obliquely upward from the nasal tip, giving a sensation of soreness and pain in the local area, sometimes radiating to the nasal root or nasal cavity.

(10) *Shuigou* (DU 26)

Definition

"*Shui*" means "tears"; "*gou*," "ditch," here referring to the philtrum groove. The point is located in the middle of the philtrum, so it is named *shuigou*, or *renzhong*.

Location

On the face, at the junction of the upper third and the middle third of the philtrum.

Methods

(i) Puncture perpendicularly 0.2–0.3 *cun*, with a pain sensation in the local area.

(ii) Puncture horizontally upward 0.5–1 *cun*, with a pain sensation, or a sense of soreness and distension, while twirling and rotating the needle.

Indications

Shock, coma, acute lumbar muscle sprain, schizophrenia, mania, hyseria, syncope.

Caution

Generally, perpendicular acupuncture is used, and horizontal puncture is applicable to severe cases. Moxibustion is unsuitable here.

Summary

Location emphasis: Intervertebra, hairline, nasal tip, midphiltrum. Points of the back are all located between vertebrae; *fengfu* (DU 16) 1 *cun* above the posterior hairline and *shangxing* (DU 23) 1 *cun* above the anterior hairline; *suliao* (DU 25) on the nasal tip; *shuigou* (DU 26) on the upper third of the philtrum.

Major indications: Mental or neurogenic diseases, limb diseases.

ACUPOINTS OF THE REN MERIDIAN[14]

(1) *Qugu* (RN 2)

Definition

"*Qugu*" is a bone name in ancient anatomy, now referring to the pubic symphysis part where the point is located.

Location

On the lower abdomen, on the anterior midline, at the midpoint of the upper border of the pubic symphysis.

Method

Puncture perpendicularly 1–1.5 *cun*, with a local sensation of soreness and distention, or sometimes a sense of soreness and numbness radiating to the perineal region. Warm moxibustion for 10–15 min is applicable.

Indications

Impotence, functional ejaculation failure, urinary retention, enuresis.

Caution

Ask the patient to urinate before acupuncture.

---

[14]Figure 28.

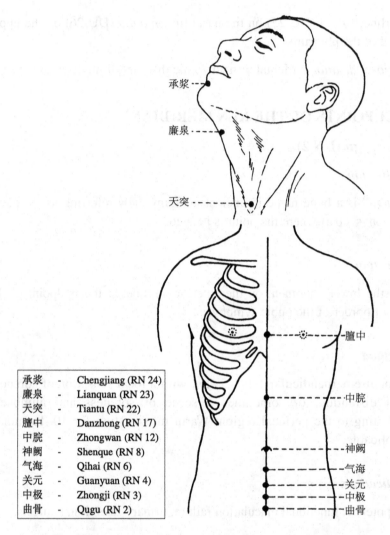

承浆
廉泉
天突

膻中
中脘
神阙
气海
关元
中极
曲骨

承浆	-	Chengjiang (RN 24)
廉泉	-	Lianquan (RN 23)
天突	-	Tiantu (RN 22)
膻中	-	Danzhong (RN 17)
中脘	-	Zhongwan (RN 12)
神阙	-	Shenque (RN 8)
气海	-	Qihai (RN 6)
关元	-	Guanyuan (RN 4)
中极	-	Zhongji (RN 3)
曲骨	-	Qugu (RN 2)

Fig. 28. Acupoints of the *ren* meridian (conception vessel).

QUESTIONS

(1) What should be paid attention to in puncturing *fengfu* (DU 16) and *qugu* (RN 2)?

(2) Describe briefly the indications and acupuncture methods of *baihui* (DU 20) and *shuigou* (DU 26).

(2) *Zhongji* (RN 3, Front–*Mu* Point of the Bladder)

Definition

"*Zhong*" means "midpoint;" "*ji*," "the end." The point is located at the midpoint of the whole body and is the ending part of the trunk, so it is named *zhongji*.

Location

On the lower abdomen, 4 *cun* below the center of the umbilicus, at the midline of the abdomen.

Method

Puncture perpendicularly 1–1.5 *cun*, with a local sensation of soreness and distension radiating to the perineal region. Three to seven cones of moxibustion are applicable, or warm moxibustion for 10–15 min.

Indications

Enuresis, urinary retention, impotence, functional ejaculation failure, menalgia, urinary tract infection.

Caution

Same as for *qugu* (RN 2).

(3) *Guanyuan* (RN 4, Front–*Mu* Point of the Small Intestine)

Definition

"*Guan*" means "hiding;" "*yuan*," "foundation of life." The point is the hiding place of nephroyin and nephroyang.

Location

On the lower abdomen, 3 *cun* below the center of the umbilicus, at the midline of the abdomen.

Method

Puncture perpendicularly 1–1.5 *cun*, with a local sensation of soreness and distension radiating to the perineal region. Five to ten cones of moxa are applicable, or warm moxibustion for 15–20 min.

Indications

Early shock, stay caducity, urinary retention, impotence, functional ejaculation failure, enuresis, uterine prolapse.

Caution

Pregnant women should avoid acupuncture and moxibustion. The others are the same as for *qugu* (RN 2).

(4) *Qihai* (RN 6)

Definition

"*Qi*" refers to primordial *qi*; "*hai*" means "meeting place." The point is the meeting place of primordial *qi*.

Location

On the lower abdomen, 1.5 *cun* below the center of the umbilicus, at the midline of the abdomen.

Method

Puncture perpendicularly 1.2–1.5 *cun*, with a local sensation of soreness and distension radiating to the perineal region. Five to ten cones of moxa are applicable, or warm moxibustion for 15–20 min.

Indications

Abdominal pain, abdominal distension, urinary retention, gastroptosis, functional uterine bleeding, menalgia, uterine prolapse.

Caution

The same as for *guanyuan* (RN 4).

(5) *Shenque* (RN 8)

Definition

"*Shen*" refers to yin and yang *qi*; "*que*" means "gateway." *Shenque* is the gateway for yin and yang *qi*.

Location

On the middle abdomen and at the center of the umbilicus.

Method

Salt or ginger moxibustion with 7–14 cones is applicable, or warm moxibustion for 15–20 min.

Indications

Acute or chronic interitis, urticaria, shock, proctoptosis.

Caution

Acupuncture is not applied to this point but penetrating puncture from *guanyuan* (RN 4) to *shenque* (RN 8).

(6) *Zhongwan* (RN 12, Front–*Mu* Point of the Stomach, Influential Point Dominating *Fu* Organs)

Definition

"*Zhong*" means "middle part"; "*Wan*," "stomach." It was believed in ancient times that the point was located in the middle of the stomach.

Location

On the upper abdomen, 4 *cun* above the center of the umbilicus, at the midline of the abdomen.

Method

Puncture perpendicularly 1.2–1.5 *cun* with a sensation of suffocation, distension and heaviness in the upper abdomen or a sensation of contraction in the stomach. Five to seven cones of moxibustion are applicable, or warm moxibustion for 10–15 min.

Indications

Peptic ulcer disease, acute or chronic gastritis, gastroptosis, gastric volvulus, hiccups, vomiting, acute pancreatitis.

Caution

As it is one of the points to which accidents often occur, puncture no deeper than 1.5 *cun*, especially for the thin and weak. For hepatosplenomegaly, avoid penetrating acupuncture to the left or the right, for fear of injuring the viscera.

(7) *Danzhong* (RN 17, Front–*Mu* Point of the Pericardium, Influential Point Dominating *Qi*)

Definition

"*Tan*" means "chest"; "*zhong*," "midpoint." The point is located at the middle of the chest.

Location

On the chest, between the nipples, at the midline of the chest, paralled to the fourth intercostal space.

Method

Puncture horizontally upward 0.5–1 *cun*, with a sensation of soreness and distension, or heaviness in the chest. Three to five cones of moxa are applicable, or warm moxibustion for 5–10 min.

Indications

Asthma, bronchitis, coronary angina pectoris, arrhythmia, acute mastitis, cyclomastopathy.

(8) *Tiantu* (RN 22)

Definition

"*Tian*" refers to celestial *qi*; "*tu*" means "chimney, pathway." The point is located on the throat, which is the pathway for celestial *qi*.

Location

On the neck and on the anterior midline, at the center of the suprasternal fossa.

Methods

(i) *Curved puncture*: Puncture perpendicularly 0.1–0.2 *cun* before inserting downward to 1–1.5 *cun* along the space between the sternum and the trachea, with a local sensation of soreness and distension, and choking and tightness in the throat.

(ii) Puncture perpendicularly 0.2–0.4 *cun*, with a local sensation of soreness and distension. Warm moxibustion for 5–10 min is applicable.

Indications

Bronchitis, diaphragmatic spasm, laryngopharyngitis, globus hystericus, disease of the vocal cords.

Caution

As it is one of the points to which accidents often occur, puncture no deeper than 0.6 *cun*, so dose curved puncture. And be more careful not to puncture left and right, for fear of injuring the subclavian artery or the apex of lung. Beginners had better choose perpendicular acupuncture.

(9) *Lianquan* (RN 23)

Definition

"*Lian*" means "upright and immaculate"; "*quan*," "spring water." The point locates beneath the tongue in which there is immaculate saliva like spring water flowing.

Location

On the neck and on the anterior midline, above the Adam's apple, at the depression above the upper part of the hyoid bone.

Method

Puncture obliquely to the lingual root 0.5–1 *cun*, with a sensation of distension and tightness in the root and the throat.

Indications

Laryngopharyngitis, aphasia, globus hystericus.

(10) *Chengjiang* (RN 24)

Definition

"*Cheng*" means "collect"; "*jiang*," "water, ingesta." The point is located on the lower lip, which collect ingesta.

Location

On the face, at the depression in the center of the mentolabial groove.

Method

Puncture obliquely 0.3–0.5 *cun* from anterior–inferior to posterior–superior, with a local sensation of distending pain. Warm moxibustion for 5 min is applicable.

Indications

Facial paralysis, mouth ulcer, sialorrhea, toothache.

Summary

Location emphasis: Fovea umbilicalis, sternum, Adam's apple, mentolabial furrow. *Qugu* (RN 2), *zhongji* (RN 3), *guanyuan* (RN 4) and *qihai* (RN 6) are located directly below the umbilicus, *shenque* (RN 8) in the middle and *zhongwan* (RN 12) directly above the umbilicus; *tanzhong* (RN 17) on the sternum; *tiantu* (RN 22) below and *lianquan* (RN 23) above the Adam's apple; *chengjiang* (RN 24) on the midpoint of the mentolabial furrow.

QUESTIONS

(1) What are the major points of the *ren* meridian on the abdomen? Describe their locations and indications.
(2) What should one be cautious about in puncturing *tiantu* (RN 22)?
(3) Describe briefly the indications and acupuncture methods of *tanzhong* (RN 17), *lianquan* (RN 23) and *chengjiang* (RN 24).

EXTRAORDINARY POINTS[15]

(1) *Yintang* (EX–HN2)

Definition

"*Yin*" means "a seal"; "*tang*," "hall." The point is located between the eyebrows, and was named *yintang* by ancient astrologers.

---

[15]Figures 29–31.

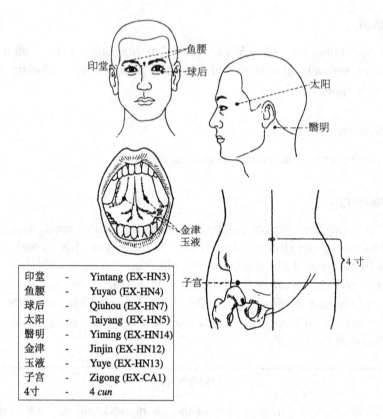

印堂	-	Yintang (EX-HN3)
鱼腰	-	Yuyao (EX-HN4)
球后	-	Qiuhou (EX-HN7)
太阳	-	Taiyang (EX-HN5)
翳明	-	Yiming (EX-HN14)
金津	-	Jinjin (EX-HN12)
玉液	-	Yuye (EX-HN13)
子宫	-	Zigong (EX-CA1)
4寸	-	4 *cun*

Fig. 29. Extraordinary points (1).

Location

On the forehead, midway between the medial ends of the two eyebrows.

Methods

(i) Puncture obliquely 0.5 *cun* with the pinching insertion method from up to down, with a distending sensation in the local area.

(ii) Puncture horizontally 1 *cun* respectively penetrating to bilateral *zanzhu* (BL 2), with a local sensation of soreness and distension. Warm moxibustion for 3–5 min is applicable.

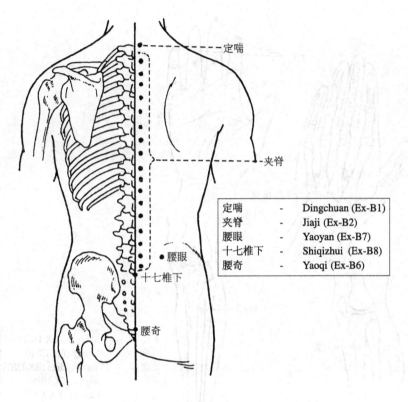

定喘

夹脊

定喘	-	Dingchuan (Ex-B1)
夹脊	-	Jiaji (Ex-B2)
腰眼	-	Yaoyan (Ex-B7)
十七椎下	-	Shiqizhui (Ex-B8)
腰奇	-	Yaoqi (Ex-B6)

腰眼

十七椎下

腰奇

Fig. 30. Extraordinary points (2).

Indications

Headache, dizziness, rhinitis, infantile convulsions, cold.

Caution

Generally, oblique puncture is applied, while horizontal puncture is for headache. Pricking with a three-edged needle for bloodletting is done for treatment of infantile convulsions and cold.

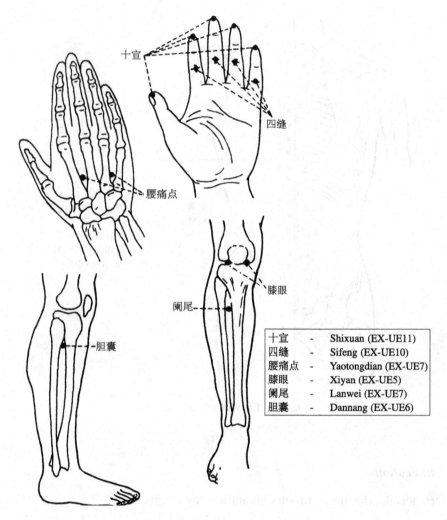

十宣	-	Shixuan (EX-UE11)
四缝	-	Sifeng (EX-UE10)
腰痛点	-	Yaotongdian (EX-UE7)
膝眼	-	Xiyan (EX-UE5)
阑尾	-	Lanwei (EX-UE7)
胆囊	-	Dannang (EX-UE6)

Fig. 31. Extraordinary points (3).

(2) *Taiyang* (EX–HN5)

Definition

"*Tai*" means "high and extreme"; "*yang*," refers to yang of yin and yang. The slight depression of the temporalis part is commonly called *taiyangxue*, where the point is located.

Location

At the temporal part of the head and on the depression 1 *cun* posterior to the midpoint between the lateral end of the eyebrow and the outer canthus.

Methods

1) Puncture perpendicularly 0.5–1 *cun*, with a local sensation of soreness and distension; or prick with a three-edge needle for bloodletting.
2) Puncture horizontally 1.5–2 *cun* toward the apex satyri, with a sensation of soreness and distension radiating to the homolateral temporalis part.
3) Puncture 2–2.5 *cun*, penetrating to *xiaguan* (ST 7).

Indications

Headache, migraine, dizziness, facial paralysis, toothache, acute conjunctivitis.

Caution

Generally, perpendicular puncture is applied. Pricking with a three-edged needle is for severe headache or acute conjunctivitis; horizontal puncture, for migraine; penetrating puncture, for sequelae of facial paralysis. The point is unsuitable for moxibustion.

(3) *Qiuhou* (EX–HN7)

Definition

"*Qiu*" means "eyeball"; "*hou*," "posterior." The point is deep behind the eyeball.

Location

On the face, at the junction of the lateral fourth and medial three-fourths of the infraorbital margin.

Method

With the patient looking up, the practitioner fixes the eyeball with the left hand and inserts the needle slightly upward–inward with the other 0.8–1.2 *cun*, with a sensation of soreness and distension or protrusion in the whole eyeball.

Indications

Juvenile myopia, optic atrophy, orbital optic neuritis, chronic simple glaucoma.

Caution

As it is one of the points to which accidents will occur, No. 32–34 fine needles should be used with slow insertion, the needle being retained as soon as the sensation arises. Avoid lifting, thrusting, twirling or rotating with a large amplitude, for fear of injury to blood vessels inducing ocular hematoma.

(4) *Jinjin* (EX–HN12), *Yuye* (EX–HN13)

Definition

"*Jin*" and "*Yu*" here mean "precious" and "valuable"; "*jin*" and "*ye*" refer to saliva, which was believed to be the essence of human body fluid. The point is located at the opening spots under the sublingual ducts of the left and right where saliva is secreted.

Location

In the mouth, on the vein on the left side (*jinjin*) and on the right side (*yuye*) of the frenulum of the tongue.

Method

Puncture perpendicularly 0.2–0.3 *cun*, with a pain sensation in the local area; or prick for blood with a three-edged needle.

Indications

Glossoncus, aphasia, mouth ulcer.

Caution

Usually, pricking needling is applied without retention of the needle.

(5) *Yiming* (EX–HN14)

Definition

"*Yi*" means "to cover"; "*ming*," "bright light." The point is able to cure eye diseases and brighten the eyes.

Location

On the nape, 1 *cun* posterior to *yifeng*, at the midpoint of the line connecting *yifeng* and *fengchi*.

Method

Puncture perpendicularly 1–1.5 *cun*, with a distending sensation on one side of the head, or distension and heaviness in the local area.

Indications

Myopia, early senile cataract, tinnitus, optic atrophy.

Caution

A satisfactory needling sensation will be achieved if the needle point is inserted toward the nasal tip.

(6) *Zigong* (EX–CA1)

Definition

"*Zigong*" means "uterus." The point is able to cure diseases of the uterus.

Location

At the lower abdomen, 4 *cun* below the center of the umbilicus and 3 *cun* lateral to *zhongji* (RN 3).

Methods

 (i) Puncture perpendicularly 1–1.5 *cun*, with a local sensation of soreness and distension.
(ii) Puncture 2.5–3 *cun* penetrating to *zhongji* (RN 3), with soreness and distension in the abdomen, sometimes a uterus tic or needling sensation radiating to the external genitalia.

Indications

Uterine prolapse; menoxenia, menalgia, pelvic inflammation.

Caution

Penetrating acupuncture is mainly applicable to uterine prolapse; perpendicular puncture, to common diseases.

(7) *Dingchuan* (EX–B1)

Definition

"*Ding*" means "conquer"; "*chuan*" refers to asthma. The point works to conquer asthma, so it is named *dingchuan*.

Location

On the back, below the spinous process of the seventh cervical vertebra, 0.5 *cun* lateral to the posterior midline.

Method

Puncture perpendicularly 0.5–1 *cun*, with the tip slightly oblique to the backbone, giving a local sensation of soreness and distension, sometimes radiating to the shoulders, the back or the chest. Three to five cones of moxibustion are applicable, or warm moxibustion for 10–15 min.

Indications

Asthma, bronchitis, urticaria, stiff neck.

Caution

Avoid deeper insertion, for fear that accidents will happen.

(8) *Jiaji* (EX–B2)

Definition

"*Jia*" means "being fixed by two opposite forces"; "*ji*," refers to the spinal column. The point is located bilateral to the spine from the first to the fifth like clamping the spine from both sides, so it is named *jiaji* — or *huatuo-jiaji*, for it was said to be discovered by the famous physician Hua Tuo of the Eastern Han Dynasty.

Location

On the back and low back, a group of 34 points on both sides of the spinal column, below the spinous processes from the first thoracic vertebra to the fifth lumbar vertebra, 0.5 *cun* lateral to the posterior midline.

Method

Puncture perpendicularly 1.5–2 *cun* slightly toward the inner side, with a local sensation of soreness and distension, or electric numbness radiating to the extremities or intercostal space. Warm moxibustion for 10–20 min is applicable.

Indications

Points on the upper breast for diseases of the heart, the lung and upper extremities; points on the pectus for diseases of the stomach and intestines;

points on the lower back for diseases of the lumbar, abdomen and lower extremities.

Caution

Perpendicular puncture is applicable to common diseases; horizontal puncture, to local muscle diseases.

QUESTIONS

(1) What are the acupuncture methods and indications of *qiuhou* (EX-HN7) and *dingchuan* (EX-B1)?

(2) Describe briefly the indications and acupuncture methods of *yintang* (EX-HN3), *jinjin* (EX-HN12), *yuye* (EX-HN13), *zigong* (EX-CA1) and *jiaji* (EX-B2).

---

(9) *Yaoyan* (EX–B7)

Definition

"*Yao*" refers to the low back; "*yan*," the eye socket, the depression. The point is located on the depression bilateral to the low back, which is commonly callled *yaoyan*.

Location

On the low back, below the spinous process of the fourth lumbar vertebra, in the depression 3.5 *cun* lateral to the posterior midline.

Methods

 (i) Puncture perpendicularly 1.5 *cun*, with a local sensation of soreness and distension.

(ii) Puncture horizontally 1.5–2 *cun*, with the tip toward the vertebrae, giving a local sensation of soreness and distension, sometimes radiating to the buttocks.

Three-to-five cones of moxa are applicable, or warm moxibustion for 10–15 min.

Indications

Acute lumbar muscle sprain, nephroptosia, chronic low back pain.

Caution

The most obvious tenderness is taken as the point for an acute lumbar muscle sprain. Horizontal acupuncture is applicable to chronic low back pain.

(10) *Yaoqi* (EX–B8)

Definition

"*Yao*" refers to the low back; "*qi*" means "peculiar." The point is located on the low back and has curative effect on some diseases, so it is named *yaoqi*.

Location

On the low back, 2 *cun* directly above the tip of the coccyx, in the depression between the sacral horns.

Method

Puncture horizontally, with the tip upward, 2–2.5 *cun* along the skin. Warm moxibustion for 10–15 min is applicable.

Indications

Mania, headache, insomnia, constipation.

(11) *Sifeng* (EX–UE10)

Definition

"*Si*" means "four"; "*feng*," "crevice." The point is located on the transverse striation of interphalangeal joints, four points on each hand, so it is named *sifeng*.

Location

Four points on each hand, on the palmar side of the seond-to-fifth fingers and at the center of the proximal interphalangeal joints.

Method

Pricking needling is applied with a thick filiform needle or a three-edged needle. Withdraw the needle rapidly before a small amount of yellow–white transparent mucus is extruded, with a pain sensation in the local area.

Indications

Infantile diarrhea, infantile malnutrition, pertussis.

Caution

During pricking, yellow–white mucus disappearing and blood flowing out show that the patients condition is getting better. Moxibustion is unsuitable here.

(12) *Shixuan* (EX–UE11)

Definition

"*Shi*" refers to ten points on both hands; "*xuan*" means "catharsis." This means that the points work to remove pathogens.

Location

Ten points on both hands, at the tips of the ten fingers, 0.1 *cun* from the free margin of the nails.

Method

Puncture perpendicularly 0.1–0.2 *cun*, or prick for blood with a three-edged needle, with a pain sensation in the local area. Warm moxibustion for 5–10 min is applicable.

Indications

Coma, syncope, heatstroke, high fever, infantile convulsions.

(13) *Yaotongdian* (EX–UE7)

Definition

It is effective in treating acute or chronic lumbar muscle sprains.

Location

On the dorsum of the hand, between the second, third, fourth and fifth metacarpal bones lateral to the midpoint of the cross striation and the metacarpophalangeal articulation, two points on each side.

Methods

 (i) Puncture perpendicularly 0.3–0.5 *cun*, with a local sensation of soreness and distension.
(ii) Puncture obliquely toward the center of the palm, two points on each side, with a sensation of soreness and distension radiating to the whole palm.

Indications

Acute lumbar muscle sprain, chronic low back pain, syncope, infantile convulsions, headache.

Caution

Oblique puncture is applicable to an acute lumbar muscle sprain; ask the patient to move the low back during manipulation. Perpendicular acupuncture is applicable to other diseases. Puncturing the point is highly effective in treating acute lumbar muscle sprains.

(14) *Xiyan* (EX–LE5)

Definition

"*Xi*" means "knee"; "*yan*," "depression." It is so named for it is located at the depressions of the bilateral knees.

Location

In the depression on both sides of the patellar ligament when the knee is flexed. The medial and lateral points are named *neixiyan* and *waixiyan*, respectively.

Methods

(i) Puncture perpendicularly 1.5–2 *cun*, from the front to the back, or from the anterior interna to the posterior externa, with a sensation of soreness and distension in the knees, radiating downward sometimes.

(ii) Puncture from the outer *xiyan* penetrating to the inner *xiyan*, with a local sensation of soreness and distension. Warm needling with one or two cones is applicable, or warm moxibustion for 10–15 min.

Indications

Swelling and pain of the knee joint, hemiplegia by stroke.

Caution

Waixiyan is *dubi* (ST 35) of the stomach meridian of foot–*yangming*. Perpendicular acupuncture is applicable to severe cases; penetrating puncture, to mild cases or patients who are afraid of needles. Warm needling is applied on the basis of perpendicular acupuncture.

(15) *Lanweixue* (EX–LE7)

Definition

It is a new acupoint beyond the meridians recently developed, and is effective in treating appendicitis, so it is named *lanwei* (the appendix in the human body).

Location

At the upper part of the anterior surface of the leg, 5 *cun* below *dubi*, one finger breadth lateral to the anterior crest of the tibia.

Method

Puncture perpendicularly 1.5–2 *cun* slightly toward the tibia, with a local sensation of soreness and distension radiating to the dorsum of the foot. Three-to-five cones of moxa are applicable, or warm moxibustion for 10–15 min.

Indications

Acute or chronic appendicitis, paraplegia, stomachache, dyspepsia.

Caution

While treating acute or chronic appendicitis, press on the point area to find the most obvious tenderness before insertion.

(16) *Dannangxue* (EX–LE6)

Definition

It is a new acupoint beyond the meridians recently developed, and is applicable to gallbladder disorders.

Location

At the upper part of the lateral surface of the leg, 2 *cun* directly below the depression anterior and inferior to the head of the fibula.

Method

Puncture perpendicularly 1.5–2 *cun*, with a local sensation of soreness and distension radiating downward sometimes. Three to five cones of moxibustion are applicable, or warm moxibustion for 10–15 min.

Indications

Acute or chronic cholecystitis, Barbados distemper, paralegia, hypochondriac pain.

Caution

As with *lanweixue* (EX–LE7), the tenderness spot must be detected before insertion in the treatment of acute or chronic cholecystitis and Barbados distemper.

QUESTIONS

(1) What are the characteristics of the locations and indications of *yaoyan* (EX–B7), *xiyan* (EX–LE5), *yaotongdian* (EX–UE7) and *yaoqi* (EX-B8)?

(2) Pricking needling is applied to both *shixuan* (EX–UE11) and *sifeng* (EX–UE10). What are the differences between their indications?

(3) What are the differences and similarities of the locations and indications between *lanweixue* (EX–LE7) and *dannangxue* (EX–LE6)?

CHAPTER 7

Techniques of Acupuncture and Moxibustion

Techniques of acupuncture and moxibustion vary a lot in the clinic, but it is the combination of various acupuncture and moxibustion techniques on some acupoints that brings about the curative effectiveness. Therefore, a good command and application of the techniques is a basic skill for an acupuncturist.

MAIN CONTENTS OF ACUPUNCTURE AND MOXIBUSTION

Techniques of acupuncture and moxibustion vary a lot, and have been innovated and increased all the time. In ancient times, the techniques were classified into three types. One technique is to stimulate the point with acupuncture apparatuses by inserting into the skin, which was called "acupuncture." Of course, a few apparatuses (like ancient round-point needles — pins) are used to press on the acupoint area to be stimulated, and they are included in this type. Another technique is to fumigate the point with ignited moxa leaves or other things; it is known as the moxibustion technique. It also includes cold moxibustion (called "medicinal vesiculation" in ancient times), which is applied to the selected points with some animal or plant medicine to cause blisters. The third technique is cupping, which is to suck or pluck on the point or complaint site with specially made containers, like a pottery cup, bamboo jar or metal can (a glass cup nowadays).

There has been great development in acupuncture and moxibustion, and a great many techniques have been created by the combination of ancient acupuncture with modern scientific technology such as electricity, optics, acoustics and magnetics, and with Western medical approaches like pharmacology, physiatry and operative surgery — among which, apart from traditional acupuncture, moxibustion and cupping, are the following three methods.

Special Acupuncture

This is new kind of needling method formed on the basis of innovating the traditional or stimulation with the common characteristic of inserting to the acupoint area, including electric acupuncture, acupoint injection, picking therapy, cutting therapy, intradermal needle embedding, acupoint catgut embedding, etc.

Special Acupoint Therapy

This is a stimulating method, placing applied physics (electricity, light, sound, magnet, heat) or chemokines (Chinese and Western medicine) on acupoints in order to regulate the organism. The common charicteristic is to stimulate on the body surface, so it is also called "noninvasive therapy," including acupoint medicinal application, iontophoresis, electrotherapy, laser irradiation, magnetotherapy, infrared radiation, etc.

Minute Needling

This is an acupuncture therapy developed in modern times. It takes a relatively small local area or organ (such as the head, ear, hand, foot, nose or eye) as a whole to prevent or cure systemic diseases. The common characteristic is that each minute method has its own set of points with different stimulations and indications. Now commonly used methods in the clinic are scalp acupuncture, ear acupuncture, eye acupuncture, face acupuncture, nose acupuncture, hand acupuncture, wrist–ankle acupuncture, foot acupuncture, hologram acupuncture, etc.

FUNCTIONS OF ACUPUNTURE AND MOXIBUSTION

Both acupuncture and moxibustion aim to regulate *qi* and blood, and balance yin and yang, by stimulating the points and provoking the functions of meridians.

Traditional acupuncture theory states that acupuncture has two major functions: regulating *qi* and concentrating *shen* (vitality). Regulating *qi* means to regulate the *qi* of meridians and *zang–fu* viscera from excess or deficiency to coordinated state or healthy state, and to harmonize *qi* and blood to circulate freely without meeting any obstruction. *Shen* in TCM is a general manifestation of the vital activities of the human body, or the mental activities in a narrow sense. Regulating and concentrating the vitality by acupuncture functions promotes the effectiveness of regulating *qi* and strengthens the circulation of *qi* and blood in meridians, just like what was said in *Neijing* (*The Inner Classic*) — "concentration of *qi* makes it circulate freely"; on the other hand, regulation and concentration of *qi* itself means to regulate the whole of the vital activities, which was emphasized in *Neijing*, like "the key point of acupuncture is to concentrate on the vitality."

The functions of moxibustion are similar to those of acupuncture in general, but moxibustion is used to cure diseases by means of warmth and heat stimulation, which is able to warm meridians, dissipate cold and circulate blood for those with blood stasis due to coagulated cold, and to recover depleted yang and relieve prostration for those with yang deficiency. What is more, moxibustion has the function of disease prevention and healthcare since it improves and consolidates yang *qi* so as to reinforce the defensive function of the human body.

There have been further studies on the functions of acupuncture and moxibustion, and a great deal of clinical observation and experimental research has proven that:

(1) Acupuncture and moxibustion involve the stimulating spots: puncturing acupoints is more effective than puncturing nonpoint spots, and puncturing local points more effective than puncturing distant points.
(2) Acupuncture and moxibustion involve the quality and quantity of needling methods: the effectiveness varies with different methods like

moxibustion, electroacupuncture or needling, with different stimulation intensity or length of moxibustion.

(3) Acupuncture and moxibustion involve the functional state of the main body: it has little effect on healthy bodies but significant effect on the bodies of dysfunction and illness.

REQUIREMENTS OF ACUPUNCTURE AND MOXIBUSTION

Locate Precisely the Position

To achieve effectiveness, acupuncture and moxibustion must be applied to a certain position that refers to two aspects: one is the correct acupoint, and the other is the depth of insertion. For example, different positions of different depths were mentioned in *Neijing,* like puncturing the skin, tendon, flesh, channel or bone. In addition, different stimulation methods have different requirements for the positions.

Select Different Manipulations

The ultimate goal is to prevent or cure diseases with acupuncture and moxibustion, but different manipulations will lead to different effectiveness. Only with proper manipulation can satisfactory effect be achieved. Generally speaking, acupuncture is more widely used, while moxibustion is applicable to disorders arising from cold or cases with yang deficiency and weak constitution; electroacupuncture to relieving pain; point injection to eliminating inflammation; and scalp acupuncture to brain diseases like hemiparalysis. How to select the proper manipulation is also relative to the host factors. For example, mild stimulation is applicable to the old and the weak, and painless and safe stimulation like laser irradiation to children.

Use the Correct Stimulating Dose

The stimulating dose includes the intensity and the length of stimulation. Generally speaking, the stronger or the longer the stimulation is, the larger the dose will be, and vice versa. The dose depends on the patient's constitution and condition. Supply a large dose to the strong, and a small one to the weak; a large dose to those unresponsive to stimulation, and a small one to the sensitive; a large dose to acute and sthenic syndromes, and a small one to chronic and deficiency syndromes. In short, nothing is absolute, and different problems should be analyzed with different approaches.

QUESTIONS

(1) What are the main contents of acupuncture and moxibustion?
(2) What are the functions and requirements of acupuncture and moxibustion?

CHAPTER 8

Prevention and Management of Possible Accidents in Acupuncture Treatment

Acupuncture accidents are accidental injuries owing to either the practitioner or the sufferer during acupuncture, moxibustion or other acupoint stimulation. Slight injuries may cause pain, and severe ones may lead to lifetime physical disability or even death. The following will be introduced here: causes, classification, precautions, and accidents commonly seen in the clinic.

CAUSES OF POSSIBLE ACCIDENTS

The causes involve the practitioner and the patient, but the former takes the main responsibility.

Causes Concerning the Practitioner

(1) Incorrect points location and imperfect manipulations. Accidents may happen because of neglect of the knowledge of anatomy, with only deep insertion, or insertion in a wrong direction; or inserting aimlessly or promiscuously, damaging the organs.
(2) Infection caused by improper sterilization of needles or selected region for needling; a bent needle due to an eroded base; or other injuries caused by overthick needles.
(3) Too-strong electroacupuncture stimulation or out-of-specification of the apparatus resulting in broken needles.
(4) Absence of responsibility of the practitioner during treatment — another important factor in possible accidents.

Causes Concerning the Patient

(1) Psychologic factor, such as excessive tension, fear or agitation.
(2) Physiologic factor, such as hunger, or fatigue, which is one of the major causes of fainting during acupuncture.
(3) Constitutional factor, like inanition, or an allergic constitution.
(4) Pathologic factor, like injuries by mistake due to internal organs' pathologic changes (the lung, liver and spleen in particular) causing enlargement, a rough surface or porosity of tissue structure; for patients with hematologic disease, breaking small vessels may lead to hemophilia.
(5) Others, for example, rapid postural changes of the patients (mainly infants or mentally ill persons), may lead to needle squirm in the tissues or even needle bending; changes of the respiratory rhythm or depth may shorten the distance between the acupoint and the internal organ, and accidents tend to happen.

In general, whatever the causes are, the practitioner should take the main responsibility for the accident.

CLASSIFICATION OF ACUPUNCTURE INJURIES

The possible accidents are seen as follows.

Reactive Injury

This includes fainting reaction during acupuncture or moxibustion, anaphylactic reaction (such as allergic hives due to moxibustion) and hysteria reaction (sudden aphasia, convulsions and wild laughter).

Physical Injury

A mechanical injury is the most hazardous one; its lesion position involves internal organs, blood vessels and nerves. The degree of the injury depends on the specific organ. Generally, the most serious is the injury to the brain or the heart, which tends to cause death. A mechanical injury is the most common one in the clinic. For example, a pneumothorax by piercing is one of the most common accidents due to acupuncture.

Chemical Injury

This may arise from the development of acupoint injection therapy. Injuries vary according to different injecting sites. They include soft tissue injuries (often seen in the forearm and the hand, which may lead to hand abnormality or functional disorder), peripheral nerve injuries (radial nerve, ulnar verve and median nerve injuries; sciatic nerve injury) and vascular injuries (thromboangitis has the highest incidence). Besides improper manipulations, the causes are relevant to the physic liquor for injection, including the quality, power of hydrogen, density and dosage.

Biological Injury

This refers to secondary infection due to incomplete sterilization, i.e. causative organism (parasites, bacteria, or viruses) is brought into the patient's body by various apparatuses (filiform needle, injection needle, dermal needle, three-edged needle), causing infection like local red swelling and suppuration, or the spread of type B viral hepatitis.

In addition to the four injuries mentioned above, it is worth noting some indirect injuries. One patient was reported to have died of cerebral hemorrhage suddenly after acupuncture on points of the head, and it was found out later that the death might have been due to the nervous tension of the patient and too-strong stimulation instead of the acupuncture itself.

PREVENTION AND MANAGEMENT IN ACUPUNCTURE TREATMENT

Prevention

It is advisable to grasp the information in the book, to be cautious about selecting acupoints (especially the points noted to be dangerous), to employ the routine manipulations, to sterilize strictly both hands of the practitioner, the needles and the selected points for acupuncture, and to reinforce the sense of responsibility, improve medical ethics, keep calm and be serious in treating every patient.

Management

When accidents happen, rapid and exact judgment must be made, including the type of injury, the injury site and the degree of injury, for further treatment. It requires a comprehensive consideration of all aspects, such as inserting direction, depth, manipulation, and clinical situation of the patient. What is more, measures should be actively taken. Management of accidents consists of two kinds: (1) management in the office (such as for a mild pneumothorax, ocular hematoma, fainting during acupuncture, anaphylaxis or common infections), which requires a good command on the part of practitioners; (2) transition management (such as for a moderate or severe pneumothorax, a major visceral injury, or a bent needle that cannot be withdrawn without surgical techniques). If the accident remains unclear regarding the kind or graveness, transition management or consultation of doctors is needed.

COMMON POSSIBLE ACCIDENTS AND MANAGEMENT

Pneumothorax

This is the commonly seen accident in the clinic. It happens owing to lack of knowledge about acupuncture and anatomy. Generally speaking, a pneumothorax may be caused by too-deep puncturing on the acupoints of the chest and the back above the tenth dorsal vertebra, the ninth lateral rib and the seventh rib of the prothorax. And it may affect the patient with emphysema, even with deep needling on the acupoints of the superior belly or upper lumbar, or routine acupuncture for its overdistension of the lung and muscle atrophy.

The clinical manifestations of a pneumothorax are of three types: mild, moderate and severe. A mild pneumothorax presents with oppression in the chest, cough and dragging pain with movement; moderate and severe pneumothoraces, with stabbing pain of the costa sternales, dyspnea, severe cough, and even cold limbs or unconsciousness. The former requires a rest of 3–5 days without special management, and medicine for relieving cough or pain may be administrated according to symptoms; the latter necessitate sending the patients for surgery.

To avoid a pneumothorax, the beginner should take *jiaji* (EX-B 2) or distant points instead of acupoints of the back or the chest, especially for the patient with emphysema. If necessary, do as follows: at 1 cm lateral to the selected back–*shu* point, insert the needle at an angle of 65° toward the vertebral column until it touches the bone, and then lift the needle a little with retention, which is both safe and highly effective in the clinic.

Fainting

This is often due to nervous tension, a delicate constitution, hunger, fatigue, too-strong stimulation (too-forceful manipulation, too-long retention), stale air or noisiness in the office. The manifestations are dizziness, vertigo, palpitations, shortness of breath, fidgeting, nausea, pallor, cold sweating and a weak pulse. In severe cases, there may be loss of consciousness, fainting on the floor, excessive dripping sweat, urinary and fecal incontinence, or even convulsions. Fainting often occurs during acupuncture or minutes after the withdrawal. Fainting during cupping or moxibustion has similar manifestations.

Management

For mild cases, withdraw all the needles or cups, or stop moxibustion immediately. Then help the patient to lie down with his or her legs slightly up, and provide good ventilation. The symptoms will disappear after a short rest. If not, offer the patient some warm water. In severe cases, in addition to the above magagement, apply warm moxibustion on *baihui* (DU 20), or needle *shuigou* (DU 26) and *yongquan* (KI 1).

Ocular Hematoma

This is also a commonly seen accident in the clinic, with manifestations such as cyanosed ecchymosis on the point area or around the eyes (so-called panda eyes), which will cause otiose distress to patients as it does affect the looks.

The main causes of hematoma are too-thick needles and too-forceful manipulation. To prevent it, avoid selecting *jingming* (BL 1) and *chengqi* (ST 1), for they bleed easily. Even if it has to do, the beginner should employ shallow needling. No. 32–34 filiform needles must be used with slow insertion. Never try to lift and thrust or twirl the needles with a large amplitude. Withdraw the needle slowly and press the point for a moment with dry cotton balls.

For mild cases, no management is needed; use hot soaks to remove the ecchymosis. Severe cases often result from injury to the blood vessels or a relatively important artery or vein of the eyes, causing the loss of a large volume of blood. During the bleeding, a cold compress shoud be applied to the local area with distilled water or cold boiled water for 20 min. Then ask the patient to apply a hot compress with a hot towel two or three times a day, 20 min each time, which may be changed to once daily after the distension disappears. Generally, it takes 1–3 weeks to remove ecchymosis.

QUESTIONS

(1) Describe the causes and classification of possible accidents during acupuncture.
(2) Describe to prevent or manage possible accidents during acupuncture.
(3) Describe briefly the causes, clinical manifestations, prevention and management of pneumothoraces, fainting and eye hematoma.

CHAPTER 9

Filiform Needles

Filiform needles are widely used at present in the clinic. They are made of stainless steel. The common filiform needles have a unified gauge, which refers to the length and diameter of the needle body. The needles range from 0.5 *cun* to 4 *cun* (13–100 mm) in length, and needles measuring 1.5 *cun* and 2 *cun* are most frequently used in the clinic. The needles with regard to the diameter are of seven types, ranging from No. 26 to No. 36, and the most frequently used are No. 28 (0.4 mm in diameter), No. 30 (0.30 mm) and No. 32 (0.25 mm). The needle tip, in general, should be round and sharp; the body, straight and smooth, without rust or curves.

PREPARATIONS PRIOR TO ACUPUNCTURE TREATMENT

Preparations are divided into three parts, as follows.

Needling Practice

This is the requirement for beginners. Practise inserting, withdrawing, lifting, thrusting and rotating the needles on sheets of paper or a cotton cushion, followed by needling on the four limbs until there is no pain during insertion. A good command of manipulation is required before one applies acupuncture to patients.

Appropriate Posture of the Patient

This is significant in correct location of points, manipulation for acupuncture and moxibustion, comfort of the body, prolonged retention of the needle. Generally, the decubitus position is preferred if conditions allow. The commonly used *postures* adopted in the clinic are as follows:

(1) *Supine posture.* Suitable for the points on the head and face, neck, chest, abdomen and areas of the four limbs.
(2) *Prone posture.* Suitable for the points on the head, neck, back, lumbar and buttock regions, and the posterior region of the lower limbs.
(3) *Lateral recumbent posture.* Suitable for the points on the lateral side of the body.
(4) *Sitting erect with the elbows resting on a table.* Suitable for the points on the head, neck and breast.
(5) *Sitting in flexion*: Suitable for the points on the head, neck and back.

Besides the postures above, there are some specific postures for specific points. For example, puncturing *huantiao* (GB 30) entails stretching the leg below and flexing the leg above, in addition to the lateral posture.

Sterilization

Needle sterilization: Needles should be sterilized at high temperature (120°C) and high pressure (1.2 atmospheric pressure) for 15 min. For some other needles, like dermal and three-edged needles, soak them in 75% alcohol for 20 min or more. Given conditions, it is recommended to employ sterile needles that are used only once.

Prior to needling, the operator's fingers should first be washed with soap, and then swabbed with a 75% alcohol cotton ball.

The skin area selected for needling is swabbed round and outward with a 75% alcohol cotton ball from the needling point to its round areas.

NEEDLING METHODS

This is a vital skill for every practitioner, including insertion, manipulation and withdrawal of the needle.

Insertion

Insertion refers to the whole procedure of the tip piercing the skin to the desired depth. Generally, the needle handle is held with the thumb and index finger of the right hand, and the needle body with the middle finger. The needle is inserted into the point rapidly, aided by the thumb of the left hand holding the tip and pressing the point area, with the two hands exerting force simultaneously. The right hand is known as the puncturing hand; the left, the pressing hand.

According to the length of the needle and the location of the point, different methods of insertion are employed:

(1) *Inserting the needle aided by the pressure of the finger of the pressing hand.* This is suitable for puncturing with short needles (0.5–1 *cun*), by pressing beside the acupuncture point with the nail of the thumb or index finger of the left hand, holding the needle tip closely against the nail and then inserting the needle into the point.

(2) *Inserting the needle with the fingers stretching the skin.* Stretch the skin where the point is located with the thumb and index finger of the left hand, hold the needle with the right hand, and insert it into the point rapidly between the thumb and index finger of the left hand. This method is suitable for long needles and the points where the skin is loose.

(3) *Inserting the needle by pinching up the skin.* Pinch the skin up around the point with the thumb and index finger of the left hand, and insert the needle rapidly into the point with the right hand.

After insertion of the needle, different angles are taken according to different acupoints and pathogenetic conditions, involving perpendicular, oblique and horizontal (transverse) puncture. Perpendicular puncture is most commonly used in the clinic. In this method, the needle is inserted perpendicularly, forming a 90° angle with the skin surface. Oblique puncture is used for the points at the edge of bones, or points unsuitable for deep insertion. Generally, the needle is inserted obliquely to form an angle of approximately 45°–60° with the skin surface. Horizontal puncture is commonly used in the areas where the muscle is thin. The needle is inserted at an angle of 15°. This method also used for penetrating needling.

MANIPULATION

Needle manipulation means that needling is performed after insertion to induce a needling sensation by twirling and rotating or lifting and thrusting. The fundamental manipulation techniques are:

(1) *Lifting and thrusting*: This refers to the manner of lifting up and thrusting down the needle at the acupoint after inserting it to a certain depth. In clinical practice, it is classified into two types:

   (i) one involves lifting and thrusting in the whole acupoint area, i.e. making the needle move from the superficial to the deep, and from the deep to the superficial. The amplitude is relatively large, and this technique is similar to inserting and withdrawing the needle, so it is called the inserting–withdrawing method in some books. This type of manipulation is often employed in the comprehensive reinforcing–reducing manipulations which will be introduced in the following chapters.

   (ii) The other type refers to lifting and thrusting with a small amplitude, in which the needle is inserted and withdrawn repeatedly within a certain depth with moderate force and even amplitudes ranging from 0.1 cm to 0.5 cm, which should be regulated according to the patient's condition and constitution. The strength and speed of lifting and thrusting were believed to produce varied therapeutic effects in ancient times.

(2) *Twirling and rotating*. This refers to the manner of twirling and rotating the needle backward and forward continuously after it has reached the desired depth. Generally, hold the needle handle with the thumb and index and middle fingers of the right hand, with the thumb opposite the other fingers, or with only the thumb and the index finger, and rotate the needle clockwise or counter-clockwise with an amplitude of 180°–360°. But rotating the needle in a single direction may twine the muscle fibers and produce pain. Just like lifting and thrusting, rotating

the needle to the left or the right may produce different therapeutic effects. The two are often combined together in the clinic.

(3) *Retaining*: This means holding the needle in place after it is inserted to a given depth below the skin. The patient's age, physical constitution and pathological conditions decide the retaining and its duration of 5–10 min for short and several hours for long. In general, the needle is retained for 15–20 min. Retaining the needle is divided into still retaining and moving retaining. The former refers to retaining the needle right after the arrival of *qi* until withdrawal of the needle; the latter to repeating manipulations at intervals during the retention.

WITHDRAWAL

This refers to the manner in which the needle is withdrawn after the acupuncture treatment. On withdrawing the needle, press the skin around the point with the thumb and index finger of the pressing hand, rotate the needle gently and lift it slowly to the subcutaneous level, then withdraw it quickly and press the punctured point for a while with cotton balls to prevent bleeding or relieve the discomfort. If a stuck needle occurs during withdrawal, do not be eager to lift the needle forcefully, for fear of causing pain, bleeding, or even a bent needle. It is advisable to press the skin around the point, or puncture another point nearby before slowly withdrawing the needle. If the stuck needle is due to the change of the postures, ask the patient to return to the original position before withdrawing the needle.

QUESTIONS

(1) What is the preparation prior to acupuncture with filiform needles?
(2) What are the fundamental manipulation techniques with filiform needles?

CHAPTER 10

Introduction to Acupuncture Manipulations

Acupuncture refers to the whole procedure of needling manipulations in a broad sense, and narrowly speaking it refers to the manipulations between insertion and withdrawal of needles. Lifting–thrusting and twirling–rotating are the most fundamental and important. Many other manipulations are also available, and here the commonly used ones will be introduced.

AUXILIARY MANIPULATIONS

Auxiliary manipulations are the manipulations applied before and after insertion of needles to regulate and transmit the needling sensation that signals the arrival of *qi*. They are applied with the hands only or with the needles. They include the following.

Pressing

This means pressing an acupoint with the thumb, index finger or middle finger with even force. It is able to relieve pain induced by needling, and to facilitate the arrival of *qi* after insertion.

Massaging Along the Meridian

This refers to a procedure for promoting the needling effect by pressing with the fingers gently on the upper or lower parts of the related acupoints along the meridians and collaterals, pressing with the thumb or index finger, or tapping with the middle finger. It can promote the flow of the meridian-*qi* and remove a stuck needle.

Flicking

This is a manipulation to strengthen the needling sensation and to conduct or spread the needling sensation. It is applied with the index finger and the middle finger overlapped, or the thumb and the index finger overlapped. Gently flick the needle tail with the index finger, causing mild vibration of the needle for 7–10 times. Never flick too forcefully or too frequently, to avoid bending or sticking the needle.

Scraping

This is a manipulation to strengthen the needling sensation and to conduct or spread the needling sensation. It is applied in two ways:

(1) *Single-hand scraping.* Place the thumb on the needle tail, and then scrape the handle with the nail of the index finger or middle finger.
(2) *Double-hand scraping.* Place the thumb of the left hand on the top end of the handle, pressing a little downward; hold the needle body with two flexed index fingers, and scrape the handle slightly with the nail of the thumb of the right hand, which requires skillful manipulation and even exertion. The nail for scraping has to be round and smooth, not too long and not too short.

REINFORCING AND REDUCING MANIPULATIONS

"Reinforcing" means "replenishing and tonifying," referring to replenishing and regulating *qi* when yin–yang and *qi*-blood in some part of the body are deficient; "reducing" originally meant "discharging," here referring to eliminating the excess syndrome of yin–yang and *qi*-blood in some part. The main purpose of reinforcing and reducing is to keep the body in equilibrium. Reinforcing and reducing means to employ different manipulations during acupuncture to reinforce the deficiency and reduce the excess. There are various kinds of manipulations in acupuncture books of the past dynasties, and they are divided into two major types: simplex or basic reinforcing and reducing manipulations, and duplex or comprehensive reinforcing and reducing manipulations, most of which are rarely used in the clinic. The following are some reinforcing and reducing manipulations which are commonly used and easy to master.

Simplex Reinforcing and Reducing Manipulations

Reinforcing and reducing by twirling and rotating the needle

Derived from the basic twirling and rotating method, this is differentiated by clockwise or counter-clockwise rotation of the needle. In other words, the right rotation is the reducing method that means rotating the needle forward with the thumb, and the left rotation is the reinforcing method that means rotating the needle backward with the thumb. This technique is commonly applied to acupoints of the four limbs in treatment of locomotor system diseases. For example, reducing manipulation by twirling and rotating is suitable for pain and limb spasm, and reinforcing manipulation by twirling and rotating for numbness and weakness due to the asthenic healthy *qi*.

Reinforcing and reducing by lifting and thrusting the needle

Also derived from the basic lifting and thrusting method, the reinforcing and reducing manipulations are distinguished by heavy pressing of the needle to a deep region or forceful lifting of the needle to the superficial region. Specifically, reinforcing means to press the needle rapidly and lift it slowly, which is applicable to deficiency cold syndrome because of its warming reinforcing function, while reducing means to rapidly lift the needle and press it slowly, which is applicable to excessive heat syndrome because of its cold reducing function. It is worth noting that manipulation is often applied to acupoints of the four limbs, and that the exertions of lifting and thrusting (including the frequency and amplitude) must be different and regulated according to different conditions and constitutions.

Reinforcing and reducing according to the needling direction

This is also known as reinforcing and reducing by puncturing along and against the direction of the meridians, respectively. The needling direction depends on the running direction of the course of the 12 meridians. The three yang meridians of the hand run from the hand up to the head. The needle tip pointing downward, i.e. against the meridian course, is known as the reducing method. The needle tip pointing in the opposite direction, i.e. following the running course of the meridian, is known as the reinforcing method. The same applies to the three yin meridians of the hand running from the chest to the hand, the three yang meridians of the foot running from the head down to the foot, and the three yin meridians of the foot running from the foot up to the abdomen and the chest. During the operation, the arrival of *qi* must be achieved before one adjusts the direction of the needle tip.

Duplex Reinforcing and Reducing Manipulations

These are also known as comprehensive reinforcing and reducing manipulations, as they combine the application of basic manipulations, auxiliary manipulations, and simplex reinforcing and reducing manipulations. More then 20 methods are recorded in the acupuncture literature. The following two comprehensive methods are commonly used in the clinic.

Setting the mountain on fire

This is also known as the warm reinforcing method. When it is applied, ask the patient to naturally inhale with the nose and exhale with the mouth, and divide the predetermined depth into three layers: superficial (heaven part), middle (human part) and deep (earth part). Puncture from the superficial layer to the deep layer. Do nine times of quick pressing and slow lifting successively, first in the heaven part, then in the human, and finally in the earth. After that, lift the needle directly to the heaven part and repeat the above from the superficial layer to the deep three times inward and three times outward (actually nine times inward and three times outward), and this is one turn. Do all this several times, until the patient feels warm all over his or her body. If there is no warm feeling, forget it and retain the needle for 10–15 min. This method is generally applied to acupoints on thick muscles and applicable to paralysis, numbness, chronic enterorrhea, pathogenic cold and pain in abdomen syndromes due to deficiency cold.

Thorough heavenly cool

This is also known as the cool reducing method. Ask the patient to naturally exhale with the nose and inhale with the mouth, then insert the needle with the fingers stretching the skin. In the course of acupuncture manipulation, the needle is inserted from the deep to the superficial part. First, insert the needle directly into the deep part, lift it quickly and thrust it slowly, six times; then, lift the needle to the middle part to do the same manipulation six times. Finally, lift the needle to the superficial part to do the same manipulation six times again. After that, insert the needle directly into the deep part again to do the above manipulation. Three liftings and three insertions from the deep to the superficial part (actually nine liftings and three insertions) are one turn. Repeat the manipulation for several turns, till the patient feels cool in the punctured area or in the whole body. But usually the cool feeling is more difficult to cause than the warm feeling, so if the patient cannot feel cool, retain the needle in the point for 10–15 min. This method is mainly applicable to excessive heat syndromes like wind-stroke block syndrome, febrile diseases and manic-type schizophrenia.

QUESTIONS

(1) What are the auxiliary manipulations in acupuncture?
(2) Describe how to apply the reinforcing and reducing manipulations in acupuncture.

CHAPTER 11

Moxibustion

Moxibustion is a traditional therapy with a long history in China. It refers to the therapeutic technique (with heat stimulation) of applying ignited mugwort or other medical herbs to a certain part of the body. It is divided into two types.

MOXIBUSTION WITH MOXA WOOL

Moxibustion with moxa wool is divided into moxibustion with moxa cones, moxibustion with moxa sticks and moxibustion with apparatus. The first two will be introduced in detail, for they are most commonly used in the clinic.

Moxibustion with Moxa Cones

This is a method of moxibustion applied with moxa cones which are tapered with the tip of the cone at the top and the flat at the bottom made of moxa wool. According to the requirements of moxibustion, moxa cones vary in size — large, medium and small. The smallest one is as big as a grain of wheat; the medium-size one, a soybean; and the largest one is the size of *vicia faba*. Generally speaking, patients with strong constitutions who have caught diseases in the early stage should be given large cones; patients with weak constitutions and chronic diseases, small ones. Moxibustion with moxa cones is divided further into direct and indirect moxibustion.

Direct moxibustion

This means to place a moxa cone directly on the skin and ignite it. This type of moxibustion is subdivided into festering moxibustion and nonfestering moxibustion according to the different requirements of moxibustion.

Festering moxibustion

This is also known as scarring moxibustion. Prior to moxibustion, apply some onion or garlic juice to the site in order to increase the adhesion of the moxa cone to the skin, then put the moxa cone on the point and ignite it until it burns out. This method may lead to a local burn, blister, festering and a scar after healing, causeing great pain to the patient, and so is less used except for some intractable diseases.

Nonfestering moxibustion

Also known as nonscarring moxibustion, this is more widely used in modern times. Place a moxa cone on the point and ignite it. When the patient feels burning discomfort, remove the cone and place another one. No blister should be formed and there should be no festering or scar formation.

Indirect moxibustion

This refers to the moxibustion performed with some material placed between the smoldering moxa cone and the skin, so it is also known as separated moxibustion or insulated moxibustion, which can serve as treatment with moxibustion and treatment with drugs at the same time. The material used for separation is usually Chinese drugs in the form of slices, cakes or powder. The commonly used methods are as follows.

Moxibustion with ginger

Cut a slice of ginger about 0.3 cm thick, punch numerous holes on it and place it on the point selected. On top of this piece of ginger, a large moxa cone is placed and ignited. When the patient feels its scorching, lift the ginger up for a while before applying it again until the local skin becomes red. This method is indicated in abdominal pain and diarrhea due to a chill.

Moxibustion with garlic

Cut a slice of garlic about 0.3 cm thick, punch holes in it, and put it on the point with the ignited moxa cone above. When the patient feels the scorching, lift up the garlic a little for a while before applying it again. The moxibustion needs four or five cones in each session. Garlic is stimulatory to skin, and blisters may occur after moxibutsiton, so it is advisable to prick the large blisters with a sterilized needle and apply gentian violet onto the skin to avoid infection. This method is often applicable to scrofula, carbuncle abscess, poisonous insect bites, etc.

Moxibustion with salt

This is usually applied at the umbilicus, so it is also called moxibustion at the *shenque* point (RN 8). Fill the umbilicus with salt to the level of the skin, place a large moxa cone on top of the salt, and then ignite it. It is advisable to put a slice of ginger on the salt before moxibustion with moxa cones, lest the salt should explode when heated. This method is often used to treat acute vomiting and diarrhea, or abdominal pain.

Moxibustion with moxa sticks

Also known as moxibustion with moxa rolls, this was applied as early as in the Ming Dynasty. Moxa sticks are made by rolling moxa wool (other herbal medicines may be mixed in) into the shape of a cigar, using paper made of mulberry bark. This method is classified into mild–warm moxibustion, rounding moxibustion and sparrow-pecking moxibustion.

(1) *Mild–warm moxibustion.* Ignite one of the ends of the moxa stick, hold the stick and keep the ignited end above the selected acupoint from a distance of 3 cm, and bring a mild warmth to the local area for

3–5 min until the local skin becomes red. This method is applicable to arthromyodynia syndromes by wind and cold.

(2) *Rounding moxibustion.* This is also termed "circling moxibustion." Keep the ignited moxa stick above the selected points at a distance of 3 cm. Then move the moxa stick horizontally so as to cause a warm sensation of the skin of the acupoint area. This method is applicable to rheumatalgia, soft tissue strain and skin diseases.

(3) *Sparrow-pecking moxibustion.* Hold an ignited moxa stick with its ignited end directed at the acupoint, and move it up and down, like a sparrow pecking at food. Generally, the moxibustion is applied for 5 min and is suitable for diseases needing moxibustion with forceful stimulation.

MOXIBUSTION WITH NO MOXA WOOL

This refers to moxibustion without using moxa wool as material, including hot moxibustion and cold moxibustion.

Hot Moxibustion

This is a type of moxibustion, like moxibustion with moxa wool, referring to all kinds of moxibustion with heat energy. But, instead of moxa wool, the material for hot moxibustion includes mulberry twigs, peach twigs, bamboo shavings, and yellow wax in ancient times, and now rush-fire cauterization is most widely used.

Rush-fire cauterization is a moxibustion method in which a rush is dipped in oil and ignited for moxibustion on the point. Dip a rush about 10 cm long into vegetable oil, ignite the oiled rush, and put it on the point. Moxibustion is usually applied quickly, with the rush horizontal or oblique to the point. Not too much oil should be dipped, in case the hot oil drips cause scalding. When the burning rush touches the skin of the acupoints, a "pa" sound should be heard and the fire extinguished. This process is called a "burn," and usually one burn is used for each point, turning the local skin reddish; keep the local area clean to avoid infection. This method is mainly used to treat acute infantile diseases like epidemic parotitis.

Cold Moxibustion

Cold moxibustion, also known as medical vesiculation, or vesiculating moxibustion with herbs, is a form of moxibustion in which irritating drugs are applied to the selected points so as to cause blisters, creating effects similar to those of common moxibustion. In the clinic, the drugs commonly used for cold moxibustion include Mao Gen (*Ranunculus Japonicus*), Ban Mao (*Mylabris*), Bai Jie Zi (*Semen Sinapis Albae*), Da Suan (*Bulbus Allii*), Han Lian Cao (*Herba Ecliptae*), Tian Nan Xing (*Rhizoma Arisaematis*), Wei Ling Xian Ye (*Radix et Rhizoma Clematidis*), etc.

Bai Jie Zi (Semen Sinapis Albae) moxibustion

Grind Bai Jie Zi to powder and then mix it with cold boiled water to form a paste. Apply this to the acupoint, cover it with oil paper and fix it with an adhesive plaster. The cold moxibustion is applied for 2–4 h to make the local area congested, reddish or blistered. It is mainly used for treating facial paralysis and joint pain, and for preventing asthma in combination with other drugs.

Da Suan (Bulbus Allii) moxibustion

Pound Da Suan into a spread, and apply a proper amount of the spread to the acupoint for 1–3 h until itch, reddening and blisters occur in the local skin. This method is applicable to acute laryngitis, hemoptysis and rhinorrhagia.

INDICATIONS

Moxibustion functions to warm meridians and expel cold, and is mainly applicable to cold syndrome, yang deficiency syndrome, and all chronic diseases. In addition, it is used for healthcare. It will be introduced in the following chapters.

Among the moxibustion methods, moxibustion with moxa sticks is most frequently used, and direct moxibustion with moxa cones (especially scarring moxibustion) is inadvisable to be applied to the face, portions with obvious vessels or joints. Patients with high fever, loss of consciousness and wind-stroke block syndrome should not be treated with moxibustion.

QUESTIONS

(1) What methods does moxibustion with moxa wool include? How to use each of them?
(2) What is moxibustion with no moxa wool? And what are its contents?

CHAPTER 12

Cupping, Warm Needling and Fire Needling

CUPPING

Cupping is a therapeutic method in which a jar or a cup is attached to the skin surface to cause local congestion through the negative pressure created by introducing heat in the form of an ignited material. Also known as the sucking tube method, it was termed "horn cupping" in ancient times and was used in the Jin Dynasty. Various kinds of cupping apparatuses are available, such as a bamboo jar, pottery jar, metal (copper or iron) cup, glass cup or suction cup. Nowadays, glass cups and sucking cups are the most widely used in the clinic.

CUPPING METHODS

Two commonly used cupping methods will be introduced here.

Fire Cupping

This is a traditional cupping method which is applied by making a fire in a cup, driving away the air to create a negative pressure inside, thus producing suction by the cup on the skin. There are four types of fire cupping in common use: fire-throwing cupping, fire-twinkling cupping, cotton-attaching cupping and alcohol-fire-separated cupping.

Fire-throwing cupping

Throw an ignited ball wetted with 95% alcohol or a piece of ignited paper into a jar, and immediately place the mouth of the jar firmly against the skin on the desired location, attaching the jar to the skin. This method is applied only when the jar is required to be attached horizontally, otherwise the burning material may fall out and hurt the skin.

Fire-twinkling cupping

Clamp an alcohol cotton ball with a pair of forceps, ignite it and put it into a jar. Then, immediately take it out and place the jar on the selected point or area.

Cotton-attaching cupping

Attach an alcohol-wetted cotton slice measuring 1 cm squared to the bottom of the internal wall of a jar, ignite it, and immediately place the jar on the selected area.

Alcohol-fire-separated cupping

Place a lump of hard material (like a penicillin bottle cap), difficult to burn and conduct heat, and place an alcohol cotton ball on it. Then ignite the ball and immediately place a jar on the local area.

Among the methods above, fire-twinkling and alcohol-fire-separated cupping are frequently applied and are safe for patients, but the former requires skilled manipulation, otherwise tight suction will not be achieved; and avoid burning the mouth of the jar, for fear of injuring the skin. The latter has strong suction, though, and it requires elaborate manipulations. The method selected should be suitable for or familiar to the practitioner.

Cupping by Extracting Air

A modern cupping method, this consists of two parts: an aspirator and a plastic jar with a piston (various types). When it is applied, place the jar on the desired area, connect the piston to the air aspirator, and extract the air to form a negative pressure inside, making the cup absorbent on the skin. Pull up the plastic core when it is time to withdraw the jar. By using mechanical force instead of fire, accidents like scalding will not happen and the suction can be regulated according to the patient's constitution, condition and sucking part. It is worth promoting.

CUPPING MANIPULATIONS

Retaining Cupping

After a jar is sucked on the skin of the selected area, retain it there for 5–20 min before removing it. The retaining time may be shortened on the face or some other tenellous area and lengthened on the area with thick muscle. Generally, do not remove the jar until the local skin becomes reddish or has ecchymosis. But sometimes too-long retention may cause blisters on the cupping area; then apply gentian voilet and bind it up if necessary. Most of the cases will be absorbed to form a scab without a scar. Retaining cupping is applicable to most of the diseases which can be treated with cupping.

Quick Cupping

Also known as successive flash cupping, this is applied by placing the cup on the affected area and removing it at once. Do the same thing many times over the same area, until the skin becomes hyperemic-red. This method is mostly used for local skin numbness and miopragia of the deficiency type.

Moving Cupping

Also termed "pushing cupping," this method is suitable for cupping to an area with abundant muscle. Smear Vaseline or vegetable fat over the skin of the selected area, and cause a jar to be sucked on the area. Press the skin above the jar to stretch it tense, hold the jar with the right hand, and draw it to slide downward for a certain distance. Then, forcefully press the skin below the jar with the left hand and push it with the right hand to slide upward. Repeat this course several times, until the skin becomes red. This method is mainly used for treating muscle strain of the lumbus and the back.

Pricking-Cupping Bloodletting

Also termed "bloodletting cupping," this refers to bloodletting with a three-edged or cutaneous needle, followed by cupping, and then retaining for the jar there 10–15 min. Wipe off the blood after withdrawing the jar. This method is mainly used to treat all kinds of sprains and contusions, and muscle pain.

INDICATIONS

Cupping is applicable to rheumatalgia, sprains and contusions, cold, stomachache, abdominal pain, headache, sores and carbuncles, but not to high fever, convulsions and spasm, or areas with thin muscle, hair or cobbly bones.

WARM NEEDLING

Warm needling, also termed "burning the needle handle," is a method of acupuncture combined with moxibustion. It is a therapeutic technique of making the needle warm by burning mugwort on the handle of the needle and then inserting it into the body. It was originally mentioned in *Shang Han Lun* (*Treatise on Cold-Induced Diseases*) in the Han Dynasty.

Manipulation

After the arrival of *qi* and with the needle retained in the selected point, wrap the needle handle tightly with a unit of moxa wool. Take a moxa stick 1.5–2 cm in length and put it on the handle. Ignite it from the lower end till it burns out. Place a hard slip of paper on the point area to avoid burning the skin by dropped moxa fire.

Indications

Warm needling is mainly used to treat arthralgia and cold pain in the abdomen, and is applicable to healthcare. It is unsuitable for conditions which cannot endure retention of needles, like convulsions, spasms or tremors, and for mentally ill persons or infants. During the treatment, ask the patient not to change his or her position, so as to avoid burning the skin or clothes and bedding.

FIRE NEEDLING

Fire needling, also termed "heat needling" or "red-hot needling," is an acupuncture method of puncturing a point quickly with a red-hot needle to treat diseases. It was employed as early as in the Qin Dynasty.

Acupuncture Apparatus

This is usually a thicker needle made of stainless steel. There are two types: one is used for single needling, a No. 26 or No. 27 filiform needle 2–3 *cun* in length and 0.5–1 mm in diameter, with bamboo or sclerotin wrapped around the needle handle to avoid burning the hand; the other is for shallow puncture, with the needle body thin and short (like a dermal needle) with 3–9 needles at the top, and with a wooden handle.

Manipulations

First, locate the point or region for needling according to the pathogenetic condition, and sterilize the skin with 2% iodine tincture before swabbing away the iodine with 75% alcohol. Two needling methods are used.

Deep puncture

A long needle is employed. Hold the needle with the right hand, and fix the point with the left. Warm the needle tip and the lower portion of the needle shaft with the fire of an alcohol lamp until the color of these parts becomes red, and insert the needle accurately into the acupoint or the required area quickly and draw it immediately. Then, press the needle hole with a sterilized cotton ball. Be careful and swift in acupuncture and insert the needle to the desired depth of 0.3–0.5 *cun* (1–1.7 cm).

Shallow puncture

A needle with a wooden handle and multi-needles is employed. Burn the needle red with the fire of an alcohol lamp, then gently tap on the skin surface with the needle. This method is mainly used to treat refractory skin diseases with a large area, such as neurodermatitis and oxhide lichen. Pricking with the single needle is available for small lesions.

Indications

Rheumatalgia, crewels, elephantiasis, neurodermatitis, nevi and nodules.

Precautions

Deep puncture with fire needling must be kept away from vessels and internal organs to avoid adverse consequences. When shallow-needling, tap the skin with even and sparse force so as to avoid stripping away epidermis.

QUESTIONS

(1) What is cupping? And what does cupping involve?
(2) What are the differences of manipulations and indications between warming needling and fire needling?

CHAPTER 13

Dermal Needling, Collateral Bloodletting and Intradermal Needling

ACUPUNCTURE WITH DERMAL NEEDLES

Dermal needling is an acupuncture method of treatment using several small needles to tap shallowly on the skin of the acupoint or selected area. It is applicable to children because of its mild stimulation, and thus it is also known as infantile needling. Different from other needling methods, dermal needling is applied to not only acupoints but also the 12 meridians and the cutaneous region.

Needles

There are various kinds of dermal needles, such as the plum blossom needle, seven-star needle, temple guard needle and electric plum blossom needle. The most commonly used needle in the clinic is made up of a seven-star needle and a plum blossom needle inlaid onto the end of a long resilient handle.

Manipulation

After routine and local sterilization, hold the handle with the right hand, with the ring and small fingers fixing the end of the handle at the small thenar eminence of the palm, with the middle finger and the thumb holding the one-third part of the handle, and with the index finger pressing on the handle. Tap quickly with the tip flipping instantly after touching the skin with a frequency of proximately 100 times per minute.

The tapping force may be mild, mediate or heavy, according to the patient's physical constitution, lesion region and symptoms:

(1) *Mild stimulation*: Tapping with mild wrist force until the skin becomes reddish. It is suitable for infants or the old and weak with diseases of the head and face, deficiency syndromes or chronic diseases with a long course.

(2) *Mediate stimulation*: Tapping with a little heavy force of the wrist until the local skin becomes reddish without bleeding. It is applicable to commonly encountered diseases.

(3) *Heavy stimulation*: Tapping with a heavy strength of the wrist, with the needle raised high and a slow rhythm until the local skin becomes reddish and there appears bleeding. It is applicable to a patient with a strong constitution, the area with apparent tenderness and with abundant muscles on the back, the shoulders and the buttocks. According to the stimulation intensity and the pathogenetic condition, treatment with dermal needling may be applied once daily or once every other day 10–20 times as a course.

Tapping Areas

There are many classification methods for tapping areas, and for the sake of beginners, here three types will be introduced: global tapping area, local tapping area and acupoint tapping area. The last one, like other stimulations, refers to tapping on the skin around the selected point. The first two are as follows:

(1) *Globle tapping area*: Three lines bilateral to the spinal column on the back; the first line is 1 cm from the spinal column, second 2 cm and the third 3–4 cm. Most of the diseases are treated by tapping on these areas.

(2) *Local tapping area*: Including the affected area, tenderness spot, paresthesia area and matters of positive reaction (like subcutaneous nodes or something of trabs shape found by touching).

During the operation, the three types of areas can be employed by combination. For example, for treating stomachache, tap on the two sides of the spinal column and then tap on the selected acupoint, the tenderness spot or something of positive reaction.

Indications

Headache, hypertension, myopia, neurasthenia, diseases of the gastrointestinal tract, local dermatoses like neurodermatitis.

During the treatment with dermal needling, the needles must remain in good condition. If the tip hooks hair or the needle gets rusty, repair or exchange it immediately. Sterilize the needles in 75% alcohol or some other disinfection liquid. A sterilized needle used only once is preferred. The tapping area must be sterilized too. The method is not suitable for those with wounds or ulcers on the skin.

COLLATERAL PRICKING

Collateral pricking is also called the bloodletting method, or three-edged needling since the three-edged needle is common used.

Needles

Now, in the clinic, the three-edged needle and thick filiform needle are most commonly employed. Three-edged needles are of the large, medium and small types, and the 0.5 *cun* filiform needle No. 26 is preferred.

Manipulations

(1) *Spot pricking*. During the operation, press and push the site to be pricked to cause local congestion, hold the site with the left hand, with the thumb and index finger of the right hand gripping the handle, and the belly of the middle finger supporting the lower portion of its shaft, exposing approximately 0.1–0.2 cm from the tip of the needle; direct the tip precisely at the spot to be punctured and withdraw it immediately. Then, squeeze out a few drops of blood by pressing the skin around the punctured hole, and press over the hole with a sterilized dry cotton ball until the bleeding stops. This is the most widely used method in the clinic.

(2) *Clumpy pricking*. Prick around a small area with a three-edged needle repeatedly to cause a little bleeding. This method, often combined with cupping, which is the prick-cupping method, is mostly used for acute or chronic soft tissue injuries.

(3) *Scattered pricking*. Similar to clumpy pricking, scattered pricking is performed on a larger area with a bigger distance. According to the size of the focus, prick the area 10–20 times. This method is mainly applicable to erysipelas, neurodermatitis, etc.

(4) *Breaking pricking*. This is a method developed from spot pricking, and is mainly applicable to certain diseases on the relevant part of the skin, which are manifested by tenderness, sleepiness, papules and subcutaneous nodes. These may occur on different parts of the body and are commonly seen on the back, two sides to the line between the seventh and fifth cervical vertebrae. If it is a papule, it may be slightly prominent above the skin, 2–4 mm in diameter, usually grayish-white, dark-red, and brown or light-red. During the operation, after local sterilization, press and fix the skin with the left hand, hold a three-edged needle of small size, prick and break the skin quickly, insert the needle deep to the subcutaneous tissue, tilt the shaft of the needle and then gently move it upward to break some of the fibrous tissue. After that, wipe off the blood and cover the skin with an aseptic dressing and fix it.

Indications

Collateral pricking is applicable to sunstroke, apoplectic coma, shock, acute gastroenteritis, acute conjunctivitis, headache, neurodermatitis, acute tonsillitis, lumbar muscle strain, erysipelas, furuncles, etc. Breaking pricking is also used to treat some chronic diseases. Collateral pricking requires strict sterilization, is forbidden for hematologic diseases, and should be used cautiously for the weak, the anemic, or pregnant women. Generally, the bleeding should be about 10 ml at most.

ACUPUNCTURE WITH INTRADERMAL NEEDLES

Acupuncture with intradermal needles, also called needle-embedding therapy, is a treatment method that inserts and leaves a small needle beneath the skin so as to give the body a long-lasting continuous stimulation. It was developed from the retention of filiform needles and has a certain clinical effectiveness.

Needles

There are two types of intradermal needles widely used in the clinic: the thumbtack type and the grain-like type. The former is more widely used, because of its convenience and safety.

Manipulation

Since the needle is retained beneath the skin for a relatively long time, ear points are often employed so as not to affect the normal movements of the human body.

(1) *Grain-like needle.* After sterilization, hold the needle handle with a pair of forceps, insert the needle perpendicularly directly into the acupoint to the dermis. Then, horizontally puncture in the direction along the skin and embed the needle shaft 0.5–0.1 cm inside the skin. Finally, fix the handle of the needle left outside on the skin with an adhesive plaster. This method is often applied to body acupoints or penetrating acupuncture of ear points.

(2) *Thumbtack needle.* After sterilization, hold the exterior ring with a pair of forceps, direct the needle tip at the acupoint and insert it into the point, make the flat-expanded handle of the needle lie flat on the skin and fix it with an adhesive tape.

The embedding duration depends on the pathogenetic condition and the climate — no longer than two days in summer and three-to-four days in winter.

Indications

It is mainly applied to diseases of recurrent attacks, like neuropathic headache, migraine, intercostal neuralgia, trifacial neuralgia, sciatica, biliary colic, stomachache and angina pectoris, as well as some chronic diseases, like hypertension, asthma, menoxenia and enuresis.

Be sure to do the sterilization before the manipulation. It is better to employ a disposable needle, or a needle soaked in 75% alcohol and taken out with a pair of sterilized forceps. If the patient complains of stabbing pain or difficulty in moving, withdraw the needle and embed it again. In summer too much perspiration may cause infection, so withdraw the needle immediately if the patient feels pain in the embedding area.

QUESTIONS

(1) What are the characteristics of the tapping method and the tapping area with dermal needles?

(2) What are the four methods of collateral pricking? And what are the indications and precautions?

(3) Describe how to manipulate the acupuncture with the intradermal needle.

CHAPTER 14

Electroacupuncture, Acupoint Application, Acupoint Injection and Acupoint Laser Irradiation

ELECTROACUPUNCTURE

Electroacupuncture is a needling method widely used in the clinic. It combines filiform needling and the impulsive current on acupoints or a certain area to enhance the curative effect.

Apparatus

The apparatus for electroacupuncture is called the electroacupuncture stimulator or electroacupuncture therapeutic apparatus. The buzzer electric stimular to used previously has been replaced by the transistor electroacupuncture stimulator since the late 1960s. There are many types of apparatus. The commonly used one in the clinic is the modulating pulse electroacupuncture apparatus, like the G6805 type with both ac and dc, which has three different waves: continous wave (with a regular and lasting waveform), irregular wave (formed by the electric pulse changing from low frequency to high frequency) and intermittent wave (an irregular wave with periodic intermissions). A beginner should use the simple regular pulse wave electroacupuncture apparatus, such as the BT701 type, which has four pairs of output circuits connecting eight acupoints with the continuous wave. There is a turn button regulating the frequency, and four buttons regulating the intensity neon light indicating switching on and off and the frequency. The apparatus is easy to master and simple to operate.

Manipulation

Prior to using the electroacupuncture apparatus, besides reading carefully the instruction book to know its features and requirements, careful examination must be made to ensure that it is in good condition. That to say, clamp two wetted absorbent cotton balls to a pair of output circuits respectively, and press the balls with the index finger and middle finger of the left hand. Then switch on the apparatus with the right hand and reinforce the current gradually to experience the sensation personally and get familiar with the apparatus.

(1) After the needle is inserted into a certain acupoint and the needling sensation is felt, adjust the output potential instrument of the electroacupuncture apparatus to zero, then connect the two out wires with the two needle handles, select the required waveform and frequency, and gradually amplify the output current to the tolerance of the patient. During the treatment, the patient will be adaptive to the stimulation and feel the stimulation getting weaker. At the time, increase the output current appropriately. The stimulation continues for 1–20 min or longer, for 0.5–1 h.

(2) When the treatment is finished, the output potential instrument is adjusted back to zero, the electricity supply is cut off, the wires are taken away and the needles are withdrawn. Observe whether the filiform needle becomes dark, thinner or damaged, and if there is such an occurrence, stop using the type of electroacupuncture apparatus.

The point combination for electroacupuncture is the same way as for the filiform needles, but generally it requires acupoints in pairs because a single point cannot make the current circuit achieve the stimulation goals. If only one acupoint is needed, and connect one output wire to the needle, and the other wire to the wetted gauze that is placed on the skin of the same side.

Indications

Generally, the electroacupuncture may be applied to whatever the filiform needle is applicable to, especially pain and paralysis. But the stimulation is stronger than that of filiform needling, so fainting must be prevented during the operation. It is inadvisable to apply this method to dying patients, pregnant women, or individuals with fatigue, hunger or drunkenness.

ACUPOINT APPLICATION

This is a therapy for treatment of diseases by applying medicinals to certain acupoints. Some stimulating medicinals, such as Maogen (buttercup), Banmao (*Mylabris*) and Baijiezi (*Semen Sinapis*), may be pounded or ground into powder and applied to desired points to induce blisters or suppuration in the local area like moxibustion sores, and this is termed "natural moxibustion," which has been introduced in a previous chapter. If the medicinals are applied to Shenque (RN 8) to treat diseases by being absorbed through the umbilical region or stimulating the umbilical region, such a method is called umbilical compress therapy.

Common Medicinals for Application

Applicators include *Bingpian* (*Borneolum Syntheticum*), Shexiang (*Moschus*), Dingxiang (*Flos Caryophylli*), Huajiao (*Pericarpium Zanthoxyli*), ginger, green onion, Rougui (*Cortex Cinnamomi*), Xixin (*Radix et Rhizoma Asari*), Baizhi (*Radix Angelicae Dahuricae*), Zaojiao (*Fructus Gleditsiae*), which are for dredging channels and activating collaterals, as well as Sheng Nanxing (raw *Rhizoma Arisaematis*), Sheng Banxia (raw *Rhizoma Pinelliae*), Chuanwu (*Radix Aconiti*), Caowu (*Radix Aconiti Kusnezoffii*) Badou (*Fructus Crotonis*), Fuzi (*Radix Aconiti Lateralis Praeparata*) and Daji (*Radix Euphorbiae Pekinensis*), which have strong smells and potency. Common solvents (or excipients) are water, distillate spirit or yellow wine, vinegar, ginger pop, honey, albumen and Vaseline. Besides, drug infusion may be available.

Dosage Forms

Pills

Grind medicinals into fine powder, and mix and stir it even with water, honey or medicine liquor to make pills of various sizes.

Pulvers

Grind medicinals into fine powder and stuff it onto the umbilical region for treatment.

Pastes

Grind medicinals into fine powder, make it into a paste with water, vinegar, alcohol, albumen or ginger pop, and apply it to the desired acupoint covered with gauze and fixed with an adhesive tape.

Unguentum

Make the selected medicinals into an emplastrum or ointment for application.

Cake

Grind medicinals into fine powder, stir it even with an appropriate amount of water to make medicine cake of various sizes, and apply the cake to the affected area of the acupoint covered with gauze and fixed with an adhesive tape. Alternatively, pound rhizomes or leaves of fresh plants to make into medicine cakes heated for application.

Manipulation

Point selection

The points for application are selected less but qualified, generally involving acupoints of the affected area, Ashi points or experienced points, among which *shenque* (RN 8) and *yongquan* (KI 1) are more frequently employed.

Application method

According to the selected acupoints, adopt the proper posture, suitable for better application. Prior to operation, fix the point, and clean the skin around the point with warm water or alcohol cotton balls. To avoid moving or dropping, whatever the medicinal forms are, they must be fixed with adhesive tape, or covered with gauze or oil paper before fixing them with adhesive tape. At present, there are specially made dressings for application, convenient and simple to operate or fix. If a replacement is needed, wet dry sterilized cotton balls in warm water or plant oil of any kind, or paraffin oil to wipe out the medicinal on the skin surface, and perform the application again. Generally, medicinals with mild stimulation are replaced once every 1–3 days; those without solvent may be replaced once every 5–7 days; and those with strong stimulation may be replaced from several minutes to hours, according to the patient's reaction or the degree of effervescence. Another application should not be made until the local skin returns to normal.

Indications

It is applicable to many kinds of diseases involving the departments of internal medicine, surgery, gynecology, pediatrics, ophthalmology and otorhinolaryngology. In the clinic, it is mainly used to treat cold, chronic bronchitis, bronchial asthma, coronary artery disease, diarrhea, facial paralysis, insomnia, hypertension, cervical osteoarthritis, menstruation disorder, uterine prolapse, infantile diarrhea, enuresis, adolescent myopia, allergic coryza and toothache.

Medicinals prepared with solvents must be used with the preparation, to avoid evaporation. During the operation, select the area for application with fewer movements. Medicinals with strong stimulation should not be retained for long. If a blister appears, smear gentian violet on it. If a skin allergy occurs, determine the causes. Change to another medicinal if the allergy is due to the medicine, and change to gauze if that is due to the adhesive tape. Avoid applying medicinals with strong stimulation or toxicity to pregnant women or infants.

Acupoint Injection

Also known as hydroacupunctrue, this is a needling therapy where injecting certain Chinese or Western medicines are injected into the acupoint or special spot. It has the double effectiveness of acupuncture and medication.

Instruments: Injectors of 1 ml, 2 ml, 5 ml, 10 ml and 20 ml or disposable syringes. Ordinary points are injected with long pinheads of No. 5 for dentistry, points of the eye with No. 4 pinheads, and points of deep parts with long pinheads for blocking.

Commonly used physic liquor: 0.20%–2% procaine hydrochloride, vitamins B1, B2, K3 and C, atropine, physiological saline, water for injection, various kinds of antibiotics, γ-aminobutyric acid, acetylglutamine, adenosine triphosphate, *Danshen* injection (*Salviae Miltiorrhiza*), Danggui injection (*Angelicae Sinensis*), Yuxingcao injection (*Herba Houttuyniae*) and Yemugua injection (*Fructus Chaenomelis*).

Manipulation

Preoperative preparation

Sterilize the injectors and the local skin, and examine the liquor; never use those with ampules damaged, overdue or deteriorated. Check the name and dosage, make hypersensitive tests in advance for those which may cause an allergy like procaine or penicillin, and they should not be applied to patients with positive reaction.

Injecting method

Insert the needle quickly and push it slowly to the desired depth, lifting and thrusting it till the arrival of *qi*, then pump back the wick-in-needle. If there is no back-streaming of blood, inject the liquor. Generally, push into the liquor at a moderate speed but slowly for the weak and patients with chronic diseases. And push quickly for patients with strong constitutions or acute diseases. If the liquor is too much, injection by layering from deep to superficial should be employed. The dosage for injection to different acupoints depends on the patient's condition and constitution, the drug concentration and the acupoint area, mostly ranging from 0.3 ml to 1 ml, sometimes from 5 ml to 20 ml. The manipulation is applied once daily or once every other day 7–10 times as a course.

Indications

Acupoint injection is widely used in the clinic and is applicable to various systemic diseases, but is more commonly used for pain and inflammatory diseases, such as trifacial neuralgia, sciatica, lobar pneumonia or acute appendicitis. During the injection, never use drugs with high concentration or too- strong stimulation. For some parts like the joint cavity and some points like *hegu* (LI 4) of infants in particular, this method should not be employed.

ACUPOINT LASER IRRADIATION

Also known as laser acupuncture and light needling, this is a needling therapy where the acupoint is irradiated with laser beams. It is a product of the combination of modern laser technique and traditional acupuncture, and was widely accepted by acupuncturists of many countries instantly after its appearance in the mid-1970s as it causes no injury or pain, and is simple and safe to operate.

Instruments

Many laser apparatuses for irradiation are available, and in the clinic the most commonly used is the H-N laser therapeutic apparatus with small power, which consists of a discharging tube, an optical resonator and a laser light emitter, with an output power of 1–25 milliwatts, a wavelength of 632.8 nm (1 nm = 10 angstroms) and a depth for penetration of 10–15 mm.

Manipulation

Prior to treatment, check the apparatus. Ask the patient to take a proper posture, and adjust the apparatus to direct the laser beam to the acupoint. Turn on the power switch, and the apparatus emits an orange beam. The irradiating distance is about 20–30 mm, and at most 100 mm, and the echogenic spot should be limited to 3 mm in diameter. If optical fiber is employed for irradiation, hold the fiber with one hand, directing it to the acupoint. The manipulation is applied for 2–5 min, to 2–4 points each time, 10 times as a course, with an interval of 7–10 days between courses.

Indications

In the clinic it is mainly applicable to migraine, headache, rhinitis, bronchitis, asthma, stomach ulcer, duodenal ulcer, hypertension, chronic colitis, menalgia, neuralgia of various kinds and dermatoses. Because there is no pain during the treatment, laser irradiation therapy is popular with child patients, and is highly effective for infantile enuresis, infantile diarrhea, infantile pneumonia and infantile paralysis.

Safe as it is, fainting may occur during the acupuncture, with symptoms and management similar to those of body acupuncture. In addition, the practitioner must wear laser-protective eyeglasses during the operation.

QUESTIONS

(1) Give an introduction to specific manipulations of electroacupuncture.
(2) What are the precautions when acupoint injection is applied?
(3) What are the indications of acupoint laser irradiation therapy?
(4) What are the medicinals commonly used for acupoint application?

CHAPTER 15

Ear Acupuncture

Ear acupuncture is a medical method to diagnose and treat diseases by detecting and stimulating specific areas on the auricle (otopoints). It is a unique therapy among so many needling methods in acupuncture, and has its own stimulation region with the most acupoints on the small auricle, second only to the number of body acupoints. What is more, ear acupuncture has the quaternity advantage of diagnosis, prevention, treatment and healthcare. Originating in ancient China, it has in modern times undergone great development and become a consummate therapy. Professor P. Nogier in France published his otopoints figure in the mid-1950s, which greatly promoted the development of ear acupuncture (Figs. 32 and 33).

MAIN STRUCTURE OF THE AURICLE[1]

The auricle is a part of the ear and otopoints are the specific spots for diagnosis and treatment. The following is the anatomical structure of the auricle surface.

Distribution of the Anterior Surface[2]

(1) Helix: the prominent tip of the auricle border.
(2) Helix crus: a portion of the helix which transverses into the auricular cavity.

---

[1]Figures 32 and 33.
[2]Figure 32.

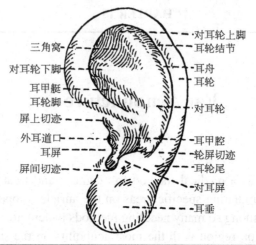

三角窝	-	Triangular fossa	耳轮结节	-	Helix tubercle
对耳轮下脚	-	Inferior of the antihelix	耳舟	-	Scapha
耳甲庭	-	Cymba concha	耳轮	-	Helix
耳轮脚	-	Helix crus	对耳轮	-	Antihelix
屏上切迹	-	Supratragic notch	耳甲腔	-	Cavum concha
外耳道口	-	Opening of the external auditory meatus	轮屏切迹	-	Notch between antitragus and antihelix
耳屏	-	Tragus	耳轮尾	-	Helix cauda
屏间切迹	-	Intertragic notch	对耳屏	-	Antitragus
对耳轮上脚	-	Superior of the antihelix	耳垂	-	Earlobe

Fig. 32. Anterior structure of the auricle.

(3) Helix tubercle: the small tubercle on the posterior–superior aspect of the helix.

(4) Helix cauda: the lower end of the helix, at the junction of the helix and the earlobe.

(5) Antihelix: the inner ridge opposite the helix.

(6) Superior and inferior of the antihelix: the upper and lower branches of the antihelix.

(7) Triangular fossa: the triangular depression between the two crura of the antihelix.

(8) Scapha: the depression between the helix and the antihelix.

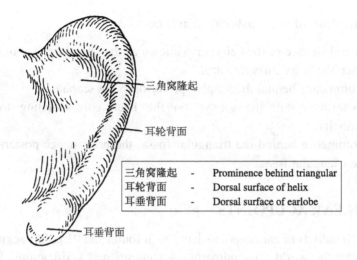

三角窝隆起	-	Prominence behind triangular
耳轮背面	-	Dorsal surface of helix
耳垂背面	-	Dorsal surface of earlobe

Fig. 33. Posterior structure of the auricle.

(9) Tragus: the valviform prominence in front of the auricle.

(10) Antitragus: the upper part of the ear lobe, the projection opposite the tragus.

(11) Supratragic notch: the notch between the superior border of the tragus and the crus of the helix.

(12) Intertragic notch: the notch between the tragus and the antitragus.

(13) Notch between the antitragus and the antihelix: the depression between the antitragus and the antihelix.

(14) Auricular concha: the depression surrounded by the antitragus, vaulted antihelix and inferior border of the inferior crura of the antihelix. It has two parts: cymba concha (the part of the auricular cavity above the helix crus) and cavum concha (the part of the auricular cavity below the helix crus).

(15) Earlobe: the inferior part of the auricle which does not contain cartilage.

(16) Opening of the external auditory meatus: the exit of the external auditory meatus in the cavum concha covered by the tragus.

Distribution of the Posterior Surface

(1) Dorsal surface of the helix: also known as the lateral surface of helix since the helix curls forward.
(2) Prominence behind the scapha: posterior to the scapha.
(3) Posterior canal: the groove on the back corresponding to the antihelix.
(4) Prominence behind the triangular fossa: the prominence posterior to the triangular fossa.

MAIN EAR ACUPOINTS[3]

So far, hundreds of ear acupoints have been found and 91 points acknowledged by the world after numerous screenings and verifications. Here, only 41 points will be introduced; they are the most commonly used in the clinic.

There is a certain regularity in the distribution of ear points, especially those on the anterior surface of the auricle like a fetus lying at an inverse site in the uterus, with its head downward and its buttocks upward; that is to say, points corresponding to the head and face on the tragus and earlobe; points to the upper limbs on the scapha; points to the trunk on the helix; points to the lower limbs and the buttocks on the superior and inferior crura of the helix; points to the cavitas pelvis on the triangular fossa; points to the alimentary canal around the crus of the helix; points to the belly cavity on the cymba concha; points to the thoracic cavity on the cavum concha; and points to the pars nasalis pharyngis on the tragus. The locations and indications of the commonly used otopoints in the clinic are seen in the following table:

---

[3] Figure 34.

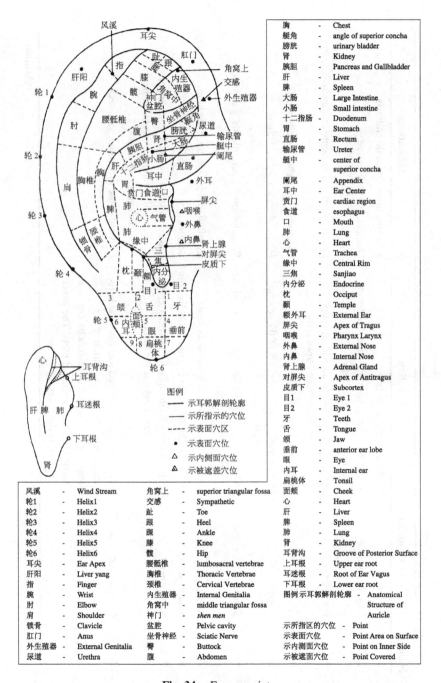

胸	-	Chest
艇角	-	angle of superior concha
膀胱	-	urinary bladder
肾	-	Kidney
胰胆	-	Pancreas and Gallbladder
肝	-	Liver
脾	-	Spleen
大肠	-	Large Intestine
小肠	-	Small intestine
十二指肠	-	Duodenum
胃	-	Stomach
直肠	-	Rectum
输尿管	-	Ureter
艇中	-	center of superior concha
阑尾	-	Appendix
耳中	-	Ear Center
贲门	-	cardiac region
食道	-	esophagus
口	-	Mouth
肺	-	Lung
心	-	Heart
气管	-	Trachea
缘中	-	Central Rim
三焦	-	Sanjiao
内分泌	-	Endocrine
枕	-	Occiput
颞	-	Temple
额外耳	-	External Ear
屏尖	-	Apex of Tragus
咽喉	-	Pharynx Larynx
外鼻	-	External Nose
内鼻	-	Internal Nose
肾上腺	-	Adrenal Gland
对屏尖	-	Apex of Antitragus
皮质下	-	Subcortex
目1	-	Eye 1
目2	-	Eye 2
牙	-	Teeth
舌	-	Tongue
颌	-	Jaw
垂前	-	anterior ear lobe
眼	-	Eye
内耳	-	Internal ear
扁桃体	-	Tonsil
面颊	-	Cheek
心	-	Heart
肝	-	Liver
脾	-	Spleen
肺	-	Lung
肾	-	Kidney
耳背沟	-	Groove of Posterior Surface
上耳根	-	Upper ear root
耳迷根	-	Root of Ear Vagus
下耳根	-	Lower ear root

图例

— 示耳郭解剖轮廓
— 示所指示的穴位
---- 示表面穴区
• 示表面穴位
△ 示内侧面穴位
▲ 示被遮盖穴位

风溪	-	Wind Stream	角窝上	-	superior triangular fossa
轮1	-	Helix1	交感	-	Sympathetic
轮2	-	Helix2	趾	-	Toe
轮3	-	Helix3	跟	-	Heel
轮4	-	Helix4	踝	-	Ankle
轮5	-	Helix5	膝	-	Knee
轮6	-	Helix6	髋	-	Hip
耳尖	-	Ear Apex	腰骶椎	-	lumbosacral vertebrae
肝阳	-	Liver yang	胸椎	-	Thoracic Vertebrae
指	-	Finger	颈椎	-	Cervical Vertebrae
腕	-	Wrist	内生殖器	-	Internal Genitalia
肘	-	Elbow	角窝中	-	middle triangular fossa
肩	-	Shoulder	神门	-	shen men
锁骨	-	Clavicle	盆腔	-	Pelvic cavity
肛门	-	Anus	坐骨神经	-	Sciatic Nerve
外生殖器	-	External Genitalia	臀	-	Buttock
尿道	-	Urethra	腹	-	Abdomen

图例 示耳郭解剖轮廓 - Anatomical Structure of Auricle
示所指区的穴位 - Point
示表面穴位 - Point Area on Surface
示内测面穴位 - Point on Inner Side
示被遮面穴位 - Point Covered

Fig. 34. Ear acupoints.

Number	Name of Otopoint	Location	Indications
1	Ear center	On the crus of the helix	Hiccups, hives, infantile enuresis
2	External genitalia	On the helix, level with the upper border of the inferior antihelix crus	Orchitis, pruritus vulvae
3	Ear apex	At the upper part of the auricle and superior to the helix when folded toward the tragus	Fever, hypertension, acute conjunctivitis, styes
4	Node	At the node of the helix	Dizziness, headache, hypertension
5	Wind stream	At the junction of 2/5 and 3/5 of the scapha, anterior to the node	Hives, allergic coryza, asthma
6	Shoulder	Divide the scapha into five equal parts and the fourth is the shoulder	Scapulohumeral periarthritis, gallstones
7	Knee	At the 1/3 of the superior antihelix crus	Swelling and pain of the knee joint
8	Sciatic nerve	At the middle 2/3 of the inferior antihelix crus	Sciatica
9	Sympathetic	At the junction of the inferior antihelix crus and the inner margin of the helix	Gastrointestinal spasm, angina pectoris, calculi of the ureter, vegetative nerve functional disturbance
10	Cervical vertebrae	On the antihelix, a curved line from the helix-tragic notch to the bifurcation of the superior and the inferior antihelix crus can be divided into five equal parts. The lower 1/5 of it is the point.	Cervical spine syndrome, stiff neck

(Continued)

(Continued)

Number	Name of Otopoint	Location	Indications
11	Thoracic vertebrae	The same as the above	Thoraxicohypochondriac pain, mastitis, postpartum insufficient lactation
12	*Shen men*	At the lateral 1/3 of the triangular fossa, at the bifurcating point between the superior and the inferior crura of the antihelix	Insomnia, dream-disturbed sleep, pain, menopausal syndrome
13	Internal genitalia	At the lower 1/3 of the triangular fossa	Menalgia, irregular menstruation, leukorrhegia, dysfunctional uterine bleeding, seminal emission, premature ejaculation
14	External ear	On the supratragic notch close to the helix	Inflammation of the external auditory canal, otitis media, tinnitus
15	External nose	At the center of the tragus	Rhinitis, simple obesity
16	Apex of the tragus	At the tip of the upper prominence on the border of the tragus	Fever, toothache
17	Adrenal gland	At the tip of the lower protubercle on the border of the tragus	Hypotension, cold, rheumatic arthritis
18	Pharynx–larynx	On the upper half of the medial part of the tragus	Laryngopharyngitis, tonsillitis
19	Internal nose	On the lower half of the medial part of the tragus	Rhinitis, nasal sinusitis, rhinorrhagia
20	Apex of the antitragus	At the tip of the antitragus	Asthma, parotitis, cutaneous pruritus

(Continued)

(Continued)

Number	Name of Otopoint	Location	Indications
21	Central rim	Between the tip of the antitragus and the helix notch	Enuresis, oticodinia
22	Temple	In the middle of the lateral aspect of the antitragus	Migraine
23	Subcortex	On the medial side of the antitragus	Neurasthenia, pseudomyopia, hypertension, diarrhea, pain
24	Heart	In the depression of the middle cavum concha	Anisorhythmia, angina pectoris, neurasthenia
25	Lung	Around the center of the cavum concha	Cough and dyspnea, dermatosis, constipation, smoking cessation
26	Spleen	At the posterior–superior aspect of the cavum concha	Abdominal distension, diarrhea, constipation, anorexia, dysfunctional uterine bleeding
27	Endocrine	At the base of the cavum concha in the intertragic notch	Dysmenorrhea, irregular menstruation, climacteric syndrome
28	Mouth	At the lower 1/3 of the helix crus	Stomatitis, smoking cessation, cholelithiasis
29	Stomach	Around the area where the helix crus terminates	Gastritis, peptic ulcer, gastrospasm, insomnia, cholelithiasis
30	Duodenum	At the posterior 1/3 of the superior aspect of the helix crus	Peptic ulcer, cholelithiasis
31	Large intestine	At the medial 1/3 of the superior aspect of the helix crus	Diarrhea, constipation

(Continued)

(Continued)

Number	Name of Otopoint	Location	Indications
32	Liver	Posterior–inferior to the cymba concha	Hypochondriac pain, dizziness, menoxenia, hypertension
33	Pancreas and gallbladder	At the posterior–superior part of the cymba concha between the two points of the liver and kidney	Cholecystitis, cholelithiasis, acute pancreatitis
34	Kidney	Below the bifurcating point between the superior and the inferior antihelix cruses	Enuresis, low back pain, nephritis, menoxenia, emission, premature ejaculation
35	Teeth	On the first of the ear lobe sections. The way of dividing the ear lobe is: from the lower border of the cartilage of the intertragic notch to the lower border of the ear lobe, draw three horizontal lines with an equal distance between each, and then, crossing the second horizontal line, draw two vertical lines by which the area is vertically and equally divided. From inferior to exterior, and superior to inferior, the auricular lobe is divided into sections numbered 1–9.	Toothache, periodontitis, hypotension
36	Eye	On the fifth of the ear lobe sections	Acute conjunctivitis, pseudomyopia, styes and other eyes diseases

(Continued)

(Continued)

Number	Name of Otopoint	Location	Indications
37	Cheek	Around the junction of the fifth and sixth of the ear lobe sections	Peripheral facial paralysis, trifacial neuralgia
38	Internal ear	On the sixth of the ear lobe sections	Tinnitus, deafness, endolymphatic hydrops
39	Tonsil	On the eighth section	Tonsillitis, pharyngitis
40	Root of the ear vagus	At the root at the junction of the back side of the ear and the mastoid process, corresponding to the place of the helix crus	Cholelithiasis, arrhythmia
41	Groove of the posterior surface	Also called the groove for lowering blood pressure, through the back side of the superior antihelix crus and the inferior antihelix, in the depression as a "Y" form	Hypertension, cutaneous pruritus

---

QUESTIONS

(1) Restate the anatomical structure of the auricle surface.
(2) Review the locations and indications of the 41 ear points introduced.

DETECTION OF EAR ACUPOINTS

When an internal organ or a part of the body is diseased, reactions can be detected at the corresponding areas on the auricle, such as cholecystopathy corresponding to the pancreas and gallbladder areas, or lung diseases to the lung area. Clinical practice has proven that stimulating these reaction points yields good therapeutic results. But the reaction points may be different from person to person, since the shape and size of the auricle vary in different individuals. Therefore, detecting reaction points is necessary and should be combined when one is selecting the point to be punctured.

There are three commonly used detecting methods. One is direct observation or observation with the naked eye or microscopy, which is to observe under the natural light any change in the form or color of the corresponding area on the auricle. Another method is detection of electrical changes, referring to detecting any change of the resistance and electric potential in the corresponding areas on the auricle with the specially made electronic apparatus. Both methods depend either on the experience or on the apparatus, so beginners had better employ the third one — detection of the tender spot, which is applied as follows.

Select an ear point according to the patient's condition, and press it evenly with a filiform needle or a toothpick from the outside to the center. When the sensitive spot is pressed, the patient will have reactions such as frowning, blinking, calling out in pain or evading. Then press it a little more forcefully and make a mark for acupuncture. If tender spots cannot be detected on the auricles of a few patients, massage the area before detecting again.

METHODS FOR THE COMPATIBILITY OF EAR ACUPOINTS

There are four methods for the compatibility of ear acupoints.

According to Syndrome Differentiation of *Zang–Fu* Viscera

This is to select acupoints according to the traditional theory of TCM. For example, it is believed that "the lung governs the skin and hair," so the point of the lung is employed to treat skin diseases; or "the essence of the kidney lies in the hair," so the kidney may be employed to treat alopecia areata.

According to Modern Medical Theory

Quite a few ear points are named after modern medicine, such as subcortex, sympathetic, adrenal gland, endocrine, and root of the ear vagus, whose functions are coincident with modern theory. For example, the point of the adrenal gland is able to regulate the adrenal glands.

According to the Corresponding Area

This is the most simple and widely used method in the clinic. It involves selecting the corresponding points according to the affected part.

According to Clinical Experiences

Clinical practice has found that there are ways to combine points to treat a certain disease or some diseases, such as the point of the ear apex for hypertension and the ear center for diaphragmatic spasm.

In actual practice, the above-mentioned methods are often used comprehensively. For example, to treat hypertension, the sympathetic is employed according to Western theory, the heart is added to *zang–fu* theory or the ear apex to clinical experiences.

METHODS FOR STIMULATION OF EAR ACUPOINTS

There are more than 30 kinds of stimulating methods for ear points; here, only 3 will be introduced.

Puncturing with a Filiform Needle

Filiform needles of stainless steel, Nos. 28–32, are usually employed. First, give a routine local sterilization to the point by smearing with 2%

iodine tincture, before deiodination with cotton balls wetted in 75% alcohol. When the needle is inserted, fix the auricle with the thumb and index finger of the left hand, with the middle finger supporting the back of the ear for the purpose of controlling the insertion depth and relieving the pain of puncturing. Then, hold the needle with the thumb and the index and middle fingers of the right hand, and insert it into the sensitive point. The depth depends on the thickness of the different parts. Reach the ear cartilage but do not penetrate it, inducing a needling sensation that presents itself as pain mostly, and soreness, distension, coolness and numbness sometimes. The needle is retained for 20–30 min. Finally, support the ear back with the left hand and withdraw the needle with the right hand, and press the needle hole with sterilized dry cotton balls to avoid bleeding. Acupuncture is applied to one side or both sides, once daily or once every other day.

Needle Embedding

Embed the intradermal needle in the ear point — usually the thumbtack needle. First, give a strict sterilization to the local skin, and fix the auricle with the left hand to make the skin tense. Hold a pair of forceps with the right hand to clamp the needle ring, and insert it gently into the selected point and fix it with an adhesive tape. Generally, needle embedding is applied to one side, and to both sides if necessary. The patient is to press the point himself or herself, three or four times. The needle is retained for 2–4 days. The duration may be shortened in summer and lengthened in winter. Avoid wetting or soaking the embedding area, and make an examination if local distension or discomfort arises. The method is unsuitable for cases with inflammation of the skin of the ear or chilblains in the local area.

Pressing

Also known as pressing otopoints with beans or ear point sticking, this is a simple and safe method. The materials for pressing commonly used are *Vaccaria segetalis* seeds, mung beans and magnetic beads (with the intensity of 180–380 G). After the selection of the point, wipe clean the local skin with 75% alcohol and wipe it with sterilized dry cotton balls. Clamp a small square of adhesive tape (about 7×7 cm^2) with the material and place it closely on the point. Then press it until the auricle becomes red and hot, during which the thumb and the index finger are put respectively interior and exterior to the auricle so as to hold the pressing material. Repeat pressing the point for half a minute each time, for each point. And press the point three or four times every day, and replace the plaster once or twice each week.

INDICATIONS

Ear acupuncture is widely used in the clinic and has been applied to prevention, treatment and healthcare for more than 150 diseases according to statistics, including diseases of pain such as headache, migraine, trifacial neuralgia or sciatica; inflammatory diseases like acute conjunctivitis, tonsillitis or laryngopharyngitis; allergic disorders like hives or allergic coryza; and functional disorders like anisorhythmia, hypertension or neurasthenia. In recent years in particular, ear acupuncture has been more significantly effective in dealing with smoking cessation, weight reduction, dermatoses (like juvenile acne or chloasma) and athletic syndrome.

Ear acupuncture is usually safe but is unsuitable for patients with chilblains broken, infection, ulcer and eczema on the external ear. Pregnant women, especially those with a history of habitual abortion, are forbidden from having ear acupunture.

POSSIBLE ACCIDENTS AND MANAGEMENT
IN EAR ACUPUNCTURE

If one follows the operating instructions, accidents will not happen with ear acupuncture. Infection of the auricle due to improper sterilization is most commonly seen in the clinic. Because the auricle has bad blood circulation, the infection will spread to the ear cartilages and, in severe cases, cause auricle atrophy and abnormality by distension of the auricle, or chondronecrosis. In order to avoid such accidents, make sure to sterilize the needles, and disposable needles are preferred; then do double sterilizations to point areas with iodine tincture prior to alcohol; finally, during pressing with drugs, do not perform twisting manipulation, which may injure the epidermis to cause inflammation.

Auricle infection is superficial in the early stage, characterized by red swelling of local skin accompanied by a small amount of effusion with mild pain, which can be managed by applying 2.5% alcohol to the local skin 2–3 times a day, or paste ointment to eliminate inflammation for 4–5 days. If it develops into ear chondritis with obvious red swelling, heat and pain in the local area, or even abscess in severe cases, often accompanied by systemic symptoms like fever, headache, poor appetite and WBC increase, immediately turn the patient to surgery. Never ignore the sterilization, especially for beginners.

QUESTIONS

(1) What are the methods for the compatibility of ear acupoints?
(2) What are the stimulating methods of ear acupuncture and how to manipulate?

CHAPTER 16

Scalp Acupuncture

Scalp acupuncture is a therapeutic method where specific areas or lines of the scalp are needed. It was suggested as early as the 1950s but only popularized after the 1970s. A great deal of practice has proven that this method has a unique effect on many diseases in the brain, as well as being convenient and simple to operate.

COMMON STIMULATION AREAS FOR SCALP ACUPUNCTURE[1]

In contrast to the selection of body acupuncture, acupoints for scalp acupuncture have six different systems with different characteristics, particularly standard nomenclature of Chinese scalp acupuncture lines, Jiao Shun-fa's nomenclature and Fang Yun-pen's nomenclature. But it is hard for beginners to get a good command. In clinical practice, Jiao's system is more influential, safer and suitable for beginners; it is introduced in this chapter, and the standardization project is applied as an appendix at the end.

Prior to selecting the points, determine the following two reference lines on the scalp:

(1) The anterior–posterior median line — The vertical line connecting the center of the glabella and the midpoint of the lower border of the external occipital protuberance.
(2) The eyebrow-occipital line — The horizontal line connecting the midpoint of the upper border of the eyebrow and the highest prominence of the external occipital protuberance.

---

[1]Figure 35.

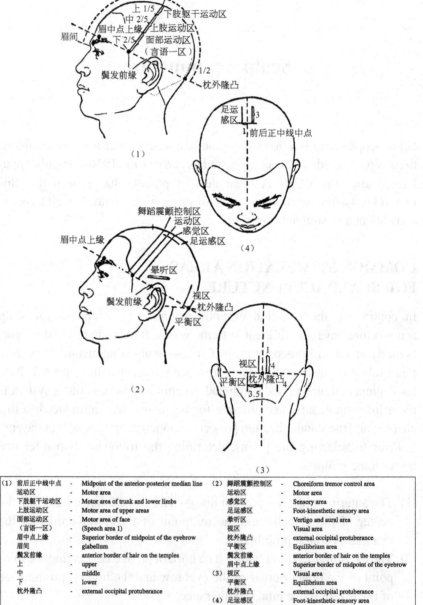

(1)	前后正中线中点	-	Midpoint of the anterior-posterior median line	(2)	舞蹈震颤控制区	-	Choreiform tremor control area
	运动区	-	Motor area		运动区	-	Motor area
	下肢躯干运动区	-	Motor area of trunk and lower limbs		感觉区	-	Sensory area
	上肢运动区	-	Motor area of upper areas		足运感区	-	Foot-kinesthetic sensory area
	面部运动区	-	Motor area of face		晕听区	-	Vertigo and aural area
	（言语一区）	-	(Speech area 1)		视区	-	Visual area
	眉中点上缘	-	Superior border of midpoint of the eyebrow		枕外隆凸	-	external occipital protuberance
	眉间	-	glabellum		平衡区	-	Equilibrium area
	鬓发前缘	-	anterior border of hair on the temples		鬓发前缘	-	anterior border of hair on the temples
	上	-	upper		眉中点上缘	-	Superior border of midpoint of the eyebrow
	中	-	middle	(3)	视区	-	Visual area
	下	-	lower		平衡区	-	Equilibrium area
	枕外隆凸	-	external occipital protuberance		枕外隆凸	-	external occipital protuberance
				(4)	足运感区	-	Foot-kinesthetic sensory area
					前后正中线中点	-	Midpoint of the anterior-posterior median line

Fig. 35. Common stimulation areas for scalp acupuncture.

Motor area

The upper point of this area is 0.5 cm posterior to the midpoint of the anteroposterior median line, and the lower point is at the junction of the eyebrow-occipital line and the temporal hairline (if the temporal hairline is not obvious, the point 0.5 cm anterior to the junction of the eyebrow-occipital line and the line ascending vertically from the midpoint of the zygomatic arch is taken as the lower point). The line connecting these two points represents the motor area.

Indications

The upper one-fifth of the motor area is applicable to paralysis of the lower limbs; the middle two-fifths, to paralysis of the upper limbs; the lower two-fifths, to central facial palsy, motor aphasia and sialorrhea.

Sensory Area

This is the line parallel with and 1.5 cm posterior to the motor area.

Indications

The upper one-fifth of the sensory area is applicable to pain, numbness and paresthesia of the contralateral leg and low back; the middle two-fifths, to pain, numbness and paresthesia of the contralateral upper limbs; the lower two-fifths, to contralateral numbness, pain and migraine.

Choreiform Tremor Control Area

This is the line parallel with and 1.5 cm anterior to the motor area.

Indications

Chorea, paralysis agitans.

Vertigo and Aural Area

This is the line with its midpoint 1.5 cm above the apex of the auricle, extending horizontally 2.0 cm forward and backward.

Indications

Vertigo, tinnitus, decrease in the hearing ability.

Foot-Kinesthetic Sensory Area

This comprises two straight lines, beginning at the points 1 cm respectively lateral to the midpoint of the anteroposterior median line, and extending 3 cm backward, parallel with the anteroposterior median line.

Indications

Contralateral numbness, pain and paralysis of the lower limbs.

Visual Area

This comprises two straight lines, beginning at the point 1 cm lateral to the external occipital protuberance and extending 4 cm upward, parallel with the anteroposterior median line.

Indications

Cortical disturbance of vision, cataract.

Equilibrium Area

This comprises two straight lines, beginning at the point 3.5 cm lateral to the occipital protuberance and extending 4 cm downward, parallel with the anteroposterior median line.

Indications

Cerebellar disturbance of equilibrium.

    Besides the above-mentioned seven areas which are the most frequently used ones, there are another seven areas: vasomotion area, speech area 2, speech area 3, praxia area, stomach area, thoracic area and genetic area, which are less used and omitted here.

PREPARATIONS PRIOR TO ACUPUNCTURE

Needles

Generally, employ Nos. 28–30 filiform needles 1.5–2 *cun* in length and made of stainless steel. Beginners may use 1 *cun* needles if they have difficulty inserting the needles, while 0.5–1 *cun* needles are suitable for infants.

Area Determination

It is of great significance to determine the area for scalp acupuncture. Beginners should determine exactly the area with a measuring tape and mark it with gentian violet. Ask the patient to assume a sitting position, divide his or her hair, and sterilize the area thoroughly.

MANIPULATIONS

Insertion

Keep from the hair follicle, cicatrix, and local infection, lest pain should occur. Beginners may insert the needle quickly with the fingernail-pressure needle-inserting method at an angle of 15°–30° with the scalp. Rapid insertion may relieve pain, and is done as follows. Pinching the lower end of the needle (2 cm from the tip) with the thumb and index finger of the right hand, direct the tip at the area of insertion accurately and keep the fingertip 5–10 cm away from the scalp. Then, swiftly insert the needle by sudden and forceful palmar flexion of the wrist into the scalp or the muscular layer.

After insertion, hold the lower half of the needle handle with the thumb and index finger of the right hand, with the middle finger supporting the distal end, and push the needle to the underlayer of the epicranial aponeurosis. Then, the finger will feel the decrease in the resistance. Push the needle 0.5–1.5 *cun* deep along the direction of stimulation, followed by manipulation. But be sure to control the angle; the needle may be inserted into the muscular layer at a too-small angle, while pain will occur if one punctures the periosteum at a too-large angle. To relieve pain during puncture, ask the patient to hold his or her breath after deep inspiration.

Manipulation

Scalp acupuncture requires twirling and rotating instead of lifting and thrusting. For the sake of convenience in manipulation, pinch the needle hand with the facies volares of the thumb and the facies radialis of the index finger, and twirl the needle by continuous and alternate flexion and extension of the metacarpophalangeal joint of the index finger at a frequency of about 200 times per minute, which is difficult for beginners to master and therefore needs practice for a long time. Twirl the needle for 1–2 min every time. Retain the needle for 15–30 min, during which twirl it once every 5–10 min. If there is difficulty twirling the needle, replace it with an electric needle with the frequency of 200–300 times per minute, with a continuous wave and the intensity tolerable to the patient.

Two more methods are available. One is withdrawing–reducing manipulation, referring to the following needling method. The needle is quickly inserted to the selected line through the skin to the scalp to the subfascial layer, then pushed horizontally and thrust slowly to the original depth again. This course is repeated three times to induce the needling sensation. The other method is entering–reinforcing manipulation, which is, contrary to the previous method, applied by rapid thrusting and slow lifting. The depth of lifting and thrusting is limited within 0.1 *cun* with rapid movement.

Withdrawal

Withdraw the needle to the subcutaneous layer, and pull it out quickly. Since there are abundant vessels, withdrawal should be followed instantly by pressing over the needle hole with a sterilized cotton ball for a moment to prevent bleeding.

The manipulation is applied once daily or once every other day 10 times as a course, with an interval of 5–7 days between courses.

INDICATIONS

It is mainly applicable to cerebrovascular diseases. The total effective rate in treatment of hemiplegia induced by stroke (cerebral hemorrhage or cerebral infarction) is 90% or higher. The acupuncture is also effective in treating posttraumatic brain syndrome, infantile cerebral palsy, infantile atelencephalia, paralysis agitans, chorea, tinnitus and chronic pain of various kinds. In recent years, it has been used for senile dementia and infantile disturbance of intelligence.

PRECAUTIONS

Prevent needling fainting, since the stimulation caused by scalp acupuncture is strong.

A sticking needle may occur during the operation, so lengthen the retaining time and ask the patient to relax; gently massage the skin around the needle and withdraw it slowly.

In patients with stroke induced by cerebral hemorrhage with coma, fever and unstable blood pressure in the acute stage, scalp acupuncture should not be done until the patient's condition and blood pressure have improved. It is inadvisable to use this type of acupuncture on patients who have high fever or heart failure.

QUESTIONS

(1) Get familiar with the stimulation areas for scalp acupuncture.
(2) What are the manipulations and indications of scalp acupuncture?

APPENDIX: CURRENTLY USED STIMULATION AREAS FOR SCALP ACUPUNCTURE[2]

The following originated from the standard nomenclature of Chinese scalp acupuncture lines, which was instituted by China and recommended to the world by the WHO:

(1) *Middle line of the forehead*: 1 *cun* long from *shenting* (DU 24), on the anterior median line, 0.5 *cun* above the hairline, straight downward, belonging to the *du* meridian.

   Indications: Mental disorders and diseases of the head, nose, eye, tongue and throat, such as loss of consciousness, insomnia, headache, nasal congestion, red eyes and sore throat.

(2) *Line 1 lateral to the forehead*: 1 *cun* long from *meichong* (BL 3), 0.5 *cun* above the hairline, straight downward, belonging to the bladder meridian of foot–*taiyang*.

   Indications: Disorders of lung and heart which are located in the upper–*jiao*, such as cough, chest pain, cold, shortness of breath, insomnia, dizziness, palpitation and pectoral stuffiness pain.

(3) *Line 2 lateral to the forehead*: 1 *cun* long from *toulinqi* (GB 41), straight downward, belonging to the gallbadder meridian of foot-*shaoyang*.

   Indications: Disorders of the spleen, stomach, liver and gallbladder which are located in the middle *jiao*, such as stomachache, gastric stuffiness, enterorrhea, abdominal distension, and hypochondriac pain.

(4) *Line 3 lateral to the forehead*: 1 *cun* long from the point 0.75 *cun* medial to *touwei* (ST 8), straight downward, belonging to the gall-bladder meridian of foot–*shaoyang* and the stomach meridian of foot–*yangming*.

   Indications: Disorders of the kidney and urinary bladder which are located in the lower *jiao*, such as emission, impotence, uroschesis, frequency of micturition, and enuresis.

---

[2]Figure 36.

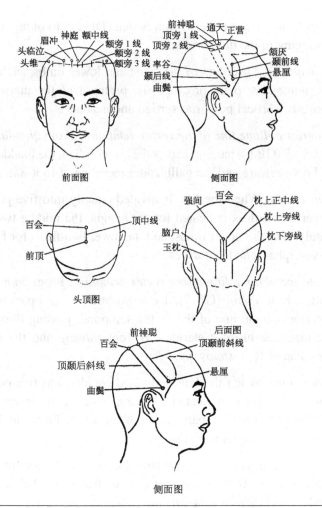

前面图

側面图

头顶图

后面图

側面图

前面图	-	The front:	顶旁2线	-	Line 2 Lateral Vertex	玉枕	-	Yuzhen (BL 9)
头维	-	Touwei (ST 8)	率谷	-	Shuaigu (GB 8)	枕上正中线	-	Upper-Middle Line of Occiput
头临泣	-	Toulinqi (GB 15)	颞后线	-	Posterior Temporal Line	枕上旁线	-	Upper-Lateral Line of Occiput
眉冲	-	Meichong (BL 3)	曲鬓	-	Qubin (GB 7)	枕下旁线	-	Lower-Lateral Line of Occiput
神庭	-	Shenting (DU 24)	颔厌	-	Hanyan (GB 4)	側面图	-	The side:
额中线	-	Middle Line of Forehead	颞前线	-	Anterior Temporal Line	曲鬓	-	Qubin (GB 7)
额旁1线	-	Line 1 Lateral to Forehead	悬厘	-	Xuanli (GB 6)	顶颞后斜线	-	Posterior Oblique Line of Vertex-Temporal
额旁2线	-	Line 2 Lateral to Forehead	头顶图	-	The vertex:	百会	-	Baihui (DU 20)
额旁3线	-	Line 3 Lateral to Forehead	百会	-	Baihui (DU 20)	前神聪	-	the front point of Sishencong (EX-HN 1)
側面图	-	The side:	前顶	-	Qianding (DU 21)	顶颞前斜线	-	Anterior Oblique Line of Vertex-Temporal
正营	-	Zhengying	顶中线	-	Middle Line of Vertex	悬厘	-	Xuanli (GB 6)
通天	-	Tongtian (BL 7)	后面图	-	The back:			
前神聪	-	the front point of Sishencong (EX-HN 1)	百会	-	Baihui (DU 20)			
			强间	-	Qiangjian (DU 18)			
顶旁1线	-	Line 1 Lateral Vertex	脑户	-	Naohu (DU 17)			

Fig. 36. Currently used stimulation areas for scalp acupuncture.

(5) *Middle line of the vertex*: From *baihui* (DU 20) to *qianding* (DU 21), belonging to the *du* meridian.

Indicatfions: Disorders of the waist and lower limbs, such as paralysis, numbness, pain, proctoptosis, prolapse of the uterus, infantile enuresis, cortical polyuria, vertigo and headache.

(6) *Anterior oblique line of the vertex–temporal*: From *qianding* (DU 21) to *xuanli* (GB 6), passing across the *du* meridian, the bladder meridian of Foot–*taiyang* and the gallbladder meridian of foot–*shaoyang*.

Indications: When the line is divided equally into five portions, the upper one-fifth is indicated for paraplegia, the middle two-fifths for paralysis of the upper limbs, and the lower two-fifths for facial palsy, motor aphasia and sialorrhea.

(7) *Posterior oblique line of the vertex–temporal*: From *baihui* (DU 20) obliquely to *qubin* (GB 7), 1 *cun* posterior to and parallel with the anterior oblique line of the vertex–temporal, passing through the *du* meridan, the bladder meridian of foot–*taiyang* and the gallbladder meridian of foot–*shaoyang*.

Indications: When the line is divided equally into five portions, the upper one-fifth is indicated for paresthesia of the lower limbs, the middle two-fifths for paresthesia of the upper limbs, and the lower two-fifths for facial paresthesia.

(8) *Line 1 lateral vertex*: 1.5 *cun* lateral to the middle line of the vertex, 1.5 *cun* long from *chengguan* (BL 6) backward, belonging to the bladder meridian of foot–*taiyang*.

Indications: Disorders of the waist and legs, such as paralysis, numbness and pain.

(9) *Line 2 lateral vertex*: 0.75 *cun* lateral to line 1 lateral to the vertex, 1.5 *cun* long from *zhengying* (GB 17) backward, belonging to the gallbladder meridian of foot–*shaoyang*.

Indications: Disorders of the shoulder, upper arm and hand, such as paralysis, numbness and pain.

(10) *Anterior temporal line*: From *hanyan* (GB 4) to *xuanli* (GB 6), belonging to the gallbaldder meridian of foot–*shaoyang*.

Indications: Migraine, motor aphasia, peripheral facial paralysis and disorders of the mouth.

(11) *Posterior temporal line*: From *shuaigu* (GB 8) to *qubin* (GB 7), belonging to the gallbladder meridian of foot–*shaoyang*.

Indications: Migraine, vertigo, tinnitus and deafness.

(12) *Upper-middle line of the occiput*: From *qiangjian* (DU 18) to *naohu* (DU 17), belonging to the *du* meridian.

Indications: Eye problems and lumbar vertebra pain.

(13) *Upper-lateral line of the occiput*: 0.5 *cun* lateral and parallel to the upper-middle line of the occiput, belonging to the bladder meridian of foot–*taiyang*.

Indications: The same as for the upper-middle line of the occiput.

(14) *Lower-lateral line of the occiput*: 2 *cun* long line from *yuzhen* (BL 9) to *tianzhu* (BL 10), belonging to the bladder meridian of foot–*taiyang*.

Indications: Disorders due to problems of the cerebellum, such disequilibrium, and pain in the back of the head.

CHAPTER 17

Eye Acupuncture and Wrist–Ankle Acupuncture

Eye acupuncture and wrist–ankle acupuncture are both effective for certain diseases and simple to master for beginners.

EYE ACUPUNCTURE[1]

Eye acupuncture, originally used in the 1970s, is a therapy with micro-acupuncture needles formed through observations and practice on tens of thousands of patients by acupuncturist Peng Jing-shan on the basis of the records about "diagnosing diseases by observing the eyes" in ancient times. It is easy to master as there are only a few acupoints, and safe to operate for hypodermic needling.

Eye Acupuncture Area

There are 8 meridian areas and 13 point sections. The point sections are included in the meridian areas.

Division of meridian areas

Looking straight ahead, make a horizontal line via the center of the pupil, extending through the exterior and the interior canthus; and make a vertical line via the pupil center, extending through the upper and lower orbits, and thus four quadrants are formed. Lead out lines from both sides to divide each quadrant equally into two areas, which are the 8 meridian areas.

---

[1]Figure 37.

279

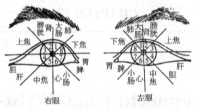

右眼	-	Right Eye: 1	中焦	-	middle jiao 6
大肠	-	large intestine	心	-	heart
肺	-	lung 2	小肠	-	small intestine 7
膀胱	-	bladder	脾	-	spleen
肾	-	kidney 3	胃	-	stomach 8
上焦	-	upper jiao 4	下焦	-	lower jiao
胆	-	gallbladder	左眼 Left Eye - (同上 the same as the above)
肝	-	liver 5			

Fig. 37.   Acupoints for eye acupuncture.

Denomination and location of point sections

Among the 8 meridian areas, the upper *jiao*, middle *jiao* and lower *jiao* take up one area respectively, and the remaining areas are divided into two point regions, in total 13 sections, which are named after *zang* and *fu* in TCM. Namely: section 1 — lung and large intestine; section 2 — kidney and bladder; section 3 — upper *jiao*; section 4 — liver and gallbladder ; section 5 — middle *jiao*; section 6 — heart and small intestine; section 7 — spleen and stomach; section 8 — lower *jiao*.

The needling spot for eye acupuncture lies in the middle of each section, one fingerbreath *cun* between the external orbit and the pupil. The sensitive spot of the superior orbit is at the lower border of the eyebrow, while the sensitive spot of the inferior orbit is 2 *fen* from the border of the orbit. In total there are 13 spots called points around the orbit.

Indications

Each point section represents the function of its corresponding organ, indicating for diseases of the very organ; but the upper *jiao* represents organs above the diaphragm, including the head and face, upper limbs, chest and back, heart and lung; the middle *jiao* represents the function of the organs above the umbilicus and below the diaphragm, including the back and the low back, and the upper abdomen; the lower *jiao* represents organs below the umbilicus, including the lower back, cavitas pelvis, urogenital system and lower limbs. Experience supports the view that eye acupuncture is mainly applicable to functional and painful diseases.

Manipulation

Point selection: Three methods

Selection along meridians

Observing carefully the meridian areas and point sections on the bulbar conjunctiva, select the point where there is any vessel or color change with lesions on the corresponding organ.

Selection according to the eyes

Whatever the diseases are, select the point where there is any obvious change in vessel forms and color in meridian areas.

Selection according to the disease

Puncture the point in a certain area according to its corresponding organs. For example, to treat hemiplegia induced by stroke, apply acupuncture to the upper *jiao* and lower *jiao,* because they represent the upper limbs and lower limbs, respectively.

Needling methods

The No. 28 filiform needle, 0.5 *cun* long, is employed. Before insertion, press and fix the eyeball with the left hand to make the skin within the orbit tense. Hold the needle with the right hand and insert it gently, either perpendicularly or horizontally. Puncture perpendicularly till the periosteum and horizontally along the skin from the border of the meridian area and within the selected area, to a depth of 2–4 *fen*. After insertion, lift, thrust, twirl and rotate the needle slightly until the arrival of *qi*, which is generally the needling sensation of electrification, soreness, numbness and hotness.

The needle is retained for 10–15 min, during which it is manipulated once every 5 min by slightly twirling and rotating at an amplitude of no more than 10°.

Indications

Eye acupuncture is mainly applicable to hemiplegia induced by stroke (cerebral hemorrhage or cerebral infarction), and especially effective in patients with a course of no longer than three months and without deformities of the body. Also, it is used to treat toothache, headache, acute sprains and contusions, sciatica, menalgia and gastrointestinal spasm. When eye acupuncture is being applied, avoid injuring the eyeball. Puncture section 8 of the left eye and section 4 of the right eye not too deep, lest that should injure by mistake the angular artery to cause bleeding. One should be cautious about applying eye acupuncture to patients with fleshy eyelids, obvious palpebral veins and local lesions.

WRIST–ANKLE ACUPUNCTURE

Wrist–ankle acupuncture is a therapy for systemic diseases that involves puncturing a specific acupoint of the wrist or the ankle. It was formed and developed in the light of the theory of the cutaneous region of the meridian theory, and was generalized in the clinic in the early 1970s. It is popular with both practitioners and patients because of simple selection of points, simple operation, little injury to the body, and safety and effectiveness for some diseases.

Acupoint Location

There are 12 stimulating points in total — 6 in the wrist and 6 in the ankle (Fig. 38).

Points in the wrist

These are located at the circle about two fingerbreaths proximal to the transverse crease of the wrist. They are, in order, called upper 1–6 from the ulnar side to the radial side of the dorsal surface.

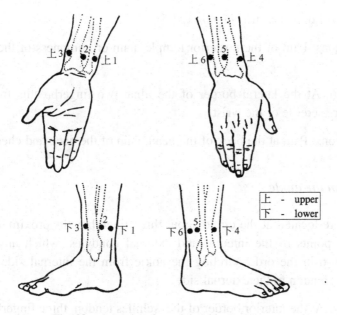

Fig. 38. Acupoints for wrist–ankle acupuncture.

Upper 1: Two fingerbreaths anterior to the ulna margin of the lateral little finger; a depression appears when one is pressing.

Indications: Frontal headache, eye disease, in affection of the nose, facial paralysis, anterior tooth swelling and pain, cough, cough and dyspnea, epigastric pain, palpitations, insomnia, depressive psychosis.

Upper 2: Equivalent to *neiguan* (PC 6).

Indications: Headache, toothache, breast pain, chest pain, astma and numbness of fingers.

Upper 3: Lateral to the radial artery, two fingerbreaths from the transverse crease of the wrist, and exterior to the border of the radius margin.

Indications: Hypertension, chest pain.

Upper 4: With the palm facing inward, at the radial border of the radius.

Indications: Vertex headache, ear disorders, chest pain, stiff shoulder

Upper 5: Equivalent to *waiguan* (SJ 5).

Indications: Pain of the posterior temple, pain or numbness of the upper limbs.

Upper 6: At the lateral border of the ulna, two fingerbreaths from the transverse crease of the wrist.

Indications: Pain at the back of the head, pain of the neck and chest.

Points in the ankle

These are located at the circle about three fingerbreaths proximal to the highest points of the internal and external condyles, which are called lower 1–6 in the order circling the ankle from the internal side of the Achilles tendon to the external side.

Lower 1: At the interior border of the Achilles tendon, three fingerbreaths proximal to the highest point of the internal condyles.

Indications: Upper abdomen pain, menalgia, enuresis, heel pain.

Lower 2: At the center of the medial surface, close to the posterior border of the interior side of the shin bone, three fingerbreaths proximal to the highest point of the internal condyles.

Indications: Lateral hypochondriac pain, abdominal pain, allergic colitis.

Lower 3: 1 cm medial to the anterior spine of the tibia, three fingerbreaths proximal to the highest point of the internal condyles.

Indications: Pain at the medial border of the knee joint.

Lower 4: At the posterior border of the tibia and the anterior border of the fibula, three fingerbreaths proximal to the highest point of the external condyles.

Indications: Numbness in the lower limbs, pain, paralysis.

Lower 5: At the posterior border of the fibula, three fingerbreaths proximal to the highest point of the external condyles.

Indications: Pain in coxalgia, sprain of the ankle joint.

Lower 6: At the lateral border of the Achilles tendon, three fingerbreaths proximal to the highest point of the external condyles.

Indications: Acute or chronic low back pain, sciatica.

Among the points mentioned above, upper 3 and lower 3 are the least-used in the clinic.

Manipulation

Point selection

Employ points of the wrist for diseases above the diaphragm and points of the ankle for those below. If the disease involves both, select both upper and lower points. For example, upper 5 and lower 4 may be employed for treating hemiplegia; if the disease has no clear location, such as insomnia, points of both sides are employed. Select and combine the points according to the specific indications of each point.

Needling

For the operation, select 1.5-*cun*-long No. 30 filiform needles. No special postures are required but the decubitus position is more suitable for puncturing points of the ankle. Give a routine sterilization to the selected point, tense the needle with the thumb and index finger of the left hand, and hold the needle handle with the thumb and the index and middle fingers of the right hand, with the thumb below the other fingers. Swiftly insert the needle at 30° angle formed by the skin and the needle shaft through the skin. Then, horizontally push the needle along the superficial layer of subcutaneous tissue. If it feels soft under the needle and no pain is caused to the patient, this manipulation is better. If the patient complains of soreness, numbness, distension or pain, this indicates that the needle has been too deep by inserted into the subfascial layer or the direction of the needle has been along a vertical line, and the needle should be withdrawn to the superficial layer and pushed shallowly for another try. Generally, the needle is pushed for about 1.4 *cun*. But if the disease is located at the hand or foot, the direction of needling may be downward. Never twirl, rotate, lift or thrust the needle after insertion. Retain it for 30 min. This acupuncture is done once every other day, or once daily for acute cases, 10 times as a course.

Indications

So far, wrist–ankle acupuncture has been applied to more than 50 diseases. It is highly effective in relieving pains like vascular cephalgia, lumbar sprains, toothache and menalgia; and also effective in treating arrhythmia, facial spasm, facial paralysis, asthma, enuresis, hysteria and stroke hemiplegia.

Note: If there are thick blood vessels or obvious pain occurs due to insertion, shift the insertion point vertically instead of horizontally.

QUESTIONS

(1) What stimulation areas do eye acupuncture and wrist–ankle acupuncture have respectively?

(2) Describe the manipulations and indications of eye acupuncture and wrist–ankle acupuncture.

CHAPTER 18

A General Introduction to Acupuncture Treatment

Just like drug therapies, acupuncture treatment follows general principles, involves effective formulas of acupuncture points and employs optimal needling techniques. This chapter will mainly address treatment principles and selection coupled with combination of points.

TREATMENT PRINCIPLES OF ACUPUNCTURE

The principles of treatment are essential to selection of points and methods of needling. They can be summarized into the following four aspects.

Treating Both the Root and the Branch

The root is the nature and the primary, and the branch is the symptom and the secondary; the etiological factors are the root, and the clinical manifestations are the branch; the chief complaints are the root, and the accompanying symptoms are the branch; and the conditions of the internal organs are the root, while the conditions of the body surface are the branch. Under general circumstances, the root should be treated first. Sometimes the root and the branch should be taken into account simultaneously. However, the branch should be prioritized in the case of an emergent condition. (Under certain circumstances, the symptoms are very critical, and it is necessary to observe the principle of "in an urgent condition, treat the branch.") For example, a patient with hemiplegia suddenly develops an acute episode of bronchitis after exposure to cold. According to the aforementioned principles, the hemiplegia is the root, while the bronchitis is the branch. Nonetheless, bronchitis requires emergent treatment by needling *kongzui* (LU 6), *fengmen* (BL 12) and *feishu* (BL 13). This will be followed by treatment of hemiplegia when the acute symptoms of bronchitis are under control.

Reinforcing Deficiency and Reducing Excess

Deficiency means that the body resistance is insufficient and weak, while excess means that pathogenic factors are excessive and strong. Reinforcing deficiency is to strengthen the body resistance and the *zang–fu* organs, while reducing excess is to dispel pathogenic factors. The reinforcing method in acupuncture therapy focuses on "treating deficiency with supplementation" and "treating the sinking with moxibustion." Deficiency refers to the deficiency of *qi*, blood, yin and yang. The reinforcing method is used to boost *qi* and assist yang, replenish blood and enrich yin with acupuncture and moxibustion. The "sinking" refers to uterine or rectal prolapse due to *qi* deficiency, which can be warmed and supplemented with moxibustion by lifting the sunken *qi*. The reducing method emphasizes "treating excess with drainage" and "treating blood stagnation by bleeding," which means that the excessive and strong pathogenic factors should be treated with the reducing method by bloodletting. In addition, other methods such as reinforcing and reducing simultaneously, reinforcing prior to reducing or reducing prior to reinforcing can be employed according to different syndromes.

Treatment of Diseases According to Climatic and Seasonal Conditions, Geographical Locations and the Individual Conditions

The climatic and seasonal conditions, the geographical locations, the patient's age and constitution and other factors must be taken into consideration when one is determining an appropriate method in acupuncture treatment. For instance, treatment of malaria is usually performaed 2–3 h before its attack, and dysmenorrhea is usually treated before the menstrual periods. For another example, weak stimulation of the needle should be given to the elderly and those with a weak constitution, while shallow needling should be given to infants.

THERAPEUTIC METHODS

Acupuncture and moxibustion is a therapy that involves needling or moxibustion at certain points of the human body. The selection and combination of points are summarized as follows.

Point Selection

Selection of points is the first step in acupuncture treatment. It has three categories, namely selection of adjacent points, selection of distal points and selection of points according to symptoms.

Selection of adjacent points

This refers to selecting points in or around the affected area. For example, *jingming* (BL 1) and *chengqi* (ST 1) are selected for eye diseases; *yingxiang* (LI 20) for nose diseases; *xiaguan* (ST 7) and *jiache* (ST 6) for toothache; *zhongwan* (RN 12) and *liangmen* (ST 21) for epigastric diseases, *quchi* (LI 11) for elbow pain and *dubi* (ST 35) for knee pain. When there is an ulcer, wound or scar in the affected area, select adjacent points instead. This is a relatively easy method for beginners.

Selection of distal points

"Distal" refers to a location far from the affected area. Generally, these points are located below the elbows and knees. For example, *hegu* (LI 4) and *neiting* (ST 44) are selected for toothache, *neiguan* (PC 6) and *gongsun* (SP 4) for stomachache and *yuji* (LU 10) for asthma. In distal selection, points on the lower body should be selected for the upper problems, and vice versa. For example, *baihui* (DU 20) is selected for rectal prolapse. Point selection is performed according to the channel theory and the respective functions of points.

Selection of points according to symptoms

This refers to the selection of the corresponding points according to various symptoms. Unlike the previous two methods involving the location of affected areas, this selection method is more indicated for systemic conditions such as fever, insomnia and spontaneous perspiration. For example, *dazhui* (DU 14) is selected for fever, or *hegu* (LI 4) and *fuliu* (KI 7) for spontaneous perspiration. In addition, selection by pressing the tenderness spots is covered in this category; for example, *lanweixue* (EX-LE7) is selected by pressing the tenderness spot for appendicitis.

Point Combination

Point combination refers to selecting two or more acupoints to form a proper acupuncture prescription according to different symptoms. It also includes single-point prescriptions, for example needling *shuigou* (DU 26) for sudden syncope or moxibustion to *zhiyin* (BL 67) for fetal malposition. The following is an introduction to five common ways of point combination.

Front and back point combination

"Front" refers to the chest and abdomen; "back," refers to the back and low back. Generally, points located on the front and the back, corresponding to the disease, can be selected. For example, *liangmen* (ST 21) on the front and *weishu* (BL 21) on the back are selected to treat stomachache. Besides, it is typical to combine the back–*shu* points and the front–*mu* points. For instance, *dachangshu* (BL 25) and *tianshu* (ST 25) are selected for diarrhea.

Exterior–interior-related channel point combination

"Exterior" refers to yang channels; "interior," yin channels. The combination of the yang and yin channel points is used to enhance the curative effects. For example, *yanglingquan* (GB 34) is combined with *taichong* (LR 3) to treat cholecystalgia (biliary colic) or *zusanli* (ST36) with *gongsun* (SP 4) for gastric diseases.

Upper and lower point combination

"Upper" refers to the upper limbs and the area above the waist; "lower," the opposite. This is most commonly used in clinical practice. For example, *jiache* (ST 6) and *xiaguan* (ST 7) on the face are combined with *neiting* (ST 44) on the foot for toothache, or *jingming* (BL 1) with *guangming* (GB 37) for eye diseases.

Right and left point combination

This refers to the combination of points on both sides of the body, and has three categories. One is the combination of the points sharing the same name, such as *hegu* (LI 4) on both sides selected for headache, or *zusanli* (ST 36) for stomachache. Another is the combination of different points on both sides. For example, facial points on the affected side combined with *hegu* (LI 4) on the healthy side are selected for trigeminal neuralgia, or *taiyang* (EX-HN 5) on the affected side with *yanglingquan* (GB 34) on the healthy side for migraine. The third category is that points on the left side should be selected for the diseases on the right side and vice versa. For example, *jianyu* (LI 15) and *jianliao* (LI 14) on the right are selected for shoulder periarthritis on the left, or points on the healthy side are selected to treat hemiplegia following stroke. This method was named "contralateral needling" in *Neijing* (*Canon of Internal Medicine*), and has proven to be clinically effective.

Adjacent and distal point combination

This is in fact a comprehensive use of both adjacent and distal point selection. For example, selecting *zhongwan* (CV 12) for stomachache is adjacent selection and selecting *neiguan* (PC 6) is distal selection, while the combination of the two points is within this category. Meanwhile, this is also a general summary of the previous four methods.

Therapeutic Method

An acupuncture prescription includes point selection and method application, and how to perform acupuncture and moxibustion correctly is critical, requiring one to:

Select an appropriate point for stimulation

Previously, a variety of point stimulations have been introduced, such as filiform needling, moxibustion, electroacupuncture, acupoint injection, ear acupuncture, scalp acupuncture, eye acupuncture and wrist–ankle acupuncture, which, according to their different indications, may be used alone or in combination to get a better curative effect. For example, scalp acupuncture or eye acupuncture may be used for stroke hemiplegia; electroacupuncture or ear acupuncture, for pain disorders; acupoint injection, for inflammatory diseases.

Regulate the effective stimulation intensity

This includes reinforcing–reducing manipulation with filiform needles, electroacupuncture frequency, waveform, intensity, dosage and concentration of the point injection. Therefore, during treatment with acupuncture and moxibustion, proper stimulation intensities should be adopted flexibly in order to achieve the best results.

Take the proper acupuncture time

Acupuncture time is very important. Firstly, the proper time should be chosen. For example, treatment of malaria, as previously mentioned is usually done 2–3 h before its attack. Secondly, in accordance with the characteristics of the diseases, acute cases should be treated 2–3 times a day, and chronic cases once a day or every two days. In addition, the course system should be established and treatment can be stopped for a period of time between courses.

QUESTIONS

(1) What are the treatment principles of acupuncture and moxibustion?
(2) Describe how to select acupoints and combine prescriptions.

CHAPTER 19

Acupuncture and Moxibustion
for Infectious Diseases

INFLUENZA

Overview

Influenza, commonly referred to as flu, is an acute infection of the respiratory tract caused by the influenza virus. The early symptoms are nasal congestion, runny nose, sore throat and coughing, followed by fever, chills, headache, fatigue and general discomfort. It was said that acupuncture and moxibustion had a significant effect on flu, in many reports in the 1950s. Typically, flu is transmitted through the air by droplets; so, if it is not controlled, flu pandemics will occur. Many acupuncturists apply acupuncture and moxibustion to prevent or control flu, with satisfactory results.

Prevention and Treatment

Body acupuncture (1)

Selection of points: Zusanli (ST 36).

Manipulation: Bilateral *zusanli* (ST 36) are selected. A No. 28 filiform needle 1.5 *cun* in length is inserted to a depth of 1.2 *cun*. When the patient feels soreness and distension, lifting and thrusting coupled with twirling at a moderate intensity is applied to allow the needling sensation to radiate toward the dorsum of the foot. Withdraw the needle instantly in 1–2 min. The acupuncture is performed only once; alternately, another treatment may be carried out in the second month during the peak period of influenza.

Body acupuncture (2)

Selection of points: Commonly used points — *dazhui* (DU 14), *hegu* (LI 4) and *fengchi* (GB 20). Supplementary points — *zusanli* (ST 36), and *quchi* (LI 11).

Manipulation: Commonly used points are selected first, and supplementary points should be used if fatigue and fever are significant. For *dazhui* (DU 14), the needle is inserted obliquely to a depth of 1–1.2 *cun*, with a local feeling of soreness and distension; for *fengchi* (GB 20), the needle is inserted toward the tip of the nose to 1.5 *cun*, until the needling sensation is felt; for *hegu* (LI 4), the needle is inserted slightly upward to a depth of 1.2–1.5 *cun*, to the degree of a strong sensation of soreness and distension. *Zusanli* (ST 36) and *quchi* (LI 11) are punctured till the arrival of *qi*. The reducing manipulation is applied by lifting and thrusting the needle to propagate the sensation to the arm and the dorsum of the foot. The needles are retained in each point for 1–2 min, once a day, or twice if necessary.

Moxibustion

Selection of points: Commonly used points — *dazhui* (DU 14). Supplementary points — *feishu* (BL 13) and *weizhong* (BL 40).

Manipulation: Only *dazhui* (DU 14) is employed at each session, and sparrow-pecking moxibustion with moxa stick is given for 15–20 min, until the local skin becomes reddish. If the effect is not present, supplementary points are employed (BL 40 on both sides) using a moxa stick for moderate moxibustion on each point for 15 min, two or three times daily.

Remarks

The firST body acupuncture, mainly for the prevention of influenza, was applied in the flu pandemic to 1908 healthy people only once, with the result that not a single incident occurred during the period.

The latter two methods are used to treat influenza. The second method — body acupuncture (2) — has a significant (antipyretic) cooling effect, with 53.08% of 373 cases returning to normal temperature in 24 h and 28.95%

in 48 h after only-once needling. However, this method requires skilled operation, and more caution is needed for *dazhui* (DU 14) and *fengchi* (GB 20), which are dangerous points. In contrast, moxibustion is relatively safe and more appropriate for beginners although its efficacy is inferior to that of the previous method.

BACILLARY DYSENTERY

Overview

Bacillary dysentery is an enteric infectious disease caused by *Bacillus dysenteriae*. Clinically, it is characterized by rapid onset, abdominal pain, bulge, and stools containing mucus, pus and blood, several times a day to more than 10 times, accompanied by fever, nausea, vomiting, loss of appetite and left-lower-quadrant tenderness. Acupuncture therapy for this disease firST appeared in *The Systematic Classic of Acupuncture and Moxibustion* in the Jin Dynasty, but scientific observations and a great number of experimental studies have been carried out in the laST 40 years. It has been proven statistically by thousands of cases that, with acupuncture and moxibustion, the cure rate is above 90%, the symptoms are removed in a shorter time, and the fecal bacteria negative rate is higher than for those taking medicine. Acupuncture has an effect on various types of bacillary dysentery, especially Freund's. Acupuncture for toxic bacillary dysentery, though effective, will not be discussed here, since that very dangerous disease should be treated with drug therapies.

Treatment

Body acupuncture

Selection of points: tianshu (ST 25), shangjuxu (ST 37) or *zusanli* (ST 36).

Manipulation: Two points are employed at each session. *Tianshu* (ST 25) is required, and *shangjuxu* (ST 37) and *zusanli* (ST 36) are used alternately. The insertion may be a bit deep, and the reducing manipulation is applied by lifting and pressing — combined with twirling — the needle for 1 min, with the intensity increasing accordingly. The needles are retained for 30–60 min, during which repeatedly manipulating the needles is advisable so as to increase the stimulation. Seriously ill cases are punctured once every 8 h; mild cases, once or twice daily. After the symptoms are relieved, needle once a day till total recovery. Acupuncture for this disease is more effective without taking the course into account.

Point injection

Selection of points: Commonly used points — *tianshu* (ST 25) and *shangjuxu* (ST 37). Supplementary points — *zusanli* (ST 37), *guanyuan* (CV 4), *qihai* (CV 6).

Manipulation: Select any one of the following: 12.5% chloramphenicol injection 2 ml and 1% procaine injection 2 ml; vitamin B1 injection; angelica injection. Two or three points on one side are employed at each session. Dental needle V and a 2–5 ml syringe are inserted into the point (an allergy teST is needed prior to procaine injection) by slightly thrusting and lifting at the arrival of *qi* to strengthen the needling sensation, but be sure not to stir blindly or carelessly. Withdrawing without blood is followed by injecting quickly 0.5 ml into each point, usually once a day, or twice if necessary. Alternate the points on both sides.

Ear acupuncture

Selection of points: Common points — *dachang* (the large intestine) and the lower portion of the rectum [at the anterior portion of the helix, level with the Ot (otopoint) large intestine]. Supplementary points — subcortex and sympathetic.

Manipulation: Common points are all employed, and one supplementary point is added according to different symptoms. When the sensitive points are found, a filiform needle is inserted by rapid twirling and rotating, with the intensity tolerable to the sufferer, and retain for 15–45 min. Continued manipulations are applied intermittently until the abdominal pain and the desire to have BM are significantly reduced or removed. Sufferers with severe symptoms should be applied to twice a day, and then once a day after the disease is controlled, with points on both ears alternated.

Remarks

Among the three methods mentioned above, body acupuncture is the most effective and widely used. But, for *tianshu* (ST 25), the needling should not be inserted too deep, in case of injuring the organs; meanwhile, compound reinforcing–reducing manipulation is required to be mastered. Point injection is applicable to those who have intramuscular injection experience. The injection dose is large not, but an obvious needling sensation is necessary. Ear acupuncture is the easiest of the three and effective if used appropriately, but the needling sensation is intolerable to some sufferers, so it is advisable to explain to the patients in advance. In short, which method is preferred depends on the operator's proficiency in needling and the features of the individuals.

QUESTIONS

(1) LiST the three methods for preventing influenza with acupuncture and moxibustion.
(2) Describe how to manipulate body acupuncture and ear acupuncture for bacillary dysentery.

BACTERIAL FOOD POISONING

Overview

This is an acute infectious toxic disease caused by eating food contaminated by bacteria and their toxins. It comprises many types, including staphylococcal food poisoning and halophilic bacterial food poisoning. The former, induced by the staphylococcal enterotoxin, is characterized by rapid onset, severe gastrointestinal symptoms (especially severe vomiting that may cause dehydration and exhaustion), etc.; the latter is often related to the consumption of unclean pickled objects, with the manifestations of rapid onset, severe abdominal pain, watery or yellow paste diarrhea, even bloody or watery stools. Acupuncture and moxibustion for the two types is so effective that a total cure rate of more than 96% is achieved, and all symptoms are relieved in ten or tens of minutes.

Treatment

Acupuncture and moxibustion

Selection of points: Commonly used points — *neiguan* (PC 6), *zhongwan* (CV 12) and *zusanli* (ST 36). Supplementary points — *tianshu* (ST 25) is added for diarrhea, *shenque* (CV 8) for blood pressure dearease and cold extremities, and *chengshan* (BL 57) for spasm of the calf.

Manipulation: Generally, common points are selected, and supplementary points should be added in cases with severe symptoms. Insert the needle till the arrival of *qi*, and thrusting and lifting or twirling and rotating is applied for 1 min. Strengthen the stimulation to a degree an obvious sensation of soreness and distension is felt. *Chengshan* (BL 57) is needled till the arrival of *qi*. The needles are retained for 20–30 min, during which manipulate them once every 5 or 10 min. *Shenque* (CV 8) is applied with sparrow-pecking moxibustion for 15–60 min, according to the pathological conditions. If the result is not satisfactory, another acupuncture treatment should be performed after 4–6 h.

Bloodletting method

Selection of points: Commonly used points — *zhongchong* (PC 9) and *shaoshang* (LU 11). Supplementary points — *shenque* (CV 8) and *zusanli* (ST 36).

Manipulation: Common points are employed, and the supplementary points should be added in cases of obvious diarrhea. Spot pricking with a three-edged needle is applied to bilateral *zhongchong* (PC 9) and *shaoshang* (LU 11), and press the site to cause local congestion until the blood becomes reddish or dark-purple. The three-edged needles are inserted into *shenque* (CV 8) on the four sides of the point to a depth of 0.1–0.2 *cun*, followed by cupping on the desired area with a big jar until *shenque* (CV 8) congests to a heart shape and the blood flows linearly. The 26th–28th filiform needle is inserted into *zusanli* (ST 36) till the arrival of *qi*, with the needle retained for 20–30 min.

Remarks

Of the two methods above, the first is mainly used for staphylococcal food poisoning; it was applied to 116 patients with the result of total recovery, most of whom returned to normal within 10–30 min, and others within 2 h. However, much attention should be paid to the insertion intensity and the retention time, which may be respectively strengthened and lengthened according to the pathological conditions of each patient. The second method is for halophilic bacterial food poisoning. It was once compared with Western medicine treatment, and the cure rate and the effective rate were 60th found to be higher. Of course, those with severe vomiting and diarrhea should be given an infusion to prevent dehydration, and those in whom acupuncture is ineffective should be treated with Chinese or Western medicine.

ACUTE JAUNDICE HEPATITIS

Overview

Acute jaundice hepatitis, one kind of acute viral hepatitis, is clinically manifested by rapid onset, poor appetite, being tired of oil, fatigue, abdominal discomfort, hepatalgia, nausea and vomiting. Fever, followed by dark urine, and jaundice on the sclera and skin accompany them in some cases. Acupuncture and moxibustion for this disease was first recorded in *The Systematic Classic of Acupuncture and Moxibustion*, to which ancient practitioners attached great importance. Now, extensive clinical observations and experimental researches have been carried out and have made great achievements. It has been proven that acupuncture therapy, no matter whether a long-term or a short-term effect, in adults or infants, is superior to herbal therapy and Western medication in restoring appetite, degrading jaundice and improving liver functions, besides offering a lower recurrence rate and a high cure rate.

Of course, there are indications for acupuncture therapy in treating acute jaundice hepatitis, recognized now as the following: (1) the ordinary type without any folder diseases; (2) the course of the disease being within two weeks; (3) one with typical clinical symptoms mentioned above; (4) one with a swelling liver, local tenderness and percussion pain; (5) one with two or more abnormal items in the liver function test.

Treatment

Body acupuncture

Selection of points: Common points — *zhiyang* (DU 9), *yanglingquan* (GB 34) penetrating toward *yinlingquan* (SP 9), or *taichong* (LR 3) toward *yongquan* (KI 1). Supplementary points — *quchi* (LI 11) is added for fever, *qimen* (LR 14) for hypochondriac pain, *neiguan* (PC 6) for nausea and *tianshu* (ST 25) for abdominal distension.

Manipulation: Common points are the main points; two pairs of points are used alternately, one pair each time. Supplementary points are added according to different symptoms. Reducing manipulations are applied by thrusting and lifting or twirling and rotating, with stronger stimulation within the limit of the patient's tolerance. The needles are retained for 20 min, during which manipulation is carried out two or three times, 1–2 min each time, once a day, and a second manipulation may be added in severe cases.

Electroacupuncture

Selection of points: Common points — *zusanli* (ST 36), *taichong* (LR 3) and *yongquan* (KI 1). Supplementary points — *ganshu* (BL 18), *danshu* (BL 19), *yanglingquan* (GB 34) and *zhiyang* (DU 9).

Manipulation: Commonly used points are employed at each session. After a needling sensation is induced, the two lines of the electric acupuncture apparatus are attached to the filiform needles, with the two output leads connected to the same side of the body with an alternately dense and sparse wave (also termed an "irregular wave"). The power switch is turned on, and the output current is gradually increased until tolerable soreness, numbness, distension or muscle vibration is induced in the patient. The duration of electrical stimulation is usually 10–20 min. If the effect is not obvious, supplementary points are employed, with two electrodes of a pair connected to *ganshu* (BL 18) and *danshu* (BL 19) on the same side after the arrival of *qi* for 15–20 min, once or twice per day; the reST of the points remain unconnected.

Ear acupuncture

Selection of points: Commonly used points — liver, pancreas and spleen. Supplementary points — stomach is added for a poor appetite, *shenmen* and subcortex for hepatodynia and subcortex and large intestine for abdominal distension.

Manipulation: Commonly used points are required; supplementary points are optional, according to different symptoms. Four-to-six points are employed at each session, with manipulation on only one side. A No. 28 filiform needle, 0.5 *cun* long, is inserted swiftly after the sensitive point is found, for half a minute, with the needle retained for 1 h, once a day. The right and the left are applied to alternately.

Remarks

Of the three methods above, body acupuncture is the most widely used, with affirmative effect. It was applied to more than 400 cases, and a cure rate of 84.3%–100% was achieved. Electroacupuncture is relatively easy and is suitable for those who are not skilled at manipulation techniques. The clinical cure rate reaches about 85%. Ear acupuncture is inferior to the previous two methods in curative effect, but is easy to operate, and is often changed to *Semen Vaccariae* seeds for ear acupuncture as an auxiliary method to body acupuncture. The combination tends to achieve much better results for improving the symptoms and boosting the recovery.

QUESTIONS

(1) What are the two acupoint stimulations for treating bacterial food poisoning?

(2) Which acute hepatitis can be treated with acupuncture and moxibustion? What are the acupoint stimulations?

MALARIA

Overview

Malaria is an infectious disease caused by parasites, characterized by paroxysms of shivering chills and high fever occurring at regular intervals, and mostly found in late summer and early autumn. It starts with sudden chills, body weakness, headache, thirsty, dysthesia, and then manifests high fever (body temperature up to 40°C) and facial flushing, followed by general sweating, and the body temperature dropping to normal. It occurs cyclically and has a long period of illness which may cause splenomegaly and anemia. Subtertain malaria is a violation of internal organs with the tendency of a dangerous onset, characterized by acute high fever or irregular fever, chills, convulsions and coma. Acupuncture and moxibustion for malaria was recorded in *The Inner Classic* in detail, and reported clinically in the 1920s. It has been proven by both ancient and modern practitioners that acupuncture therapy is effective in the treatment of malaria tertiana, but poor in the treatment of pernicious malaria no matter what point stimulation is applied.

Treatment

Body acupuncture

Selection of points: Commonly used points — divided into two groups, namely (1) *dazhui* (DU 14), *houxi* (SI 3) and (2) taodao (DU 14) (on the back and at the depression below the spinous process of the firST thoracic vertebra). Supplementary points — *quchi* (LI 11) is added for fever, *neiguan* (PC 6) for cheST stuffiness and hypochondriac pain, and *taiyang* (EX-HN 5) for headache.

Manipulation: One group of points is employed at each session, with two groups used alternately, and supplementary points are added according to different conditions. Perform acupuncture treatment 2–3 h prior to the onset of the paroxysm. Needles are inserted into *dazhui* (DU 14) and *taodao* (DU 13) to a depth of 1–1.5 *cun*, till a sensation of soreness, distension and movement is felt, and then withdrawn to a nonsensory area. It is forbidden to insert the needle into the spinal canal and retain it deep inside. Acupuncture is applied to other points to induce the needling sensation in the patient, with the needles retained for 30–60 min, during which thrust, lift, twirl and rotate the needle once every 5–10 min. The stimulation intensity depends on the physical and pathological conditions of the sufferer, and it is appropriate to make it slightly stronger.

Ear acupuncture

Selection of points: Commonly used points — subcortex, endocrine, adrenal gland. Supplementary points — *shenmen* (on the ear), tenderness near the spine (found on either side of the thoracic vertebrae, mostly beside the 4th–6th thoracic vertebrae, where distension and pain may be strongly felt).

Manipulation: Commonly used points are usually employed, and supplementary points should be added in cases of unclear effect. The sensitive point having been found, insert a filiform needle 0.5 *cun* in length by twirling and rotating for 1–2 min with strong stimulation. Manipulation is applied 2 h prior to the onset of paroxysm, with the needle retained till 1–2 h after the onset predicted. During the retention, twirl the needle once every 10 min. For the tenderness near the spine, a filiform needle 1.5 *cun* long is inserted slightly toward the spine and retained till the arrival of *qi*, the same as for the above.

Remarks

The above methods are the main ones for treating malaria, especially body acupuncture, which was once applied to 500 cases and proved able to enhance the organism's ability to devour the plasmodium and effective in both malaria tertiana and pernicious malaria, with the cure rate of the former reaching 90% or more, and that of the latter about 80%. But it is difficult for beginners to guide the insertion depth to *taodao* (DU 13) and *dazhui* (DU 14). Ear acupuncture is a safe method, mainly for malaria tertiana, with a cure rate of 80%, slightly lower than for body acupuncture, which is optional (according to different conditions).

HEMOPTYSIS OF PULMONARY TUBERCULOSIS

Overview

Hemoptysis of pulmonary tuberculosis is one of the common local symptoms of pulmonary tuberculosis, which occurs in one-third or half of TB cases. It is classified as trivial, moderate or massive, depending on the amount of blood. Trivial hemoptysis (blood in phlegm) results from the increase in capillary permeability induced by the inflammation focus; moderate hemoptysis, from small vessel injury; and massive hemoptysis occurs when a comparatively macroaneurysm ruptures on the wall of the tuberculous cavity, sometimes with more than 500 ml of bright-red blood. Acupuncture treatment appeared in *Supplement to Prescriptions Worth a Thousand Gold Pieces* in the Tang Dynasty. Modern reports began in the late 1950s. Much experience has shown that acupuncture is effective in all types of hemoptysis, especially the moderate and massive ones, and 90% of the effective rate has been achieved.

Treatment

Body acupuncture

Selection of points: Commonly used points — *kongzui* (LU 6) and *chize* (LU 5). Supplementary points — *neiguan* (PC 6).

Manipulation: Commonly used points are usually employed, and supplementary points should be added if there is no obvious effect. The patient assumes the supine posture, with the whole body relaxed. The needle is inserted toward the shoulder, at an angle of 75°. Repeatedly lifting and thrusting it will make the sensation propagate to the throat or the anterior part of the chest. A better effect will be achieved if the patient feels dry in the mouth, cool in the throat, tight in the chest, etc. Manipulate the needles for 2 min every time, with a retention of 20–30 min, once every 5–10 min, once or twice daily, or two or three times for massive hemoptysis.

Acupuncture with skin needling

Selection of points: Commonly used points — the carotid pulsation area (the pulsation area of the carotid artery and its branches between submandible and clavicle). Supplementary points — *kongzui* (LU 6).

Manipulation: The skin needle (seven-star needling) is employed within the carotid pulsation area to tap up and down regularly and rhythmically like a sparrow pecking at food along the carotid of one side or both sides with moderate intension, at a frequency of 180 pulses per minute. The stimulation generally lasts for 10–30 min. Tap at *kongzui* (LU 6) like a sparrow pecking at food if the effect is not obvious with the same intension, frequency and time as the above, once or twice daily.

Electroacupuncture

Selection of points: *Neiguan* (PC 6) and *kongzui* (LU 6).

Manipulation: Employ the points on one side at each treatment session, with the filiform needle inserted till the arrival of *qi*. Connect the handle to the electroacupuncture apparatus G6805 with the continuous wave at a frequency of 180 pulses per minute and the current strength tolerable to the sufferer, for 30 min to hours. The needling is usually applied at the attack of hemoptysis.

Overview

Among the three methods, the easiest and the most effective one is skin needling, which was applied to 129 cases with an effective rate of 96%–100%, and is applicable to beginners. Pay attention to the rhythm while tapping, and it is acceptable when the local skin becomes flushed without bleeding. Body acupuncture is effective in stopping hemoptysis, but it is relatively difficult to propagate the sensation upward, which requires the cooperation of the practitioner and the sufferer. Electroacupuncture is approved for and applicable to massive hemoptysis which will stop in 30 min (a little blood still in the phlegm), and 195 cases out of 300 (65%) had no hemoptysis after 12 h, with a total effective rate of 95%. It is worth noting that hemoptysis of pulmonary tuberculosis is an emergency and must turn to other Chinese or modern therapies if the acupuncture treatment has no effect, and blood transfusion should be done if there is excessive loss of blood.

QUESTIONS

(1) Restate in detail the body acupuncture method for malaria.
(2) What are the acupoint stimulations in treating hemoptysis of pulmonary tuberculosis?

CHAPTER 20

Acupuncture and Moxibustion for Diseases of the Respiratory and Circulatory Systems

CHRONIC BRONCHITIS

Overview

Chronic bronchitis, a serious hazard to human health, is manifested clinically by chronic cough, expectoration, or being accompanied by dyspnea. The episode of attack lasts at least three months each year, for more than two years. Cough is aggravated in the early morning and the night in winter, with white and sticky mucoid sputum. Chronic bronchitis pertains to the categories of "cough" and "syndrome characterized by dyspnea" in traditional Chinese medicine, which were recorded in *Neijing* (*The Inner Classic*). Since the 1950s, acupuncture and moxibustion has been one of the commonly used treatments for chronic bronchitis. Statistics show that an effective rate of 70%–90% for 18,400 cases between 1971 and 1980 was achieved, some of which were clinically cured or controlled and most were improved in symptoms.

Treatment

Electroacupuncture

Selection of points: Commonly used points — *dazhui* (DU 14) and *taodao* (DU 13). Supplementary points — *neiguan* (PC 6) added for gasping, *fenglong* (ST 40) or *kongzui* (LU 6) for excessive phlegm, and *dingchuan* (EX-B1) for coughing.

307

Manipulation: Commonly used points are employed. The patient is in the sitting position with the head slightly lowered, and a No. 28 filiform needle, 2 *cun* long, is inserted obliquely into the selected points with the tip toward the head at an angle of 45° to a depth of 1.2–1.5 *cun* to induce a local sensation of soreness and distension. But a needling sensation radiating to the body is not needed. Being connected to the electroacupuncture apparatus, the patient may feel numb because of the electricity. The electroacupuncture is applied at a frequency of 80 pulses per minute with the continuous wave and the current strength tolerable to the patient. Supplementary points are used for the common acupuncture till the arrival of *qi*. The needles are retained at each point for 20 min, once every other day, 10 times as a course, at an interval of 3–5 days.

Acupoint application

Selection of points: Shenque (RN 8).

Manipulation: Five medicinals, Gongdingxiang (*Fog Cryophylli*) 0.5 g, Rougui (*Cortex Cinnamomi*) 5 g, Mahuang (*Herba Ephedrae*) 5 g, Cang'erzi (*Fructus Xanthii*) 3 g and Baijiezi (*Semen Sinapis*) 5 g, are ground into a fine powder and sealed in a bottle. Sterilize the naval with 75% alcohol before filling it with the powder, then place a common adhesive plaster bigger than the naval on it without the powder leaking. Replace it with another every 48 h. If there is an allergy induced by the plaster after a long time, remove the plaster and the medicinals, and clean the skin with a hot towel 2–3 h before the replacement every time. If dermatitis appears, stop mounting for a couple of days or apply ointments like fluocinolone acetonide until the dermatitis completely disappears, then apply the powder agitated with 30% alcohol. The manipulation is given 10 times as a course at an interval of one week.

Moxibustion

Selection of points: Commonly used points — *dazhui* (DU 14), *feishu* (BL 13), *tiantu* (RN 22) and *danzhong* (RN 17). Supplementary points — *chize* (LU 5), *fenglong* (ST 40) and *zusanli* (ST 36).

Manipulation: Two or three commonly used points are given ginger-separated moxibustion at each session, and one or two supplementary points moxa moxibustion. For the operation, cup the selected points [except *tiantu* (RN 22)] for 5–10 min, cut a slice of raw ginger, place a moxa cone in the size of a wheat grain on it, ignite the cone, and place the slice on the acupoint selected for moxibustion. Replace the moxa cone with another one after it is burnt out. Generally, four or five cones are used for each point. Supplementary points are given sparrow-pecking moxibustion with moxa sticks for 10–15 min at each point, until a local flush appears. The treatment is performed once every three days, four times as a course, at an interval of 5–7 days.

Remarks

Among the three methods above, the first has been applied to the most cases, in which a total effective rate of 95% was achieved, and a short-term control rate of 53% for 1500 cases. But accidents often happen to *dazhui* (DU 14) and *taodao* (DU 13), so a great deal of attention should be paid to not inserting the needle too deep. Acupoint mounting is relatively easy and safe, and the effective rate is nearly the same as for electroacupuncture. Moxibustion is inferior to the previous two methods in effectiveness and manipulation, and is applicable to beginners.

BRONCHIAL ASTHMA

Overview

Bronchial asthma is a common pulmonary allergic disease, with repeated attacks. The clinical manifestations are sudden expiratory dyspnea, prolonged expiration and an oppressed feeling in the chest. Patients tend to sit up with the hands holding ahead, the shoulders towering, sweating, irritability and wheezing sputum. Acupuncture and moxibustion for asthma was recorded in *The Classic of Nourishing Life with Acupuncture and Moxibustion* in the Song Dynasty. Many acupoint stimulations have been found in modern times, including moxibustion, magnetic therapy, point mounting, point injection, pricking therapy and cutting therapy, most of which are similar in effectiveness and the effective rate is 80%–90%.

Treatment

Body acupuncture

Selection of points: Commonly used points — *yuji* (LU 10), *feishu* (BL 13) and *dazhui* (DU 14). Supplementary points — *dingchuan* (EX-B1), *lieque* (LU 7).

Manipulation: Commonly used points are employed at each session, with one supplementary point added accordingly. *Yuji* (LU 10), punctured prior to other points, is punctured to 1 *cun* deep, the tip being obliquely toward the palm, with lifting and thrusting for drainage and powerful stimulation for half a minute. The needle is retained at the point for 20–30 min. Another manipulation is applied 5 min later. *Feishu* (BL 13) is inserted perpendicularly to 0.5 *cun*, *dazhui* (DU 14) obliquely downward to 1–1.2 *cun*, with lifting, thrusting, twirling and rotating of the needle no more than 0.1 *cun* deep. Withdraw the needle after 15 min of retention, followed by warm moxibustion with a moxa stick for 5–10 min at each point. Supplementary points are applied with the reducing method at the arrival of *qi* with medium and powerful stimulation, and the needles are retained for 20 min. Perform the manipulation once or twice during the period of onset, once every day or every other day when asthma is relieved.

Acupoint application

Selection of points: Two groups — (1) *feishu* (BL 13), *xinshu* (BL 15) and *tiantu* (RN 22); (2) *fengmen* (BL 12), *jueyinshu* (BL 14) and *danzhong* (RN 17).

Manipulation: Ointment for relieving asthma consists of Baijiezi (*Semen Sinapis*) 30%, Gansui (*Radix Kansui*) 30%, Xixin (*Radix et Rhizoma Asari*) 10%, Ganjiang (*Rhizoma Zingiberis*) 10%, Mahuang (*Herba Ephedrae*) 10% and Yanhusuo (*Rhizoma Corydalis*) 10%, which are ground into a fine powder, made into a paste with fresh ginger pop, and spread on a round sheet of vegetable parchment measuring about 10 cm². Mount to the first group with the ointment, with cotton applied around, sterilized gauze covered, and fix it with adhesive tape. Two or three hours later, when the patient feels scorching heat or slight pain, remove the ointment, and paint gentian violet on the point selected if bubbles appear. The second group is given the application in the same way after nine days. Three times is a course, one course a year. Make sure the patient does not scratch himself or herself, for fear of infection.

Ear acupuncture

Selection of points: Commonly used points — lung, adrenal gland, central rim, and sympathetic. Supplementary points — spleen, kidney, large intestine, root of the ear vagus, and *shenmen*.

Manipulation: Commonly used points are employed in an acute episode, while supplementary points are added in catabasis. A filiform needle is inserted with repeated twirling and rotating and powerful stimulation tolerable to the patient. Manipulate the needle for 1–2 min, and retain it for 20–30 min. Select points on one side each time and puncture the other side alternately, one or two times in an acute episode and once every other day in catabasis.

Remarks

The second method is mainly for preventing asthma in the way of "winter diseases, summer treatment, and vice versa," i.e. asthma in winter is treated with application in three periods of dog days, once for each period; and asthma in summer is treated in three periods of the coldest days, once every nine days. Among 4000 cases, an effective rate for prevention of 83.7%–98% has been achieved. The first and third methods aim to cure asthma, but be sure not to needle *dazhui* (DU 14), *feishu* (BL 13) or *fengmen* (BL 12) too deep. Body acupuncture is applicable to those who are skilful in manipulation, with clinical experience, while ear acupuncture is for beginners.

QUESTIONS

(1) Restate the electroacupuncture and point mounting methods in treating chronic bronchitis.

(2) What are the differences and similarities between point stimulations in treating bronchial asthma and chronic bronchitis?

ANGINA PECTORIS

Overview

Angina pectoris is the clinical symptoms caused by coronary insufficiency, cardiac rapid, transient ischemia and hypoxia. It is manifested chiefly by paroxysmal pain or an oppressed feeling in the precordial area, radiating to the left shoulder, the left arm, or even the ring finger and little finger, induced by physical exertion, overeating or emotional disturbance, and relieved quickly by rest or nitroglycerin in the mouth. The pain usually lasts for 1–5 min, and rarely more than 10–15 min. Angina pectoris belongs to the disease or syndrome categories of cardiac pain in traditional Chinese medicine, and was recorded in *Channels* in the Spring and Autumn Period. Modern reports on acupuncture and moxibustion for angina pectoris began in the late 1950s, but a large number of studies have been conducted in the past 30 years. The total effective rate for acupuncture treatment is 66%–98%, and the remission rate for ECG is 52%–67%, which shows that the effect is reliable.

Treatment

Body acupuncture

Selection of points: Commonly used points — two groups, namely (1) *xinshu* (BL 15) and *neiguan* (PC 6), and (2) *jueyinshu* (BL 14) and *danzhong* (RN 17). Supplementary points — *jianshi* (PC 5), *zusanli* (ST 36), and *shenmen* (HT 7).

Manipulation: One group of commonly used points is employed at each treatment session, and the two groups are used alternately. For back-*shu* points, insert the needle to a depth of 1.5 *cun* obliquely toward the spine, until its tip touches the spine. Thrusting, lifting, twirling and rotating are applied till the sensation of soreness and numbness reaches the chest, and scrape the needle handle for 2 min. For *neiguan* (PC 6) and *jianshi* (PC 5), the needle is inserted with the tip upward to a depth of 1–1.2 *cun*. The seeking method which involves thrusting and lifting the needle is used to transmit the sensation to the shoulder and the chest. *Danzhong* (RN 17) is given horizontal insertion, using the conventional needle technique. All the needles should be retained for 15–20 min, with manipulation once every 5 min, once daily, and two or three times a day for those suffering frequent attacks by angina.

Moxibustion

Selection of points: *Danzhong* (RN 17) and *geshu* (BL 21).

Manipulation: Both points are selected for mild-warming moxibustion with moxa sticks for 15 min, till the local skin becomes reddish. It is applied once or twice per day.

Ear acupuncture

Selection of points: Commonly used points — heart, sympathetic and endocrine. Supplementary points — subcortex, kidney, *shenmen* and central rim.

Manipulation: Three-to-five points are employed at each treatment session. For severe cases, two needles should be inserted into the heart. Once the sensitive point is found, insert a filiform needle 0.5 *cun* in length by twirling and rotating at a moderate intensity, with the needle retained for 1 h, during which an electropulse therapeutic device is connected with an irregular wave or high frequency to a degree which the sufferer can tolerate. One side is selected each time, and the two ears are applied alternately, once per day.

Remarks

Among the three methods, body acupuncture has a definite curative effect and is widely used in clinics, but it is necessary for beginners to control the inserting direction to *xinshu* (BL 15) and *jueyinshu* (BL 14). The needle should be inserted obliquely, not perpendicularly, at an angle of 45° toward with the spine until the tip is felt to reach the vertebral body, which will usually induce a needling sensation toward the chest. Moxibustion is relatively safe and easy, but has not been applied to many cases. Ear acupuncture is inferior to body acupuncture. It has been discovered that ear acupuncture will have a greater curative effect if combined with body acupuncture.

ARRHYTHMIA

Overview

Arrhythmia refers to any abnormality in the starting part of heart stroke, the heart rate and rhythm, and cardiac conduction. It is clinically classified as either impulse formation disorders or impulse conduction disorders. The common manifestations are palpitations, an oppressed feeling in the chest, shortness of breath, dizziness, even chest pain and syncope, etc. Arrhythmia, belonging to *xinji* and *zhengchong* (palpitations) in TCM, was recorded in *Channels* more than 2000 years ago. Modern clinical reports began in the 1950s, and great progress has been achieved in efficacy verification and mechanism exploration of acupuncture treatment in the past 40 years. The total effective rate of acupuncture treatment is 70%–90%, and the remission rate of ECG is 46%. But the curative effect is different for different types of arrhythmia. Generally, the effect on arrhythmia induced by the anomalous origin is superior to that induced by excited conduction anomalies.

Treatment

Body acupuncture

Selection of points: Commonly used points — two groups, namely (1) *xinshu* (BL 15) and *neiguan* (PC 6) and (2) *jueyinshu* (BL 14) and *shenmen* (HT 7). Supplementary points — *sanyinjiao* (SP 6) is added for premature beat, *zusanli* (ST 36) for tachycardia, *suliao* (DU 25) for bradycardia and *danzhong* (RN 17) and *quchi* (LI 11) for auricular fibrillation.

Manipulation: One group is employed at each treatment session, and supplementary points are added according to syndromes. The patient is in the prone position, and the needles are first inserted into the points on the back at an angle of 45° obliquely toward the spine, to a depth of 1.5 *cun* until the tip reaches the spine. On the arrival of *qi*, thrusting, lifting, twirling and rotating the needle are applied to diffuse the sensation to the chest, with reinforcing manipulation by minor twirling and rotating for 3–5 min, before withdrawing the needle. For the points on the limbs and the chest, insert the needle with the patient in the supine position and stimulate the point with moderate or strong intensity on the arrival of *qi*, with a retention of 20 min, manipulating the needle once every 5 min. The retention should last for 5–10 min for bradycardia.

Ear acupuncture

Selection of points: Commonly used points — endocrine, heart, sympathetic and *shenmen*. Supplementary points — subcortex and kidney; the ear center is added for tachycardia, and heart points (anterior to the supratragic notch, at the lower border posterior to the depression) for auricular fibrillation.

Manipulation: Three or four commonly used points are employed at each session, and one or two supplementary points added according to syndromes. Insert needles to induce the sensation with moderate and strong intensity and with a retention of 1 h. For paroxysmal tachycardia, the ear center is selected as the main point combined with two or three commonly used points, with the needles retained for 30–60 min. For auricular fibrillation, the heart point is selected as the main point combined with two or three commonly used points, with a retention of 30 min, and with mild intensity in case of needling fainting.

Electroacupuncture

Selection of points: Commonly used points — *neiguan* (PC 6), *jianshi* (PC 5), *ximen* (PC 4) and *sanyinjiao* (SP 6). Supplementary points — *zusanli* (ST 36), *xinshu* (BL 15), *danzhong* (RN 17) and *shenshu* (BL 23).

Manipulation: Two points, employed at each session, are used alternately, and supplementary points may be added if the effect is not obvious. Insert the needle to induce the sensation, then connect the G6805 electric acupuncture device with a continuous wave at the frequency of 120 beats/min. The intensity may be regulated to a degree that a sufferer can tolerate. The manipulation lasts for 15–30 min, once a day.

Remarks

Among the three methods above, body acupuncture is the first choice, with a firm effect. For 322 cases, the total curative rate for treating arrhythmia induced by the excited anomalous origin was 64.1%–84%; arrhythmia induced by excited conduction anomalies, 19%–25.5%. Ear acupuncture is easy to perform, but it needs further verification because few cases have been tested. Electroacupuncture is applicable to beginners, since it is safe for selecting points on the four limbs.

QUESTIONS

(1) How many treatment methods are there for angina pectoris with acupuncture and moxibustion? What are they?
(2) Describe how to select points and apply manipulations to treat arrhythmia with point stimulations.

HYPERLIPOPROTEINEMIA

Overview

Hyperlipoproteinemia is a metabolic disorder characterized by abnormally elevated concentrations of specific lipoprotein particles in the plasma, among which increase in cholesterol and triglyceride values is of the most clinical significance. It is closely related to the prevention of cardiovascular, endocrine, metabolic and liver diseases, especially senile diseases. There is no record in ancient books about treatment with acupuncture and moxibustion. Modern studies began in the 1950s, but not until the late 1970s did acupuncture treatment for lowering lipids draw a great deal of attention, leading to deep research on point selection, point stimulation, curative effects and mechanisms, and so on. It is definite that acupuncture and moxibustion can lower cholesterol, triglycerides, β lipoprotein and phospholipid levels in the blood.

Treatment

Body acupuncture

Selection of points: Commonly used points — *neiguan* (PC 6) and *zusanli* (ST 36). Supplementary points — *sanyinjiao* (SP 6), *taichong* (LR 3) and *taibai* (SP 3).

Manipulation: Commonly used points are generally employed, with one or two supplementary points added according to syndromes. For *neigan* (PC 6), insert the needle obliquely directed to the shoulder, and the seeking method which involves thrusting and lifting the needle is used to compel the sensation to transmit upward. Manipulate the needle by slightly thrusting, lifting, twirling and rotating for 2 min. For *zusanli* (ST 36), it is better to needle at 7–9 in the morning until the arrival of *qi* and then to manipulate the needle in the way mentioned above. The remaining points are needled as usual, with a retention of 20 min, needling once every 5–10 min. When one is withdrawing the needles, rounding moxibustion with moxa sticks is performed on *zusanli* (ST 36), once every day or every other day, for 10–15 times as a course, at an interval of 3–5 days.

Point laser irradiation

Selection of points: *neiguan* (PC 6).

Manipulation: A helium–neon laser acupuncture device is used for irradiation, with wavelength 632.8 nm, output power 2–3 mW and spot diameter 1–1.5 mm. Light-conducting fiber is put directly on *neiguan* (PC 6). Irradiation is given for 15 min each time, with the two sides applied to alternately, once a day, 10–12 times as a course, at an interval of 3–5 days.

Ear acupuncture

Selection of points: Commonly used points — liver, pancreas, gallbladder and spleen. Supplementary points — endocrine and temple.

Manipulation: Commonly used points are the main points, and supplementary points are added according to syndromes. Three or four points are employed at each session, starting with filiform insertion after the sensitive point is found, with the needle retained for 20 min. Pressing is then done five times, with *Semen vaccariae* seeds or magnetic beads (380 G) applied to the desired point. Patients are advised to press it three times a day, and apply to it once every two or three days, 15 times as a course, at an interval of 5–7 days.

Remarks

Among the three methods above, body acupuncture is the most widely used and the most effective, and it is sure to lower the cholesterol, triglyceride, β lipoprotein and phospholipid levels with a long-term effect. The effective rate is between 51.2% and 92.1%, but much attention should be paid to the manipulating technique and the insertion time. Laser irradiation is also effective, and easy to master; it is optional for those who have the devices. Ear acupuncture, especially the pill pressing, is acceptable for patients, but it is applied to relatively few cases, and needs further practice.

HYPERTENSION

Overview

Hypertension is a chronic systemic vascular disease characterized by a rise in the arterial pressure (systolic blood pressure 140 mm Hg or more, which is equal to or more than 18.7 kPa; and/or diastolic blood pressure 90 mm Hg or more, which is equal to or more than 12.0 kPa), with the clinical manifestations of headache, stretching, dizziness, insomnia, palpitations and forgetfulness. In the late stage, organs such as the heart and the brain may be damaged. Reports about acupuncture treatment for hypertension first appeared in 1953, and since then there have been many clinical observations on various acupoint stimulations, by which a total effective rate of 71%–97% has been achieved.

Treatment

Body acupuncture

Selection of points: Commonly used points — *quchi* (LI 11) and *fengchi* (GB 20). Supplementary points — *hegu* (LI 4) and *taichong* (LR 3).

Manipulation: Commonly used points are employed as the main points, and supplementary points may be added or substituted if the effect is not desirable. Points on both sides are selected, and *quchi* (LI 11) is punctured deeply, with the needle tip inserted toward *shaohai* (HT 3) to a depth of 1.5–2.5 *cun*. On the arrival of *qi*, manipulate the needle to transmit the sensation upward and downward, by thrusting, lifting, twirling and rotating the needle for 1 min. *Fengchi* (GB 20) is punctured toward the nose tip till the sensation radiates to the forehead for 1 min. *Hegu* (LI 4) is needled in the sequence of top, bottom, left and right, with the needle retained for 30–60 min after the arrival of *qi*. Manipulate the needle once every 5–10 min during the retention, once every day or every other day, six times as a course, at an interval of three days.

Ear acupuncture

Selection of points: Commonly used points — groove of the posterior, liver, heart, sympathetic and suprarenal gland. Supplementary points — *shenmen*, ear apex and kidney.

Manipulation: Three or four points are employed at each session, and supplementary points are added according to syndromes. An adhesive plaster measuring 7×7 mm² with *Semen vaccariae* seeds is stuck closely to the desired point, pressing it until the sufferer feels distension, pain and heat in the auricle. Once every two days, stick the plaster to another point on one ear, with the two ears applied to alternately, 15 times as a course.

Moxibustion

Selection of points: Commonly used points — two groups, namely (1) *zusanli* (ST 36) and *xuanzhong* (GB 39), and (2) *baihui* (DU 20) and *yongquan* (KI 1). Supplementary points — *fengchi* (GB 20), *yanglingquan* (GB 34), *zhaohai* (KI 6) and *weizhong* (BL 40).

Manipulation: Commonly used points are taken as the principal points, and supplementary points are added when the effect is not satisfactory. The first group is given direct moxibustion with moxa cones (nonscarring moxibustion) on both sides. The sufferer is in the recumbent position, with the points fully exposed. After being sterilized with 75% ethyl alcohol, the desired area is smeared with garlic juice or Vaseline ointment. Put a moxa cone of a kernel size on the point, ignited by a joss stick. When the sufferer feels burning discomfort, remove it and place another one with a pair of forceps. Repeat the course 3–5 times. The second group is given moxibustion with moxa rolls on two or three points at each session. Sparrow-pecking moxibustion is applied to *baihui* (DU 20). The moxa roll having been ignited, approach the point from a distance until the sufferer complains of burning discomfort, then lift the roll toward *baihui* from a distance. Repeat the course 10 times, between which there should be an interval so as to avoid blistering. Mild-warming moxibustion is applied to *yongquan* (KI 1) bilaterally at the same time. With the patient in the supine position, put the moxa roll ignited between 2 cm and 3 cm for moxibustion, till the patient feels warm but not burning pain. The moxibustion lasts for 15–20 min each time. Supplementary points are given mild-warming moxibustion the same way as above, once a day, 10 times as a course.

Remarks

The three methods above are all applicable, especially the otopoint pill-pressing method, which is easy and convenient, allows one to plaster continuously, and is suitable for hypertension in particular. If it is combined with body acupuncture and moxibustion, a better effect will be achieved. However, acupuncture for treatment of hypertension is obviously effective for patients at an early stage. For those taking medicine, hypotensive drugs should not be stopped suddenly, but gradually till there is a maintenance dose. It is noted that *zusanli* (ST 36) and *xuanzhong* (GB 39) are the typical principal points for preventing wind stroke, and have been proven to be effective for various strokes in modern studies. So they can be used for health purposes, even for patients at a later stage.

QUESTIONS

(1) What are the point stimulations for hyperlipoproteinemia?
(2) What are the ways to treat hypertension?

CHAPTER 21

Acupuncture and Moxibustion for Diseases of the Digestive and Blood Systems

HICCUPS

Overview

Hiccups refer to phrenospasms. They are involuntary spasms of the glottis and diaphragm. Occasional attacks of hiccups suggest a mild case and are physical in nature, but if they persist and have nothing to do with eating, they are pathological and treatment is required. The causes of hiccups are classified as reflex, central, metabolic disorders and mental.

Acupuncture therapy is mainly to treat stubborn pathological hiccups. Hiccups are one of the traditional indications for acupuncture and moxibustion, with abundant clinical material. The first report in modern times appeared in 1957, but only since the late 1980s has the acupuncture treatment for hiccups been mature, with plentiful clinical material. Many effective point selections and prescriptions have been collected through observations on differentiation prescription, differentiation point selection and employment of points previously used. Acupoint stimulations also vary greatly, including body acupuncture, acupuncture and moxibustion, ear acupuncture and eye acupuncture, with satisfactory effect. Besides, quite a few cases of stubborn hiccups have been reported to have been cured by acupuncture and moxibustion.

Treatment

Acupuncture

Selection of points: Commonly used point — *zhongkui* (EX-UE4).

Manipulation: Zhongkui (EX-UE4) is employed for needling or moxibustion. With the patient lying on his or her back, the clothes loosened and the local skin sterilized, No. 28 filiform needles 0.5–1 *cun* in length are inserted perpendicularly into *zhongkui* (EX-UE4) of both the right and the left, to a depth of 0.2 mm, twirling and rotating the needles to reinforce the stimulation. While inserting the needles, ask the patient to draw a deep breath from the nose and feel suffocated to the maximum, which may be repeated 3–5 times during the insertion. As soon as the hiccups stop, advise the patient to do abdominal breathing with the needles retained for 30 min, manipulating the needles once every 5 min. An electroacupuncture device may be used for 30 min with an intermittent wave to a degree that the patient can tolerate. Moxibustion is applicable, and is suitable for severe cases. Place a little Vaseline to *zhongkui* (EX-UE4), put a moxa cone of a kernel size on the point, and ignite it for 5–7 cones successively, once or twice a day. If there is seepage from a moxibustion scar, smear gentian violet and cover it with sterilized gauze.

Needle-like finger pressing

Selection of points: Commonly used points — *yifeng* (SJ 17) and *tianding* (LI 17). Supplementary points — *neiguan* (PC 6) and *zusanli* (ST 36).

Manipulation: One commonly used point is employed at each session, and supplementary points may be added if the curative effect is not obvious. Press hard with the thumb pulp on *yifeng* (SJ 17) till pain arises, or press toward the mandible for 1 min. If not cured for one time, repeat the pressing. *Tianding* (LI 7) is pressed with the thumb pulp or middle finger pulp for 1–3 min. *Cuanzhu* (BL 2) is pressed hard with both thumbs, with the other fingers sticking to *shuaigu* (GB 8), for 5–10 min, until a sensation of soreness and distension arises. Press with the thumb pulp on *neiguan* (PC 6), slightly at first, then heavily till the patient complains of soreness, distension and numbness at the point area, 5–10 min every time, and repeat the manipulation for obstinate cases.

Ear acupuncture

Selection of points: Commonly used points — ear center and stomach. Supplementary points — liver, spleen, sympathetic, *shenmen*, subcortex and adrenal gland.

Manipulation: Commonly used points are employed, and two or three supplementary points may be added according to symptoms. Apply shallow puncture to the ear center for drainage with a filiform needle, twirling and rotating for half a minute before penetrating needling is applied to the stomach, lifting and thrusting the needle till the arrival of *qi*, and implanting the needle with adhesive tape for 1–2 days, according to different symptoms. Supplementary points are punctured, with the needles retained for 30 min. Generally, both sides are selected.

Body acupuncture

Selection of points: Commonly used point — *xiangu* (ST 43).

Manipulation: With the patient in the supine or sitting posture, and bilateral points selected, a filiform needle 2 *cun* long is inserted toward the planter center to a depth of 1.5 *cun*, with twirling and rotating for 5 min. Meanwhile, the patient is required to inhale a deep breath and hold it as long as possible and then exhale the breath slowly with the needle retained for 30 min, during which the patient may repeat the breath-holding. Manipulate the needle once every 5 min, once a day, 10 times as a course.

Remarks

Many methods can treat hiccups, and here only four have been introduced. The first one is acupuncture and moxibustion applicable to hiccups due to different factors, with only one point selected. The finger-pressing method is used for those with a short course of disease or light symptoms, for it is convenient, practical, and may be performed at any time, without any apparatus. Ear acupuncture is for those suffering repeated attacks, and is also used after acupuncture and moxibustion to prevent recurrence. Body acupuncture is applicable to obstinate cases, but it is painful and fainting during the acupuncture must be avoided.

CHRONIC GASTRITIS

Overview

Chronic gastritis refers to various chronic inflammations involving gastric mucus due to different pathogenic factors. The main manifestations are recurrent fullness, and oppression and pain in the middle and the upper abdomen. The gastritis varies in the clinic, and acupuncture and moxibustion are applied to superficial and chronic atrophic types. Modern reports were seen in 1954, but a great number of studies about acupuncture and moxibustion for chronic gastritis did not appear until the 1980s. Now, the effective rate of various acupoint stimulations is 90%; they are especially effective for pure superficial gastritis.

Treatment

Acupoint injection

Selection of points: Commonly used points — *ganshu* (BL 18), *weishu* (BL 21) and *zusanli* (ST 36). Supplementary point — *dannang* (EX-LE6).

Manipulation: Choose one of the injections — Huanqi (astragalus), vitamin B12 (50 mcg) or vitamin C injection — or use them alternately. Two pairs of points are selected each time and *dannang* (EX-LE6) may be added if there is complicated cholecystitis. A No. 5 pinhead for dentistry and a 5 ml injector are used to insert into *ganshu* (BL 18) and *weishu* (BL 21) obliquely toward the spine, and perpendicularly into *zusanli* (ST 36) and *dannang* (EX-LE6) till the arrival of *qi*. Slightly lift and thrust the needle to cause a stronger sensation of needling before injecting the liquor. The manipulation is performed once every other day for three months as a course, at an interval of seven days between courses.

Ear acupuncture

Selection of points: Commonly used points — stomach, spleen, subcortex, duodenum and sympathetic. Supplementary points — liver and *shenmen*.

Manipulation: Three commonly used points are employed at each treatment session, and one or two supplementary points are added according to symptoms. Find the tenderness at the point area and make a mark, then stick an adhesive tape with *Vacca segetalis* seeds onto the tenderness. Ask the patient to press it 5 times a day, for 2–3 min each time. Change to another plaster on the third day, one ear each time and the two ears alternately, 10 times as a course, at an interval of 5 days.

Body acupuncture

Selection of points: Commonly used points — *zusanli* (ST 36), *neiguan* (PC 6), *pishu* (BL 20) and *weishu* (BL 21). Supplementary points — *sanyinjiao* (SP 6), *qimen* (LR 14) and *zhangmen* (LR 13).

Manipulation: Two or three commonly used points are employed at each session, and one or two supplementary points are added according to symptoms. On the arrival of *qi*, retain the needle for 15–30 min. Then withdraw it and apply warm moxibustion with moxa sticks on *pishu* (BL 20) and *weishu* (BL 21) for 10–15 min, till the local skin becomes red. The manipulation is applied once every day or every other day, 10 times as a course, at an interval of 5 days between courses.

Remarks

Acupoint injection, as the first choice among the three methods, was applied to 240 cases, for which the excellence rate was 54.6% and the total effective rate 92.9%. Pressing the auricular points is easy to perform and has a certain effect in improving chronic gastritis, though only working as a complementary therapy. Body acupuncture is mainly applicable to those with obvious symptoms and a short course of disease, but is less effective for the old.

QUESTIONS

(1) Describe in detail the acupuncture and moxibustion for treating hiccups.

(2) What are the point stimulations for treating chronic gastritis?

PEPTIC ULCER

Overview

A peptic ulcer is a chronic ulcer only seen in the contact area of the gastrointestinal tract and gastric juice. Also called a gastric or duodenal ulcer, it is clinically marked by periodic and rhythmic attacks and abdominal pain, often accompanied by belching, acid regurgitation, nausea and vomiting. This disease usually occurs to young people and people in the prime of their lives. It pertains to the concept of epigastralgia in TCM. Acupuncture and moxibustion for epigastralgia was recorded in *Neijing* (*The Inner Classic*). Modern reports appeared in the 1950s, and multiple-point stimulations since the 1970s have improved the effectiveness. Now, an effective rate of 85% has been achieved.

Treatment

Acupoint injection

Selection of points: Commonly used points — *zusanli* (ST 36), *zhongwan* (RN 12), *pishu* (BL 20) and *weishu* (BL 21). Supplementary points — *yanglingquan* (GB 34) is added for abdominal distension, *jianjing* (GB 21) for nausea and *neiguan* (PC 6) for vomiting.

Manipulation: Three or Four commonly used points are employed at each session. Vitamin B1 injection 100 mg (2 ml) and vitamin B12 injection 250 mcg (1 ml), mixed intensively with an 5 ml injector, is injected slowly into the selected points on the arrival of *qi*, 0.5 ml for each point, once a day, 10 times as a course, at an interval of 1 week.

Body acupuncture

Selection of points: Commonly used points — *zhongwan* (RN 12), *zhangmen* (LR 13), *pishu* (BL 20), *weishu* (BL 21), *neiguan* (PC 6) and *zusanli* (ST 36). Supplementary points — *gongsun* (SP 4), *sanyinjiao* (SP 6), *liangqiu* (ST 34), *qimen* (LR 14) and *yanglingquan* (GB 34).

Manipulation: Four or five commonly used points are employed at each session, and supplementary points may be added according to symptoms. On the arrival of *qi*, thrusting, lifting, twirling and rotating is applied, with the retention of the needles for 30 min. The manipulation is performed once a day, 10 times as a course, at an interval of 3 days. Generally, 3–6 courses are needed for peptic ulcers.

Moxibustion

Selection of points: Commonly used points — *zhongwan* (RN 20), *liang-men* (ST 21) and *zusanli* (ST 36). Supplementary points — *pishu* (BL 20) and *weishu* (BL 21).

Manipulation: All the commonly used points and one supplementary point (the two used alternately) are employed at each session. Pecking moxibustion with moxa sticks is applied to points of the abdomen and the back, 5–10 min for each point, until the local skin becomes hot and red. For *zusanli* (ST 36), nonscarring direct moxibustion is applied with a moxa cone, once every day or every other day, 7–9 cones each time, 30 times as a course.

Remarks

A peptic ulcer is hard to cure and the three methods are all effective in treatment. Point injection is the commonly used one and was applied to 90 cases with a total effective rate of 97.8%, significantly higher than that for patients taking or injected with Tagamet. Moxibustion is mainly applicable to patients with a weak constitution, a long course of disease, and pain worsened by catching a cold or taking cold food. Body acupuncture is for ordinary peptic ulcers. It is worth noting that whichever the method is, the patient is asked to undergo long-term treatment with stable emotion and a regular life. Catgut implantation at the acupoint is another commonly used and effective therapy, but here it is ignored due to its complicated manipulaiton.

CHRONIC ULCERATIVE COLITIS

Overview

Chronic ulcerative colitis refers to an inflammation of the colon stratum mucosum without a known cause. Common clinical symptoms include abdominal pain, diarrhea, stools with blood, pus and mucus, often accompanied by tenesmus, pain relieved after defecation, slow progression of pathological conditions, recurrence and difficulty in healing. This disease tends to grow in number in China. It belongs to the syndrome categories of *chang pi* and *li ji* (dysentery) in TCM. Records of acupuncture and moxibustion for treatment first appeared in *Zhen Jiu Jia Yi Jing* (*The Yellow Emperor's Systematic Classic of Acupuncture and Moxibustion in Three Parts*). But the disease was only identified in articles about acupuncture and moxibustion in the 1980s. At present moxibustion is the first choice in treatment and an effective rate of 90% has been achieved.

Treatment

Moxibustion

Selection of points: Commonly used points — two groups, namely (1) *zhongwan* (RN 20), *tianshu* (ST 25) and *guanyuan* (RN 4), and (2) *shangjuxu* (ST 37). Supplementary points — *pishu* (BL 20), *dachangshu* (BL 25) and *zusanli* (ST 36).

Manipulation: Either group of the commonly used points is employed, and one or two supplementary points may be added according to symptoms with different manipulations.

Group 1: Two moxibustion boxes (wooden, with a layer of wire gauze in the middle and a wooden cover) are employed. Ignite four or five moxa cones 1–3 *cun* long, before putting them in the boxes, a small and a large one. The patient takes the supine position, with the abdomen exposed. Put the small box on *zhongwan* (RN 20), and the large one on *tianshu* (ST 25) and *guanyuan* (RN 4). Cover the boxes incompletely, with a gap of 1–2 cm. The temperature is tolerable to the patient. If it is too hot, disperse the moxa cones or lift the box higher. Generally, the temperature will go down in 30 min and the moxibustion will finish in 40 min.

Group 2: Bilateral *shangjuxu* (ST 37) is given nonscarring direct moxibustion with 5–7 cones in a soybean size, and point combination moxibustion with moxa sticks in a sparrow-pecking way for 15–20 min each time till the point area becomes red. The manipulation is applied once every day or every other day, 15–20 times as a course, at an interval of 5 days.

Body acupuncture

Selection of points: Commonly used points — two groups, namely (1) four points around the umbilicus (1 *cun* above, below, and left and right of the umbilicus) and (2) *tianshu* (ST 25), *guanyuan* (RN 4) and *qihai* (RN 6). Supplementary points — *dachangshu* (BL 25), *changqiang* (DU 1), *pishu* (BL 20), *weishu* (BL 21), *zusanli* (ST 36) and *sanyinjiao* (SP 6).

Manipulation: One group is employed at each session, with the two groups alternately used, and two or three supplementary points may be added according to symptoms. With the patient in the supine position, No. 28–30 filiform needles are quickly inserted into the four points selected in the sequence of above, below, left and right, to a depth of 3–5 *cun*, with slow manipulation by twirling and rotating the needle for half a minute without retention. For *tianshu* (ST 25), *qihai* (RN 6) and *guanyuan* (RN 4), the needles are inserted to 1–1.5 *cun* deep with reinforcing manipulation by thrusting, lifting, twirling and rotating at high frequency until the needle sensation is radiated to the abdomen and the external genitalia. *Dachangshu* (BL 25), *pishu* (BL 20) and *weishu* (BL 21) are needled obliquely toward the spine to a depth of 1.5 *cun*; *changqiang* (DU 1), *zusanli* (ST 36) and *sanyinjiao* (SP 6) are needled perpendicularly to 1–1.5 *cun* deep until the arrival of *qi* by twirling and rotating. The needles are retained in each point for 15–20 min, once every 5 min. The manipulation is applied once every day or every other day, 10 times as a course.

Remarks

Both methods are commonly used in treatment, especially moxibustion as it is more effective. Without the box, sparrow-pecking moxibustion may be applied with moxa sticks for about 30 min, and is applicable to beginners due to its convenience and safety. Body acupuncture requires the achievement of *qi*, skilled manipulation and no deep insertion, for the points selected all carry danger. This disease is obstinate, recurrent and takes a long time to heal. If recurrence occurs, nonscarring direct moxibustion may be applied on *zusanli* (ST 36).

QUESTIONS

(1) What are the point stimulations for treating peptic ulcers?
(2) Describe how to apply moxibustion and body acupuncture to treat chronic ulcerative colitis.

APLASTIC ANEMIA

Overview

Aplastic anemia is a syndrome of bone marrow failure clinically manifested by worsening anemia, bleeding and infections. Acupuncture and moxibusiton is mainly applied to treat chronic cases, which are characterized by slowly occurring anemia, lassitude, dizziness, panickiness, a pale face, and other light symptoms such as infections, bleeding and fever. The syndrome belongs to the categories of *xu lao* or *xu sun* (consumptive diseases) in TCM. Acupuncture and moxibustion for treatment of *xu lao* was recorded in *Bei Ji Qian Jin Yao Fang* (*Important Formulas Worth a Thousand Gold Pieces for Emergencies*) in the Tang Dynasty. Modern reports were seen in the 1960s. The effective rate varies greatly, from about 45% to 80%, due to varied criteria.

Treatment

Acupoint injection

Selection of points: Commonly used points — *zusanli* (ST 36), *geshu* (BL 17), *shenshu* (BL 23) and *gaohuang* (BL 43). Supplementary points — *quchi* (RN 6) added for fever, *xuehai* (SP 10) for bleeding, *ganshu* (BL 18) for hepatomegaly and *pishu* (BL 20) for splenomegaly.

Manipulation: Select one of the three injections: 50% biostimulin, Dang Gui Zhu She Ye (injection of *Angelica sinensis*) and Dan Shen Zhu She Ye (injection of *Salvia miltiorrhiza*). Two pairs of commonly used points are employed and used alternately, and supplementary points are added according to symptoms. No. 5 needles for dentistry are inserted into the points selected (obliquely toward the spine to points of the back) until the arrival of *qi*. Thrust and lift the needles with medium strength before injecting the liquor, with biostimulin 2 ml and *Angelica sinensis* or *Salvia miltiorrhiza* 1 ml, into each point. The injection requires deeper insertion, quicker infusion and obvious needle sense. The manipulation is applied once every other day, or acupuncture and injection are applied alternately day by day, 10 times as a course; the next course begins after a 5-day interval.

Electroacupuncture

Selection of points: Commonly used point — *dazhui* (DU 14). Supplementary points — *shenshu* (BL 23), *zusanli* (ST 36), *gaohuang* (BL 43) and *xuehai* (SP 10).

Manipulation: The commonly used point and two supplementary points (selected alternately) are employed at each session. On the arrival of *qi*, connect to the electroacupuncture apparatus with a continuous wave at a frequency of 100 cpm, and with the strength tolerable to the patient. Thirty minutes is needed each time, once a day, 10 times as a course; the next course begins after 3–5 days.

Remarks

The two methods are the most commonly used for treating aplastic anemia, with obvious effect, but relatively few cases have been observed than for other diseases, e.g. 18 cases with point injection and only 11 with elctroacupuncture. The former cases were followed up for 2–8 years, proving long-term effectiveness by point injection. It is worth noting that both methods need a combination of Chinese and Western medicine in treatment.

THROMBOCYTOPENIC PURPURA

Overview

Thrombocytopenic purpura is a commonly seen disease in hematopathy, clinically manifested by spontaneous ecchymoses and hemorrhage from mucus and viscera, thrombocytopenia and bleeding time increase seen in chemical examination. It is either primary or secondary, the former including acute and chronic types. Acupuncture and moxibustion is mainly applied to chronic cases. The disease belongs to the categories of *zi ban* (peliona) and *xue zheng* (blood syndromes) in TCM. No classic recorded the treatment of *zi ban* with acupuncture, while ancient documents about treatment of blood syndromes appeared a lot. Modern reports were first seen in 1958. More people and more institutions have been studying the disease with acupuncture and moxibustion in the past 30 years, and an effective rate of 80% has been achieved.

Treatment

Body acupuncture

Selection of points: Commonly used points — *geshu* (BL 17), *pishu* (BL 20), *xuehai* (SP 10) and *sanyinjiao* (SP 6). Supplementary points — *yongquan* (KI 1) and *jiaji* (EX-B2) at the 11th thoracic vertebra and the 7th thoracic vertebra.

Manipulation: Mostly the commonly used points are employed. If obvious effect is not achieved, supplementary points may be added or employed. Three or four points are selected at each session. First, puncture *geshu* (BL 17) and *pishu* (BL 20), with the needles inserted obliquely toward the vertebrae at 2 cm lateral to the point, at an angle of 45°, to a depth of 1.5 *cun*. On the arrival of *qi*, reinforcing manipulation is applied by lifing, trusting, twirling and rotating the needle, and withdraw the needle after 5 min of retention. Then puncture perpendicularly *xuehai* (SP 10) and *sanyinjiao* (SP 6) in the same way and manipulate the needles three times during the retention. For supplementary points, puncture the two *jiaji* points (EX-B2) with a retention of 5–8 min after the arrival of *qi*. Puncture *yongquan* (KI 1) swiftly by twirling, rotating, lifting and thrusting the needle with powerful stimulation, without retention. The manipulation is applied once every day or every other day, 10–12 times as a course.

Moxibustion

Selection of points: *Ciliao* (BL 32) and *yaoyangguan* (DU 3).

Manipulation: Both points are given ginger moxibustion. The patient is in the prone posture, with selected points exposed completely. Smear a little paraffin oil or Vaseline on the points to prevent scalding or improve the adhesiveness. The method involves putting a slice of ginger about 0.25 cm thick on a hard slip measuring about 7×7 cm^2, and then putting a cup-like moxa cone measuring 4 mm high and 6×6 mm^2 on the ginger, igniting the cone and placing it on the points. The local area feels warm. If the patient complains of a burning pain, make a slight move. Two cones is needed for *ciliao* (BL 32) and one for *yaoyangguan* (DU 3). The manipulation is applied once a day, 10 times as a course, at an interval of 5–7 days.

Otopoint pill pressing

Selection of points: Commonly used points — spleen, liver, stomach and ear center. Supplementary points — lung and subcortex.

Manipulation: Mainly the commonly used points are employed, and supplementary points may be added according to symptoms. Sterilize the ear with 75% alcohol and massage it for 1 min, until local hyperemia appears. Stick vaccaria seeds or magnetic beads (about 380 G) on an adhesive tape measuring 7×7 mm^2, and press this on the tenderness. Ask the patient to press the point 3–5 times a day, 1 min for each point, with the two ears applied to alternately. Change the stick 3 times a week for 2 weeks as a course, at an interval of 5 days.

Remarks

The three methods are all commonly used in the treatment of thrombocytopenic purpura. Body acupuncture was applied to 59 cases, with an excellence rate of 40.7% and an effective rate of 78.0%. It is the first choice for those with practical experience, since the treatment standard is more stringent. Moxibustion and otopoint pressing, applicable to beginners, need further verification, because of their low treatment standard and relatively few cases, though their effective rates are higher (93.3% and 100%, respectively).

QUESTIONS

(1) What is aplastic anemia? What are the point stimulations in the treatment?

(2) Describe how to manipulate acupuncture in the treatment of thrombocytopenic purpura.

CHAPTER 22

Acupuncture and Moxibustion for Diseases of the Metabolic and Immune Systems

DIABETES

Overview

Diabetes is a metabolic endocrine disease, divided into primary and secondary cases. Primary diabetes is more frequent in the clinic. It shows no symptoms at the early stage, followed by polyphagia, polydipsia, polyuria, fatigue and emaciation, usually leading to diseases of cadiovascular, kidney, ocular and nervous lesions in severe cases. Primary diabetes is further divided into "insulin-dependent" (attacking from childhood with a severe syndrome) and "non-insulin-dependent" (attacking from adulthood with a light syndrome). Acupuncture and moxibustion is mainly applied to the latter. Diabetes is similar to *xiao ke* in TCM, and treatment records appeared as early as in the Spring and Autumn Period and the Warring States Period. Modern reports were first seen in 1943. It has been proven that acupuncture and moxibustion is effective for light and moderate non-insulin-dependent diabetes, and more effective for overweight and medium-sized patients than for slim ones. Besides, acupuncture and moxibustion has a satisfactory effect on diabetic complications.

TREATMENT

Body acupuncture

Selection of points: Commonly used points — *pishu* (BL 20), *geshu* (BL 17) and *zusanli* (ST 36). Supplementary points — *yixue* (EX-B3) (tender spot lateral to 6ᵗʰ–8ᵗʰ thoracic vertebrae), *diji* (SP 8), *yinlingquan*

(SP 9), *fuliu* (KI 7), *taixi* (KI 3), *sanyinjiao* (SP 6), *feishu* (BL 13) and *shenshu* (BL 23).

Manipulation: Commonly used points and two or three supplementary points are employed at each session, and supplementary points may be selected alternately. On the arrival of *qi*, press the needle swiftly and lift it slowly more than 10 times, followed by pressing slowly and lifting swiftly. The needles are retained in each point for 30 min. This is performed once more before withdrawing the needle. The manipulation is applied once a day, 10 times as a course, at an interval of 3–5 days.

Warm needling

Selection of points: Commonly used points — *pishu* (BL 20), *yishu* (EX–B3) (1.5 *cun* lateral to the posterior midline, below the 8th thoracic vertebra), *shenshu* (BL 23) and *feishu* (BL 13). Supplementary point — *geshu* (BL 17).

Manipulation: Two pairs of commonly used points are employed at each session, and *geshu* (BL 17) may be added for long courses. Prepare pure moxa cones cut to a section 1.5–2.0 cm long, and a fresh tangerine peel as thin as possible, or a softened tangerine peel. Cut the fresh tangerine peel into a $2 \times 2 \, cm^2$ piece, and then make an incision 1 cm long from the edge to the center. The points selected are given routine sterilization before inserting a filiform needle 1.5–2.0 cm long slightly obliquely toward the spinal column with lifting, thrusting, twirling and rotating till the needling sensation arises and the needles are retained in the points. The tip of the needle handle is inserted into a moxa section, penetrating the fresh peel close to the skin, with the inner side facing the skin, and a hard slip between the peel and the cone for fear that the moxa will injure the skin. Ignite the cone and withdraw the needle till the cone is burnt out. The manipulation is applied once a day, 10 times as a course, at an interval of 3–5 days between courses.

Ear acupuncture

Selection of points: Commonly used points — pancreas, gallbladder and endocrine. Supplementary points — kidney, root of the ear vagus, *shenmen*, heart and liver.

Manipulation: Commonly used points and one or two supplementary points are employed at each session. For the first course, bilateral points are selected and applied with filiform needles. On the arrival of *qi*, the needles are retained for 20–30 min. For the second course, if the symptoms are relieved, ear pressing may be applied with vaccaria seeds or magnetic beads (380 G) to one ear, twice a week, with the two ears used alternately. One course needs three months.

Remarks

Body acupuncture and warm needling are both effective in lowering blood glucose and urine glucose, and improving clinical symptoms, with a similar curative effect. But be careful not to needle the points of the back perpendicularly and deeply. Ear acupuncture is applicable to levis diabetes and effective in curing such complications as multiple folliculitis or itchy skin.

OBESITY

Overview

Obesity is a medical condition in which excess body fat caused by excessive food energy intake has accumulated to the extent that it may have an adverse effect on health. Generally, if a person's body weight is 25% higher than it should be, he or she is considered obese. The standard body weight is calculated by the formula "body weight (kg) = body height (cm) — 105" or defined by the body mass index (BMI = kilograms/meters^2). For Chinese people, if their BMI is greater than 24 kg/m^2, they are defined as obese. Obesity is classified into simple obesity, secondary obesity and other obesity, while simple obesity is subdivided into physical obesity and acquired obesity. Acupuncture treatment is mainly for simple obesity, especially acquired obesity. There is not any case treated with acupuncture in ancient books. Starting in the 1970s, it became popular in the U.S. and Japan. In China, the first report was seen in 1974 and the material concerned increased rapidly. It is affirmative about acupuncture for obesity, with a cure rate of 70%–80%.

Treatment

Ear acupuncture

Selection of points: Commonly used points — mouth, endocrine, central rim, stomach. Supplementary points — lung, spleen, *shenmen*, large intestine.

Manipulation: Three or four commonly used points and one or two supplementary points are employed at each treatment session. Sensitive points having been found, place an adhesive plaster with vaccaria seeds on the point, and press and squeeze it with the thumb and forefinger until the auricle becomes hot and red. The sufferer is advised to press it three or four times a day. One ear is applied to at each session; two ears alternately. This manipulation is repeated two or three times a week, at 10 sessions as a course, at an interval of 5–7 days.

Electroacupuncture

Selection of points: Commonly used points — *tianshu* (ST 25), *zhongwan* (RN 20) and *daheng* (SP 15). Supplementary points — *quchi* (LI 11), *hegu* (LI 4), *gaohuang* (BL 43), *neiting* (ST 44) and *sanyinjiao* (SP 6).

Manipulation: Commonly used points are employed at each treatment session, and supplementary points may be added according to the curative effect. A filiform needle 2–2.5 *cun* in length is inserted directly into *zhongwan* (RN 20), to a depth of 1.5–2 *cun*, and the other two points are punctured by piercing toward the medioventral line till the adipose layer (caution: Do not pierce the peritoneum), thrusting, lifting, twirling and rotating the needles with medium strength for 1–2 min, and the needles are retained. *Tianshu* (ST 25) and *daheng* (SP 15) are connected to an electric acupuncture device with an irregular wave to a degree the patient can tolerate. Supplementary points are punctured with the routine methods, with the needles retained on the arrival of *qi* for 15–20 min. The manipulation is given once every day or every other day, at 10 sessions as a course.

Body acupuncture

Selection of points: Jianyu (LI 15) to *quchi* (LI 11), *liangqiu* (ST 34) to *biguan* (DU 20), and *liangmen* (ST 21) to *tianshu* (ST 25).

Manipulation: No. 28 filiform needles 1–1.5 *chi* long are prepared. With all the upper points selected and the local skin sterilized, hold the needle with the right hand, with the tip touching the point, then insert the needle quickly with the help of the left hand in a twirling and pressing manner till it reaches the other point, and meanwhile manipulation is given with twirling and rotating of the needle within a range of 180°–360°, till a sensation of soreness and distension is achieved. The needle is retained for 30 min, once a day, at 6 sessions as a course, at an interval of 2–3 days.

Remarks

Of the three methods, pressing with vaccaria seeds is the most convenient and popular to the patients. Thousands of cases have proven that its effective rate is about 85%, with a lower excellence rate, and the loss of weight between 1 kg and 3 kg. Electroacupuncture is similar to the pressing method in effect but the improvement rate is significantly higher. The best method is body acupuncture, which is difficult to operate since accidents may occur due to incorrect needling. So it should be used with caution by beginners.

QUESTIONS

(1) Describe how to manipulate the stimulation of the two points in the treatment of diabetes.
(2) What are the three methods in the treatment of obesity with acupuncture and moxibustion?

GOUT

Overview

Gout is a disease caused by a set of purine metabolism disorders, and is usually seen in males. Acute gouty arthritis is the most usual way in which gout is present. It is characterized by a rapid and sudden onset, with the lower extremity joints commonly affected. It affects the patient to the peak in hours, and the joints and the soft tissue around feel hot and painful usually during the night, and do not get complete relief until after several days or weeks of recurrent attacks. Gout used to be rare in China, but it has increased in recent decades due to improvements in diet and longer life expectancy. Western medicine has specific remedies, but no radical cure for lack of etiological treatment. Acupuncture and moxibustion for gout was first seen in 1981, and new reports did not appear until 1991, with 20 articles. In treatment, besides body acupuncture, there is bloodletting with plum blossom needles or three-edged needles, fire needling, cupping, intradermal needling, ear acupuncture, and other methods combined with _tuina_, and Chinese drugs for oral use or application. Patients include those with gouty deposition as well as those with acute gouty arthritis. An effective rate is above 90%. Quite a few patients were followed up and no recurrence was found, which proved that acupuncture has a good long-term curative effect and is worth generalizing.

Treatment

Body acupuncture

Selection of points: Commonly used points — two groups, namely (1) _zusanli_ (ST 36), _yanglingquan_ (GB 34) and _sanyinjiao_ (SP 6), and (2) _quchi_ (LI 11). Supplementary points — two groups, namely (1) _taibai_ (SP 3) for gout on the medial malleolus and _qiuxu_ (GB 40) for gout on the lateral malleolus, and (2) _hegu_ (LI 4).

Manipulation: The first groups are selected for lesions in the lower limbs; the second, for lesions in the upper limbs. Commonly used points are employed as the main points, and supplementary points may be added according to symptoms. A filiform needle 10–1.5 _cun_ long is inserted and reinforcing–reducing manipulation is applied by twirling, rotating, lifting and thrusting the needle on the arrival of _qi_; reducing is applied in the acute phase, and uniform reinforcing–reducing at the convalescence stage, with a retention of 30 min in each point. Needle the points once every 10 min. The manipulation is applied once every day or every other day, 7–10 times as a course, at an interval of 3–5 days between courses.

Bloodletting

Selection of points: Commonly used points — two groups, namely (1) *ashi* point, *taichong* (LR 3), *neiting* (ST 44) and corresponding points, and (2) *quchi* (LI 11), *yangchi* (SJ 4), *yangxi* (LI 5), *taichong* (LR 3), *qiuxu* (GB 40), *taixi* (KI 3), *yanglingquan* (GB 34) and *xuehai* (SP 10). *Ashi* point — points with the most obvious red swelling, hot and painful. Corresponding points — points corresponding to the *ashi* point on the uninjured side.

Manipulation: One group only or two groups alternately are employed at each session. For the first group, select points on the affected side; for the second group, select alternately two or three points bilaterally, except for *yangchi* (SJ 4), *taixi* (KI 3) and *xuehai* (SP 10) on the affected side. For acupuncture on the first group, prick the *Ashi* point with a three-edged needle, with drops from bloodletting; then insert a No. 26 filiform needle, 1.5 *cun* long, into the corresponding point, accompanied by needling *taichong* (LR 3) and *neiting* (ST 44) at an angle of 15°, surrounding the *Ashi* point (the tips of the three needles are pointing to the bloodletting spot), with reducing manipulation, and the needles retained for 30 min. For the second group, tap the point area with fingers several times, till local congestion arises; this is followed by routine sterilization. Press the area beside the acupoint with the left hand to tense the skin when the small-size three-edged needle pricks the points swiftly to different depths according to different points; when pressing and squeezing for bloodletting, some points may be applied to with cupping, with a blood volume of 3–10 ml. Sterilize the local area, then pack and fix it with dressings. Both manipulations are applied once or twice, 3–7 times as a course, at an interval of 1 week between courses.

Fire needling

Selection of points: Commonly used points — *xingjian* (LR 2), *taichong* (LR 3), *neiting* (ST 44) and *xiangu* (ST 43). Supplementary points — *qiuxu* (GB 40), *dadu* (SP 2), *taibai* (SP 3), *xuehai* (SP 10), *geshu* (BL 17), *fenglong* (ST 40), *pishu* (BL 20), *taixi* (KI 3) and *sanyinjiao* (SP 6).

Manipulation: Two of the common used points are employed at each session, and one or two supplementary points are added according to symptoms, with thick fire needles for points on the foot and thin needles for points above the ankle joint. When one is needling points on the foot, the patient is in a standing or sitting position with layers of towels beneath the feet. Sterilize the points with iodine tincture and 75% alcohol, burn a fire needle with a spirit lamp from red to bright, and insert it swiftly to a depth of 0.3–1 *cun*, with 1–3 insertions for each point. Dark-red blood may spurt out from the pinhole while one is withdrawing the needle. Do not stop the bleeding until the blood amounts to 10–30 ml. Generally, blood is dark-red at the beginning, and it will stop when it turns light-red. If not, press to stop the bleeding. For acupoints above the ankle, with the patient in a sitting position, puncture each point once. For those with gouty arthritis at an acute episode, scattered needling is done on the inflamed area several times, until there is breilike transudation. The manipulation is applied once a week, and the patient is required to keep the pinholes clean for 48 h.

Bloodletting and cupping

Selection of points: Commonly used point — *ashi* point. Location of the *ashi* point: red swelling of the skin.

Manipulation: With the patient in a lying posture, sterilize the *ashi* point and knock hard with a seven-star needle till the skin bleeds. It is important to knock all over the skin of the red swelling. This is followed by cupping it instantly. For facets, vials of penicillin, debottomed and burnished, may be used for cupping with the degassing method. When static blood is out, withdraw the jar and wipe away the blood with dry cotton balls. The manipulation is applied with 5–10 ml of blood out of each point each time, twice a week, four times as a course.

Remarks

Among the four methods mentioned above, body acupuncture is applicable to gout at both the acute stage and the convalescent stage; for the other three, at the acute stage. Body acupuncture emphasizes manipulating skill, while the other three methods are all bloodletting and fire needling requiring clinical experience. The other three methods all focus on the *ashi* point or points around the affected area, with fewer points but a greater amount of blood. Caution: The bloodletting method is forbidden in cases with hematologic disease.

HYPERTHYROIDISM

Overview

Hyperthyroidism is due to excessive secretion of thyroxin, and is clinically marked by irritability, shortness of breath, increased sweating, polyphagia, emaciation, exophthalmia, thyroid diffusive swelling, etc. This disease is usually seen among women between 20 and 40 years old. It belongs to the category of *yingbing* (goiter) in TCM. Acupuncture and moxibustion for goiter first appeared in *Zhen Jiu Jia Yi Jing* (*The Yellow Emperor's Systematic Classic of Acupuncture and Moxibustion in Three Parts*), and the first report about modern treatment with acupuncture and moxibustion was published in 1934. More articles appeared in the 1970s and it became a hot topic in the clinical study of acupuncture and moxibustion in the 1980s. It has been proven that acupuncture and moxibustion is effective in improving not only the hypermetabolism and high circulating dynamia of hyperthyroidism, but also the endocrine exophthalmia; it has steady protective efficacy as well as obvious short-term effectiveness.

Treatment

Body acupuncture

Selection of points: Commonly used points — two groups, namely (1) *pingying* (7 *fen* lateral to cervical vertebrae No. and No. 5), *qiying* [equivalent to *tiantu* (RN 22), depending on the degree of thyromegaly] and (2) *shangtianzhu* [0.5 *cun* above *tianzhu* (BL 10)] and *fengchi* (GB 20). Supplementary points — two groups, namely (1) *neiguan* (PC 6), *jianshi* (PC 5), *zusanli* (ST 36), *sanyinjiao* (SP 6), and (2) *zanzhu* (BL 2), *sizhukong* (SJ 23) and *yangbai* (GB 14).

Manipulation: The first group of the commonly used points and of the supplementary points are applicable to various symptoms of hyperthyroidism, and the second to endocrine exophthalmia, with the commonly used points being the main points, plus two or three supplementary points according to different conditions. *Pingying* is punctured by inducing *qi*. That is to say, insert the needle to a depth of 0.5–1 *cun* and, on the arrival of *qi*, lift and thrust it slowly to send the sensation to the Adam's apple, with reducing manipulation by twirling and rotating the needle with the thumb backward; *jianshi* (PC 5) and *neiguan* (PC 6) are applied with reducing manipulation by twirling and rotating the needle with the thumb backward, accompanied by lifting gently and thrusting forcefully; *zusanli* (ST 36) and *sanyinjiao* (SP 6) are applied with reinforcing manipulation by twirling and rotating the needle with the thumb forward, also accompanied by lifting gently and thrusting forcefully. *Shangtianzhu* and *fengchi* (GB 20) are punctured to a depth of 1.2–1.5 *cun*, with the tips inserted obliquely toward the apex of the nose at an angle of 75°, by inducing *qi* with slow insertion and slow withdrawal, till the needling sensation reaches the eye area. Triple needling is applied to *zanzhu* (BL 2), *sizhukong* (SJ 23) and *yangbai* (GB 14) in the direction of the middle of the eyebrow. The needles are retained in each point for 30 min, once every day or every other day, 50 times as a course.

Acupoint injection

Selection of points: Shangtianzhu.

Manipulation: Prepare hyaluronidase 1500 units plus cortisone acetate 25 mg for injection. A No. 5 pinhead for dentistry is inserted swiftly to a depth of 1–1.5 *cun*, liftling and trusting the needle slightly, and injecting the liquor slowly, with the sensation radiating to the same eye area or the head and no blood at withdrawal. The manipulation is applied once every other day 10 times as a course, at an interval of 10 days between courses.

Acupoint laser irradiation

Selection of points: Commonly used point — *futu* (LI 18). Supplementary points — Ermen (SJ 21) and *jingming* (BL 1).

Manipulation: One of the commonly used points and one of the supplementary points are employed at each session with a helium–neon laser therapeutic apparatus, power 25 mw, wavelength 632.8 nm and facula diameter 2 mm. Commonly used points require 5–7 min of radiation each time and supplementary points 3–5 min, once a day, 10 times as a course.

Remarks

The first method is the first choice, because of its confirmed curative effect and broad applicable area, but it is complicated in manipulation, and it is especially difficult for beginners to induce the needling sensation. The second method is mainly for treatment of indocrine exophthalmia; it was applied to 50 cases involving 98 eyes, with a total effective rate of 83.7%, and it has protective efficacy. The last method is easy and safe to perform with obvious effect, but it still needs further verification as relatively few cases have been observed.

QUESTIONS

(1) Describe how to apply body acupuncture and bloodletting manipulation to gout.
(2) What characteristics are there in point selection and manipulations for the treatment of hyperthyroidism?

RHEUMATOID ARTHRITIS

Overview

Rheumatoid arthritis (RA) is a chronic systemic autoimmune disease, clinically manifested by multiple bilaterally symmetrical arthritis. It affects distal small joints of the four limbs at the early stage, and proximate interphalangeal joints are attacked most frequently, causing problems ranging from spindle-like swellings to stiffness and deformity. The disease is commonly seen in young and middle-aged people. It pertains to the concept of *li jie* (severe arthralgia) in TCM. Acupuncture and moxibustion for *li jie* may be traced back to *Neijing* (*The Inner Classic*).

Modern reports were seen in 1955 and the treatment of RA has made a progress since the 1980s. The effective rate ranges from 84.6% to 96.7%, but the recovery rate is relatively low.

Treatment

Warm needling

Selection of points: Commonly used points — *shuigou* (DU 26), *jiquan* (HT 1) and *weizhong* (BL 40). Supplementary points — three groups, namely (1) upper limbs — *baxie* (EX-UE9) (location: eight points on the dorsum of both hands, proximal to the margin of the webs between every two of the five fingers of each hand when a loose fist is made), *yangxi* (LI 5), *quchi* (LI 11), *waiguan* (SJ 5), *xiaohai* (SI 8), *jianyu* (LI 15) and *jianliao* (SJ 14); (2) lower limbs — *bafeng* (EX-LE10) (location: eight points on the instep of both feet, proximal to the margin of the webs between every two neighboring toes), *jiexi* (ST 41), *zhaohai* (KI 6), *Yanglingquan* (GB 34), *zhibian* (BL 54) and *huantiao* (GB 30); (3) back and lower back — *jiaji* (EX-B2).

Manipulation: For the commonly used points employed, *shuigou* (DU 26) is needled using the lifting and thrusting technique till there is a strong local sensation; *jiquan* (HT 1) is needled, with the upper limbs rising, by lifting and thrusting combined with twirling and rotating to make the numbness sensation radiate to the foot; *weizhong* (BL 40) is needled perpendicularly by lifting and thrusting combined with twirling and rotating until the numbness sensation reaches the foot, during which the patient takes a prostrate position with straight leg raising at about 60°. All manipulations are performed for 1 min. Of the points on the limbs, 8–10 pairs are employed at each session in the morning. On the arrival of *qi*, ignite a moxa cone 5 cm long on the needle handle. Withdraw the needle when the moxa cone burns out; *jiaji* (EX-B2) is needled in the afternoon. Fifteen pairs are employed at each session, with No. 28 filiform needles, 1.5 *cun* long, inserted obliquely toward the spine. On the arrival of *qi*, withdraw the needle a little, and fumigate the needle handle with an ignited moxa stick, and the needles are retained in each point for

15–20 min. The manipulation is applied once daily, 12 times as a course, at an interval of 3–5 days between courses.

Auxiliary moxibustion

Selection of points: From *dazhui* (DU 14) to *yaoshu* (DU 2) (location: the sacral hiatus under the fourth sacral vertebra).

Manipulation: Prepare Banshe powder 1.0–1.8 g containing Shexiang (*Moschus*) 50%, Banmao powder (*Mylabris*) 20%, Dingxiang powder (*Flos Caryophylli*) 15% and Rougui powder (*Cortex Cinnamomi*) 15%, a decorticated garlic spread 500 g and moxa wool 200 g. Moxibustion is applied on dog days. The patient is in the prone posture, with the back exposed, and routine sterilization is done on the vertebral column before applying first Banshe powder along the central line of the points selected and then the garlic spread 5 cm wide and 2.5 cm high on the powder. Finally, spread a snakelike cone 3 cm wide and 2.5 cm high with a cross-section like an isosceles triangle. Ignite the cone at the ends and the middle for moxibustion. After that, change to another cone. Generally, two or three cones are needed. Moxibustion finished, remove the garlic spread, and wipe gently with a wet towel. If there is a water vacuole, ask the patient not to scarify it, and tell him or her to tease it with a sterilized needle and wipe it with cotton wool before applying gentian violet (once every other day), covering it with a sterilized dressing, and fixing it with adhesive tape until it forms a scab and ablates by itself. Avoid raw, cold, spicy food and cold showers.

Remarks

There are many therapies with acupuncture and moxibustion for RA, but here only two have been introduced, because of their peculiarity and better effectiveness. For the first one, while needling *jiquan* (HT 1) and *weizhong* (BL 40), it is proper to feel the artery on the point area before inserting the needle beside it, which may often induce a sensation like an electric shock, during which be sure not to beat or thrust aimlessly and heavily. Withdraw the needle instantly after lifting and thrusting gently two or three times. Much importance should be attached to nursing care after manipulation for infection prevention when auxiliary moxibustion is applied.

OCULAR MYASTHENIA GRAVIS

Overview

Myasthenia gravis (MG) is an autoimmune neuromuscular disease caused by circulating antibodies that block acetylcholine receptors at the postsynaptic neuromuscular junction. It is clinically manifested by fatigability of the affected skeletal muscles, which will improve after periods of rest. Ocular MG is the most common form and also the object of acupuncture and moxibustion, with symptoms including asymmetrical ptosis (drooping of one or both eyelids) and diplopia (double vision). Modern reports about treatment with acupuncture and moxibustion first appeared in the 1950s. It is believed on the basis of abundant clinical practice that ocular MG responds well to acupuncture and moxibustion, and is likely to be cured.

Treatment

Body acupuncture

Selection of points: Commonly used points — *zanzhu* (BL 2), *yangbai* (GB 14), *hegu* (LI 4) and *baihui* (DU 20). Supplementary points — *waiguan* (SJ 5), *guangming* (GB 37) and *zusanli* (ST 36) added for eye muscle prolapse and *jingming* (BL 1) and *fengchi* (GB 20) for diplopia.

Manipulation: Three commonly used points are employed at each session, and one or two supplementary points are added according to symptoms. Needle *yangbai* (GB 14) toward *zanzhu* (BL 2) or toward the middle of the eyebrow. A No. 30 filiform needle, 1.5 *cun* long, is inserted into *jingming* (BL 1) and *zanzhu* (BL 2), lifting and thrusting slightly for half a minute to one minute on the arrival of *qi*, without retention of the needle. Points on the four limbs are punctured by swiftly insertion and slow lifting, with the needles retained in each point for 30–40 min after the arrival of *qi*. For *fengchi* (GB 20), insert the needle toward the tip of the nose to a depth of 1.5 *cun*, with the sensation radiating to the forehead or eye area, and the needles retained for 30 min. *Baihui* (DU 20) is given warm moxibustion with moxa sticks for 15 min. The performance is applied once daily for 7–10 days as a course, at an interval of 3–5 days.

Ear acupuncture

Selection of points: Commonly used points — eye, subcortex and spleen. Supplementary points — liver, endocrine, kidney and central rim.

Manipulation: It begins with filiform needling. Two or three commonly used points and one or two supplementary points are employed at each session. The tenderness in the bilateral ear acupoints having been found, insert the needle into it by twirling and rotating swiftly until a sensation of distension, heat and pain arises, with the needle retained for 30 min, during which manipulate the needle once every 5 min to strengthen the stimulation. The manipulation is applied once daily, 10 times as a course. The next course, if symptoms improve, begins with needle embedding or pill pressing on ear points, in which 3–5 points of one ear are employed, with the two ears applied to alternately. Change plasters twice a week, 10 times as a course.

Remarks

Both methods are applicable to ocular MG, especially body acupuncture, whose effect has been confirmed. But when puncturing *zanzhu* (BL 2) and *jingming* (BL 1), make sure that the fine needle is inserted slowly, to prevent ocular hematoma. A better effect may be achieved by tapping at the affected area with the skin needle after withdrawing needles in body acupuncture. Ear acupuncture was applied to fewer cases, and once ocular MG and nonocular MG cases were compared with the same method. The result was that it was effective in all ocular MG cases and ineffective in the other cases, which proved that ear acupuncture is most applicable to ocular MG.

QUESTIONS

(1) Restate the manipulation of auxiliary moxibustion.
(2) Describe how to manipulate in treatment of ocular MG with acupuncture and moxibustion.

CHAPTER 23

Acupuncture and Moxibustion for Diseases of the Neural and Mental Systems

ACUTE CEREBROVASCULAR DISEASE (WIND STROKE)

Overview

Acute cerebrovascular disease is also known as cerebral vascular accident or wind stroke. It includes cerebral hemorrhage, arteriosclerotic infarction (cerebral thrombosis), cerebral embolism and cerebral vasospasm. The first is called hemorrhagic stroke, and the other three ischemic stroke. It is clinically manifested by hemiplegia, aphasia and loss of consciousness. Cerebral hemorrhage often attacks people with hypertension who are over 50 years old, with the following symptoms: sudden loss of consciousness, hemiplegia, a pale or red complexion, vomiting, and urinary and fecal incontinence. Cerebral infarction is also common in aged people, as hemiplegia or aphasia caused by acute insufficiency of blood supply often occurs during rest or sleep. Acute cerebrovascular disease is similar to *zhong feng* (wind stroke) in TCM. Ancient practitioners accumulated much experience with acupuncture and moxibustion for wind stroke, which was recorded in *Neijing (The Inner Classic)*. Acupuncture and moxibustion in modern times is applicable to wind stroke at its convalescence stage or its sequela. The 1950s saw a report about a patient at the acute stage who was given acupuncture while being rescued. With various point stimulations, especially scalp acupuncture and ocular acupuncture, the curative effect has been increased in the past 30 years. Now, at the acute stage of cerebral hemorrhage, the effective rate in treatment with acupuncture combined with Chinese and Western medicine is 60%, and for cerebral infarction or cerebral hemorrhage at the convalescence stage, the effective rate is above 95%. Here we will focus on acupuncture treatment for wind stroke at its convalescence stage or sequela stage.

Treatment

Body acupuncture (I)

Selection of points: Commonly used points — *shuigou* (DU 26), *neiguan* (PC 6), *jiquan* (HT 1), *weizhong* (BL 40), *sanyinjiao* (SP 6) and *chize* (LU 5). Supplementary points — *fengchi* (GB 20), *yifeng* (SJ 17) and *hegu* (LI 4) added for pseudobulbar palsy.

Manipulation: Commonly used points are employed at each session. Both *neiguan* points (PC 6) are needled first by inserting the needle perpendicularly 1–1.5 *cun* deep with reducing manipulation by lifting and thrusting combined with twirling and rotating for 1 min; then *shuigou* (DU 26), with the needle tip inserted obliquely under the nasal septum to a depth of 0.5 *cun*, swiftly lifting and thrusting until tears drop or come to the eyes; at *sanyinjiao* (SP 6), the tip is inserted backward obliquely at an angle of 45° with the skin to a depth of 1–1.5 *cun* with reinforcing manipulation by lifting gently and thrusting forcefully until the patient feels abstraction in the lower limbs three times; at *jiquan* (HT 1), with the patient holding the hands up with the armpits completely exposed, insert the needle 1–1.5 *cun* deep with reducing manipulation by lifting forcefully and thrusting gently until the patient feels abstraction in the upper limbs three times; manipulation on *chize* (LU 5) is the same as for *jiquan* (HT 1); at *weizhong* (BL 40), with the patient in a supine posture with the legs rising at an angle of 90°, and the poples completely exposed, the needle is inserted 1–1.5 *cun* deep with reducing manipulation by lifting forcefully and thrusting gently until the patient feels abstraction in the lower limbs three times. When one is needling *fengchi* (GB 20), the tip is inserted toward the Adam's apple to a depth of 1.0–2.0 *cun* by quickly twirling and rotating for half a minute. *Yifeng* (SJ 17) is given the same manipulation as *fengchi* (GB 20); at *hegu* (LI 4), the tip is inserted slightly toward the metacarpal joint to a depth of 1–1.5 *cun* with reducing manipulation by lifting forcefully and thrusting gently. The performance is conducted once every day or every other day, 10 times as a course, at an interval of 3–5 days between courses.

Body acupuncture (II)

Selection of points: Commonly used points — three groups, namely (1) paralysis of the limbs and trunk — *jianyu* (LI 15), *tianding* (LI 17), *quchi* (LI 11), *waiguan* (SJ 5), *hegu* (LI 4), *huantiao* (GB 30), *yanglingquan* (GB 34), *zusanli* (ST 36) and *taichong* (LR 3); (2) facial paralysis — *jiache* (ST 6) and *dicang* (ST 4); (3) aphasia — *lianquan* (RN 23). Supplementary points — three groups, namely (1) paralysis of the limbs and trunk — *jianliao* (SJ 14), *houxi* (SI 3), *quchi* (Li 11), *fengshi* (GB 31), *zhibian* (BL 54), *kunlun* (BL 60), *jiexi* (ST 41) and *fenglong* (ST 40); (2) facial paralysis — *sibai* (ST 2) and *yingxiang* (LI 20); (3) aphasia — *tiantu* (RN 22) and *fengfu* (DU 16).

Manipulation: Commonly used points are employed as the main points, and supplementary points are added according to symptoms, with 5–8 points at each session. Generally, points on the affected side are needled, and if there is no satisfactory effect, the corresponding ones on the healthy side may be selected. *Tianding* (LI 17) is punctured perpendicularly after feeling the obvious tenderness, to make the needling sensation radiate to the fingers; *hegu* (LI 4) is punctured toward *houxi* (SI 3). Lift, thrust, twirl and rotate the needles in each point for 1–2 min, with a retention of 15–20 min. Also, one or two pairs of points are connected to the electroacupuncture apparatus with a frequency of 120 cpm and a continuous wave. This is applied once daily, 10 times as a course. If a good effect is not achieved, three-step acupuncture is performed. Step 1 is to select meridian points only on the healthy side, and ask the patient to move his or her affected limbs instantly after manipulating the needle by lifting, thrusting, twirling and rotating forcefully for 1–2 min. If there is no response, repeat the manipulation 10 min later. Repeat again after 24 h if there is still no response. If the affected limbs are able to move even a little, step 2 is applied. Points on both the affected and healthy sides are selected, giving gentle stimulation to the former points and strong stimulation to the latter ones. When the symptoms improve, apply step 3, which is to select points on the affected side with reinforcing manipulation by lifting and thrusting or twirling and rotating. The needling is applied once every other day, 20 times as a course, at an interval of 5 days.

Scalp acupuncture

Selection of points: Commonly used points — motor area and foot-kinesthetic sensory area. Supplementary points — sensory area added for paresthesia, and equilibrium area for disequilibrium.

Manipulation: Bilateral points in the equilibrium area and points on the opposite side in the other areas are employed. No. 28–30 filiform needles, 1.5–2 *cun* long, are inserted swiftly into the subcutaneous layer and further into the lower layer of the epicranial aponeurosis, with manipulation by quickly twirling and rotating at 180–200 cpm, each needle twirling for 3 min, and repeating it after 5–10 min. Repeat three times before withdrawing the needles. During manipulation, the patient is required to move his or her limbs. Sometimes it is intolerable to some patients because of its strong stimulation, and electroacupuncture may be more applicable to beginners, which is to connect the needles to the electroacupuncture apparatus with a continuous wave and a frequency of 250–300 cpm, tolerable to patients, for 15 min on switch. Scalp acupuncture is applied once every day or every other day, 10 times as a course, at an interval of 3–5 days between courses.

Eye acupuncture

Selection of points: Upper *jiao* and lower *jiao*.

Manipulation: Take points on the affected side as the main points, and the healthy side may be combined. Press gently the area around the eye with even strength, using an eyedrop stick or the handle of a three-edged needle, until there is point response, such as soreness, numbness, distension, heaviness, or feeling heat, coldness, pain, or a sensation of discomfort. Press the eyeball with fingers of the left hand to tense the orbit skin; then, a No. 32 filiform needle, 5 *fen* long, is slightly inserted 2 *fen* lateral to the orbital border. Determine the meridian area borders around the pupil and insert the needle perpendicularly or horizontally within limits along the skin, with the needle retained for 15 min, during which the patient is to move his or her limbs initiatively or passively. The manipulation is applied once daily, 10 times as a course.

Remarks

Among the four methods, the first one is named *xingnao kaiqiao fa* ("consciousness-restoring resuscitation"). It has been proven to be significantly effective for hemorrhagic and ischemic stroke by thousands of cases and experiments, with a total effective rate of 99%. The second method is a colligation of traditional acupoints and needling techniques, and it was applied to 985 cases and achieved an effective rate between 83.0% and 96.9%; scalp acupuncture and eye acupuncture are the effective methods in the clinic nowadays. Patients may choose one of them according to their own conditions. Whichever method is chosen, it is advisable to have treatment at the early stage, when the hemiplegia body shows no muscle atrophy or deformation. In particular, eye acupuncture should be avoided once deformation appears. Hemorrhagic stroke patients with unsteady condition and blood pressure should be cautions about applying acupuncture. Experience has shown that acupuncture is most effective for those with a short course (no more than one month) and incomplete paralysis. Combination of the four methods will increase the effectiveness. In treatment of aphasia, the patient is required to speak, otherwise it will be difficult for him or her to recover.

PSEUDOBULBAR PALSY

Overview

Pseudobulbar palsy is often seen in patients with wind stroke. The symptoms include dysphagia, hoarseness, slurred speech, sialorrhea, or even inappropriate emotional outbursts. Acupuncture and moxibustion for the disease has good effect, with an effective rate above 95%, no matter whether electroacupuncture or body acupuncture is applied to meridian acupoints or acupoints beyond meridians.

Treatment

Body acupuncture

Selection of points: Commonly used points — *fengchi* (GB 20), *lianquan* (RN 23) and *fengfu* (DU 16). Supplementary points — *shuigou* (DU 26), *neiguan* (PC 6), *baihui* (DU 20), *taichong* (LR 3) and *fenglong* (ST 40).

Manipulation: Commonly used points are employed, while supplementary points are taken as adjuvant for other symptoms caused by acute cerebro-vascular disease. For example, *shuigou* (DU 26) and *neiguan* (PC 6) is added for cloudiness of consciousness, *fenglong* (ST 40) for abundant and obstructed sputum, and *baihui* (DU 20) and *taichong* (LR 3) for high blood pressure. *Fengchi* (GB 20) is punctured 1–1.5 *cun* deep toward the Adam's apple, till the sensation radiates to the pars laryngea pharyngis, followed by twirling and rotating the needle for 2 min with stronger stimulation. *Lianquan* (RN 23) is punctured 1.5–2 *cun* toward the lingual root, till the needling sensation arises in the lingual root and the pars laryngea pharyngis, manipulating the needle for 1 min by lifting and thrusting combined with twirling and rotating. *Fengfu* (DU 16) is punctured perpendicularly at the same level as the mouth and ear lobule, inserting the needle slowly until distension is felt, with the needle retained in the point. Supplementary points are all punctured by lifting and thrusting combined with twirling and rotating on the arrival of *qi*. The needles are retained in each point, no matter whether it is commonly used or supplementary, for 15–20 min, during which manipulate the needles every 5–10 min. The manipulation is applied once daily, 10 times as a course. From the second course, it is applied once every other day, 15–20 times as a course.

Electroacupuncture

Selection of points: Commonly used points — *yaxue* [5 *fen* above *fengchi* (GB 20)] and *yifeng* (SJ 17). Supplementary points — *shanglianquan* (RN 23) (1 *cun* directly above the middle of the jaw) and *hegu* (LI 4).

Manipulation: All the commonly used points and one supplementary point are employed at each session. *Yaxue* is punctured bilaterally with a 1.5-*cun*-long filiform at an angle of 45°, and be careful to push the needle slowly to a depth of no more than 1 *cun*, till the arrival of *qi*; *yifeng* (SJ 17) is punctured with the tip toward the mouth, 1–1.2 *cun* deep, till the sensation radiates to the throat. *Shanglianquan* (RN 23) is punctured obliquely toward the lingual root, to a depth of 1–1.5 *cun*; withdraw the needle just beneath the skin, and insert needles obliquely 1–1.5 *cun* on both sides, until the patient feels tightness and distension in the lingual root and throat. While one is puncturing *hegu* (LI 4), the needle tip is slightly oblique toward the wrist, till the arrival of *qi*. Connect commonly used points to an electroacupuncture apparatus, each pair of electrodes to points on the same side, with a frequency of 180 cpm and the strength tolerable to patients. The needles are retained in each point for 20 min. Apply the manipulation once every day or every other day, 10 times as a course, at an interval of 5 days between courses.

Remarks

Pseudobulbar palsy is caused by recurrent attacks of acute cerebrovascular disease. Acupuncture is applicable to cases at the stable stage or convalescence stage. Both of the methods above have obvious effect in improving dysphagia, choking cough and salivation, but be sure to follow closely the operating instructions, and control the direction and depth of needling to avoid accidents while puncturing *fengchi* (GB 20), *fengfu* (DU 16) and *Yaxue*.

QUESTIONS

(1) What are the two body acupuncture methods for acute cerebrovascular disease? Restate in detail consciousness-restoring resuscitation.

(2) Describe how to apply scalp acupuncture and eye acupuncture in treatment of acute cerebrovascular disease.

(3) What should one be cautious about in applying body acupuncture and electroacupuncture to pseudobulbar palsy?

PARALYSIS AGITANS

Overview

Paralysis agitans, also known as Parkinson's disease (PD), is clinically manifested by tremor, rigidity, and slowness of movement. It is common in males aged 50–60. Tremor at the onset typically appears in only one arm or leg, becoming bilateral later; owing to increased muscle tone, the rigidity can be uniform (lead pipe rigidity) or ratchety (cogwheel rigidity); less movement and step difficulty result in festination and a masklike facial expression. PD is similar to *chan zheng* (tremor syndrome) in TCM. Treatment with acupuncture and moxibustion has no record in the classics. It did not draw any attention until the 1970s, when acupuncture was applied to the points of the head in a hospital in Shanghai. Quite a few clinical essays about acupuncture for PD have been published in the past 30 years, including individual cases and observation summaries on multiple cases. Methods about acupuncture stimulation vary a lot, including scalp acupuncture, body acupuncture, electroacupuncture and acupoint injection. The effective rate is about 80%. The acupuncture therapy for PD is not mature, but may after all be accepted as a worthy one with no side effects since PD is so troublesome in the Chinese or Western medical field.

Treatment

Electroacupuncture

Selection of points: Commonly used points — *naokong* (GB 19). Supplementary points — *qianding* (DU 21), *baihui* (DU 20), *chengling* (GB 18), *xuanlu* (GB 5), *tianchong* (GB 9) and *tongtian* (BL 7).

Manipulation: Commonly used points are employed each time, and supplementary points are selected alternately, three or four points each time. Insert a No. 28–30 filiform needle obliquely along the scalp to a depth of 1–1.5 *cun*, twirling and rotating till a sensation of distension and heaviness arises in the local area. Then connect to the electroacupuncture apparatus with a continuous wave, frequency (120–150 cpm) and strength tolerable to patients for 20 min on switch. The manipulation is applied once daily, 15 times as a course, at an interval of 3–5 days between courses.

Scalp acupuncture

Selection of points: Commonly used points — choreiform tremor area. Supplementary points — motor areas, vertigo and aural areas.

Manipulation: For cases with tremor, commonly used points are employed; for cases with tremor and enhancement of muscle strength, the motor area is added; for cases with dizziness resulting from medications, combine the vertigo and aural areas. In the early stage, when patients have unilateral tremor or enhancement of muscle strength, the unilateral point area on the head is employed, while in the later stage, when bilateral symptoms appear, bilateral areas are employed. And different diseased regions need corresponding point areas. For example, two-fifths of the motor area is selected for symptoms on the upper limbs. A No. 28 filiform needle is inserted quickly and pushed to the depth required, before twirling it at a frequency of 200–240 cpm for 1 min, with the needle retained for 15–20 min. Twirl and rotate the needle once every 5 min, and repeat that before withdrawing the needle. A better effect will be achieved if a sensation of heat, numbness and distension arises in the contralateral body. Alternatively, electroacupuncture can be applied at a frequency (250–300 cpm), continuous wave and strength tolerable to patients for 20–30 min. The operation is performed once every day or every other day, 15 times as a course. The next course begins after an interval of 5–7 days.

Scalp and body acupuncture

Selection of points: Commonly used points — choreiform tremor area (head points), *baihui* (DU 20), *fengchi* (GB 20) and *dazhui* (DU 14). Supplementary points — *quchi* (LI 11), *zusanli* (ST 36), *hegu* (LI 4) and *sanyinjiao* (SP 6).

Manipulation: Commonly used points are employed at each session and supplementary points alternately, two points each time. Six needles 1 *cun* long are inserted in sequence along the point line, followed by switching on an impulsive current with a continuous wave, and a frequency of 250–300 cpm. For the remaining points, uniform reinforcing–reducing manipulation is applied by lifting and thrusting combined with slight twirling and rotating after the arrival of *qi*. The needles are retained in each point for 30 min. Perform the operation once every day or every other day, 10 times as a course. From the fourth course, it is applied twice a week.

Body acupuncture

Selection of points: Commonly used points — *sishencong* (EX-HN1) or *sizhongxue* (1 *cun* away from the four points of *sishencong*), *fengchi* (GB 20), *wangu* (SI 4), *tianzhu* (BL 10) and *yamen* (DU 15). Supplementary points — *fuliu* (KI 7) added for thirst and a red tongue tip, *mingmen* (DU 4) and *shenshu* (BL 23) for rigidity and soreness of lower vertebrae, *zusanli* (ST 36) for constipation and a yellow tongue coating, and *shanglianquan* (RN 23) for speech disorder.

Manipulation: Three or four commonly used points are employed at each session, and supplementary points are added according to symptoms. A No. 30 filiform is inserted into *sishencong* (EX-HN1) or *sizhongxue* 1 or 1.5 *cun* deep, with the tip toward *baihui* (DU 20), and *fengchi* (Gb 20) is punctured 1.5 *cun* deep toward the contralateral eye area, and other points are applied to with routine acupuncture. Reinforcing–reducing manipulation is applied by twirling and rotating the needles, in which reducing is to commonly used points *zusanli* (ST 36) and *shanglianquan* (RN 23) without retaining the needles, while reinforcing is to *fuliu* (KI 7), *mingmen* (DU 4) and *shenshu* (BL 23) with the needles retained for 30 min, during which reinforcing–reducing manipulation by twirling and rotating the needles is applied once every 10 min. Acupuncture is performed once every other day, 10 times as a course, and the second course begins after 7 days' rest.

Remarks

The four methods are all effective for PD, to different degrees. Cases of rigidity respond to electroacupuncture much better than cases of tremor, which shows that electroacupuncture is applicable to patients with ridigity as the main symptom. Scalp acupuncture has an obvious effect in the early stage of treatment. The third method may be applied at different stages but has a better effect in improving movement reduction and stepping difficulty. Body acupuncture is for patients with obvious concomitant symptoms, but much attention should be paid to the manipulation. During the acupuncture, medication is vital and cannot be reduced with the improvement of the disease.

ACUTE INFECTIOUS POLYRADICULONEURITIS

Overview

Acute infectious polyradiculoneuritis is a symmetric injury to peripheral nerves induced by infections. It is manifested by flaccid paralysis of the four limbs, sensation disorders, pachyderma without complete analgesia, sometimes facial palsy, or even breathing difficulty in grave cases. There was not much information about acupuncture for this disease until recent years. Generally, whichever point stimulations are used, they require combination with Chinese and Western medications, especially in severe cases. At present, a combined therapy for the disease has achieved a good effect, with an effective rate above 85% — superior to single medications.

Treatment

Acupoint injection

Selection of points: Commonly used points — *dazhui* (DU 14), *jiaji* (EX-B2) (T2–S4), *jianyu* (LI 15), *quchi* (LI 11), *biguan* (ST 31), *yangling-quan* (GB 34), *xuanzhong* (GB 39), *huantiao* (GB 30) and *waiguan* (SJ 5). Supplementary points — *ganshu* (BL 18), *pishu* (BL 20), and *mingmen* (DU 4) added for general asthenia and trunk paralysis; *dicang* (ST 4), *jiache* (ST 6) and *zanzhu* (BL 2) for facial paralysis.

Manipulation: Prepare the injection mixed with an adenosine triphosphate (atp), a coenzyme A, a vitamin B1, a vitamin B12, and a galanthamine. Common used points are taken as the main points, and supplementary points as adjuvant. Divide the points into two groups — one for acupuncture and the other for injection, with the two groups used alternately. For acupuncture, reducing manipulation is applied by lifting and trusting or twirling and rotating 100 times in each point. Mild stimulation is applicable to cases of high excitability; strong stimulation, low excitability. Except for infants, the needles are retained for 20–30 min in each point. For point injection, take the No. 5 pinhead used in dentistry, and swiftly lift and thrust the needle till the arrival of *qi*. Push into the injection when there is no back-streaming of blood 0.5 ml at each point. In the early stage, acupuncture and injection can be performed simultaneously, and then alternately with the improvement of the disease. The manipulation is applied once a day, 10 times as a course, at an interval of 3 days. It may be changed to once every other day from the second course.

Acupuncture with thick needles

Selection of points: Commonly used points — *quchi* (LI 11), *hegu* (LI 4), *baxie* (EX-UE9), *yanglingquan* (GB 34), *xuanzhong* (GB 39) and *bafeng* (EX-LE10). Supplementary points — *shousanli* (LI 10) and *qiuxu* (GB 40).

Manipulation: Commonly used points are taken as the main points, and supplementary points as adjuvant, two or three points at each session. A tailor-made thick needle (0.8–1 mm in diameter and 3–8 *cun* in length) is quickly inserted into the point, first superficially and then deeply, with slow pressing and swift lifting, twirling and rotating combined with lifting and thrusting. The needle is manipulated repeatedly until there arises a sensation of being electrified, once every 10 min, and it is retained for 30 min. Then withdraw the needle, and no pressing with sterilized cotton balls is needed if there is no capillary hemorrhage. Acupuncture with thick needles is a strong stimulation which is applicable to treatment twice per week, 10 times as a course.

Remarks

Prior to acupuncture therapy, it is proper for patients to take hormones, vitamins, antibiotics or Chinese drugs to clear away heat, remove toxic substances and promote blood circulation in order to stabilize their condition and enhance the curative effect. Of the two methods introduced here, the first is preferred for its confirmed effectiveness, and the second is not suitable for infants or weak people because of its strong needling sensation, and should be applied with gentle, slow and careful manipulation in case vessels or nerves are injured.

QUESTIONS

(1) Describe in detail how to manipulate scalp acupuncture for treatment of paralysis agitans (or Parkinson's disease).

(2) What are the two acupuncture therapies for treatment of acute infectious polyradiculoneuritis?

FACIAL NERVE PALSY

Overview

Facial nerve palsy, also called Bell's palsy, is characterized by unilateral (few bilateral) sudden paralysis of the facial muscles, loss of the forehead wrinkles, flattening of the nasolabial groove, a drooping eyebrow, the corner of the mouth being pulled down, deviation of the face to the healthy side, inability to frown, bulge the cheeks, close the eyes, etc. It is similar to *kou pi* (deviated mouth) in TCM. Acupuncture therapy was recorded in *Nei jing*. Modern reports about the treatment of facial palsy with acupuncture and moxibustion began in the 1920s. In the early manipulation, traditional techniques were preferred, and in the past 50 years new point stimulations have been introduced into the treatment. At present, a total effective rate of 95% has been achieved and acupuncture is believed to enhance the recovery rate, shorten the convalescence period and prevent sequelae, although the disease tends to be spontaneously cured.

Treatment

Body acupuncture

Selection of points: Commonly used points — *dicang* (ST 4), *shuigou* (DU 26), *sibai* (ST 2), *taiyang* (EX-HN5), *sizhukong* (SJ 23), *yifeng* (SJ 17) and *jingming* (BL 1). Supplementary points — *hegu* (LI 4) and *neiting* (ST 44).

Manipulation: Four or five commonly used points and one supplementary points are employed at each session. Penetrating needling can be applied to points on the face. Choose needles according to the distance between the points to be penetrated. Usually, the points for penetrating needling are *dicang* (ST 4) to *sibai* (ST 2), and *taiyang* (EX-HN5) to *sizhukong* (SJ 23). Insert the needle quickly and push it slowly, with the needle and the skin at an angle of 10°–15°, but with no lifting, thrusting, twirling or rotating. If penetrating needling is performed, push the needle a further 0.3 *cun* after the tip reaches the corresponding point. For *yifeng* (SJ 17), insert the needle obliquely upward till the needling sensation arrives at the face; for *jingming* (BL 1), shallow needling is applied with a 0.5-cun-long filiform needle to a depth of 0.1–0.2 cun. Supplementary points are punctured perpendicularly with shaking on a small scale till the arrival of qi, followed by retention of the needles for 20–30 min, during which manipulate the needle once or twice by twirling or rotating. The whole manipulation is applied once every day or every other day, 10 times as a course, at an interval of 5–7 days.

Electroacupuncture

Selection of points: Commonly used points — qianzheng (EX-HN16) (0.5 cun anterior to the earlobe), *dicang* (ST 4), *shuigou* (DU 26), *yangbai* (GB 14), *yifeng* (SJ 17) and *xiaguan* (ST 7). Supplementary points — *hegu* (LI 4), *xingjian* (LR 2), *waiguan* (SJ 5) and houxi (SI 3).

Manipulation: Two or three commonly used points and one or two supplementary points are employed at each session. Prior to the acupuncture, apply *tuina* manipulation to the affected side in the direction of the sulcus auriculae posterior, with the finger pulp or the palm of the left hand. The methods are as follows. Puncture *yangbai* (GB 14) downward to the middle of the eyebrow, and puncture *yingxiang* (LI 20) upward to the infraorbital for the loss of forehead wrinkles; for flattening of the nasolabial groove and the corner of the mouth being pulled down, puncture *dicang* (ST 4) to *jiache* (ST 6), and puncture *taiyang* (EX-HN5) deeply. For cases with a long course, puncture both *xiaguan* points (ST 7). The remaining points are given routine acupuncture. Connect to the electroacupuncture apparatus with intermittent wave and strength till there is a slight abstraction in the face. For cases in the early stage, it is on switch for 5–10 min; for cases of more than 15 days, it may be prolonged to 15 min. The electroacupuncture is applied once every day or every other day, 10 times as a course, at an interval of 3–5 days between courses.

Needling and cupping

Selection of points: Commonly used points — two groups, namely (1) *ashi* point (1 *cun* below and posterior to the middle of the inferior border of the malar bone) and (2) *dicang* (ST 4), *jiache* (ST 6) and *taiyang*

(EX-HN5). Supplementary points — *jingming* (BL 1), *chengjiang* (RN 24), *tinghui* (GB 2) and *sizhukong* (SJ 23).

Manipulation: The two groups of commonly used points are employed alternately. Supplymentary points are taken as the reaching points for penetration, according to the requirements of the main points. No. 28–30 filiform needles are inserted into the *ashi* point subcutaneously toward *jingming* (BL 1), *dicang* (ST 4) and *jiache* (ST 6) by twirling and rotating; withdraw the needle after 1–2 min of manipulation. Cupping is given to the *ashi* points for about 10 min. For the second group, insert the needle into *dicang* (ST 4) subcutaneously toward *sizhukong* (SJ 23) and *sibai* (ST 2), with the needle retained for 20 min. The manipulation is applied once every other day, 16 times as a course, with the two groups selected alternately.

Remarks

Among the three methods above, penetrating needling is taken as the main therapy, combined with electroacupuncture or cupping, and an effective rate of 97% has been achieved. In the course of the acupuncture, pay attention to the following three problems: (1) while performing penetrating needling, avoid puncturing too deep, and it is better to place the needle between muscle fibers; (2) electroacupuncture is more effective if it is applied 15 days from the onset; (3) cupping should not last too long, in case ecchymosis is left on the face for a long time.

FACIAL SPASM

Overview

Facial spasm, also known as facial tics, is characterized by involuntary contractions of the face on one side. If tends to be intermittent and irregular, and varies in degree. It usually begins with occasional contractions of the muscles around the eyes, then slowly progresses to involve the entire face. It is often seen in female adults. This disease belongs to *jin ti rou* in TCM; its treatment with acupuncture and moxibustion was recorded in

Bei Ji Qian Jin Yao Fang (*Important Formulas Worth a Thousand Gold Pieces for Emergencies*) in the Tang Dynasty. Modern documents began to appear in the middle of the 1960s but did not draw much attention until the 1980s. At present, the effective rate of various acupuncture therapies is around 80%, but the recovery rate is still relatively low.

Treatment

Body acupuncture

Selection of points: Commonly used points — *waiguan* (SJ 5), *hegu* (LI 4), *neiguan* (PC 6). Supplementary points — *fengchi* (GB 20) and *wangu* (SI 4).

Manipulation: One or two commonly used points and one supplementary point are employed at each session with the respiration technique. It requires a quiet environment room temperature (20°C–25°C), with the patient undressed. A No. 28 or No. 30 filiform needle is quickly inserted into the selected point area to a depth of 0.5 *cun*, with the tip slightly toward the heart. Lift and thrust the needle lightly and swiftly on the arrival of *qi* to send the sensation upward; lift slowly and thrust quickly for 1 min. For supplementary points, press the area beneath the point with the index finger of the left hand, and insert the needle with the right hand to a depth of 1.5 *cun*, transmitting the sensation around the eyes. The needles are retained in each point for 20 min, during which they are manipulated once every 5–10 min. The operation is performed once every day or every other day, 10 times as a course.

Cluster needling

Selection of points: Commonly used points — *ashi* point (the starting point of facial spasm). Supplementary points — *sibai* (ST 2), *zanzhu* (BL 2), *yingxiang* (LI 20) and *jiache* (ST 6).

Manipulation: Apply No. 15–30 filiform needles, 0.5–1.5 *cun* long, to the *ashi* point with shallow puncture densely, with the needles in alignment or with scattered needling (0.5–1 cm between needles). The skin around the tip should protrude like a monticule, with the needle body hanging. Two or three supplementary points are given shallow puncture, with the needles retained for 20–30 min. The manipulation is applied once daily, 10 times as a course.

Remarks

Both of the methods above are effective and unique in the treatment of facial spasm. The key point of the first therapy, also called the respiration technique, lies in the transmission of the needling sensation to the face, which is a bit difficult for beginners. The more the needling, the easier the respiration, and the more effective for cases with a short course. The second therapy focuses on cluster needling, followed by shallow needling without the needle body dropping, during which some patients will complain of slight pain, and sometimes slight heat or dermahemia in the area punctured.

QUESTIONS

(1) Describe briefly the acupoint stimulations in treatment of facial nerve palsy.
(2) Describe how to manipulate cluster needling in treatment of facial spasm.

TRIGEMINAL NEURALGIA

Overview

Trigeminal neuralgia (TN) refers to recurrent, short-lasting, paroxysmal, severe pain in the trigeminal region. It is clinically manifested by a sudden attack of facial pain described as intense, sharp, like an electric shock, lancing, stabbing, burning or tearing. Episodes usually begin with the absence of signs and are strictly limited to the sensation area of the trigeminal region. Pain, usually unilateral, lasts from a few seconds to 2 min and can be triggered by facial activity or touching a point on the cheek (described as a trigger point). Modern articles about treatment with acupuncture and moxibustion first appeared in 1955. At present, the effective rate for treatment of TN with body acupuncture is above 85%, similar to that of other point stimulations, and the protective efficacy has been strengthened.

Treatment

Body acupuncture

Selection of points: Commonly used points — *yuyao* (EX-HN4) (in the middle of the eyebrow, directly above the pupil), *sibai* (ST 2) and *xiaguan* (ST 7). Supplementary points — *jiachengjiang* (1 *cun* lateral to *chengjiang* (RN 24), at the anterior maxillary foramen of the mandible).

Manipulation: For pain in branch I of the trigeminal nerve, *yuyao* (EX-HN4) is punctured obliquely downward to a depth of 0.3–0.5 *cun* until the sensation of an electric shock is transmitted to the eyes and the forehead, followed by lifting and thrusting the needle 20–50 times. For pain in branch II, *sibai* (ST 2) is punctured obliquely upward at an angle of 45° to a depth of 0.5–0.8 *cun*, followed by lifting and thrusting the needle 20–50 times until the sensation of an electric shock is transmitted to the upper lip and upper teeth. *Xiaguan* (ST 7) is selected for pain in branches II and III or only in branch III, and perpendicularly punctured 1.5 *cun*, lifting and thrusting the needle 20–50 times until the electric shock sensation is transmitted to the tongue and the lower mandible. If *xiaguan* (ST 7) fails to achieve a satisfactory effect, *jiachengjiang* is available, and it is punctured obliquely downward an angle of 30° to a depth of 0.5 *cun*, followed by lifting and thrusting 20–50 times until the electric shock sensation is transmitted to the lower lip. All the acupoints mentioned above are selected from the affected side. If no needling sensation is needed, adjust the direction and depth of the needle carefully. The manipulation is applied once every other day, 10 times as a course, or once daily for severe cases.

Acupoint injection

Selection of points: Commonly used point — *ashi* point (trigger point). Supplementary points — *yuyao* (EX-HN4) and *yangbai* (GB 14) added for pain in branch I; *sibai* (ST 2), *yingxiang* (LI 20) and *yifeng* (SJ 17) for pain in branch II; *dicang* (ST 4), *jiache* (ST 6) and *yingxiang* (LI 20) for pain in branch III.

Manipulation: Prepare 654-2 injection or water for injection. Commonly used points and two or three supplementary points on the affected side are employed at each session. Locate the *ashi* point, the trigger point which induces pain in the trigeminal nerve, and it is given an intradermal injection with 0.1 ml injection water using a No. 4 needle, which makes the local skin protrude in the form of a white heap (not subcutaneous injection). The other acupoints are punctured with a No. 5 needle from dentistry until the sensation of an electric shock or something else arises. Then lift the needle a little, push into 654-2 injection, 5–10 ml at each point. The manipulation is applied once daily, or once every other day or twice a week for cases of infrequent seizures, 10 times as a course.

Electroacupuncture

Selection of points: Commonly used points — *yuyao* (EX-HN4) for pain in branch I; *sibai* (ST 2) and *xiaguan* (ST 7) for pain in branch II; *dicang* (ST 4) for pain in branch III. Supplementary points — *yangbai* (GB 14), *shuigou* (DU 26), *chengjiang* (RN 24) and *yingxiang* (LI 20).

Manipulation: Points are selected according to pains in different branches, and one or two supplementary points may be added as adjuvant, all on the affected side. On the arrival of *qi*, connect to the G6805 electroacupuncture apparatus with a continuous wave, frequency (150–600 cpm) and strength tolerable to the patient. This lasts for 10–20 min on switch with the needles in the points, during which the current flow may be enhanced once or twice according to the patient's response, in order to retain the strong needling sensation. The manipulation is applied once daily, or twice for severe cases, 10 days as a course.

Remarks

Among the three therapies above, body acupuncture has been applied to as many as 1000 cases, with a total effective rate of 99.2%, out of which 540 cases were followed up for half a year, and 39.49% of the patients experienced a returned pain, showing that body acupuncture has a long-term effect and may be taken as the first choice. But the key point during the manipulation lies in the sensation of an electric shock that needs careful searching and feeling. Point injection and electroacupuncture therapies relieve pains in many people, but the former should avoid needling too deep during injection into the trigger point, while the latter requires a certain amount of electric stimulation.

VASCULAR MIGRAINE

Overview

Vascular migraine (or migraine) is one of the common types of acute headaches. It is clinically manifested by transient disorders of brain functions like optical illusion and hemiscotosis before the onset, progressing to unilateral headache with pulsating drilling pain, prickling pain or dull pain. Severe cases may experience dizziness, perspiration, nausea, vomiting, panickiness, constipation and other symptoms, which may last several hours, with periodic episodes at an interval of weeks. The disease is named *piao tou tong* (migraine) in TCM, and *Bian Que Xin Shu* (*The Teachings of Bian Que*) recorded prescriptions for it with acupuncture and moxibustion. Quite a lot of experience in the treatment of migraine with acupuncture and moxibustion has been accumulated in modern times. Generally, it is advisable to apply traditional penetrating needling, while bloodletting and cupping therapy is also available. An effective rate of 90% has been achieved.

Treatment

Body acupuncture

Selection of points: Commonly used points — *taiyang* (EX-HN5) (directly above the ear apex, 1.5 *cun* from the hairline) penetrating to *shuaigu* (GB 8) (1.5 *cun* into the hairline, directly above the ear apex) and *fengchi* (GB 20). Supplementary points — *taichong* (LR 3) and *hegu* (LI 4).

Manipulation: Commonly used points are employed at each session, and one or two supplementary points may be added according to conditions. Insert a 2.5-*cun*-long filiform needle perpendicularly into *taiyang* (EX-HN5) 1 *cun* deep, and withdraw it just the subcutaneous layer on the arrival of *qi*, followed by inserting the needle toward *shuaigu* (GB 8) by twirling and rotating to a depth of 1.5–2.2 *cun* combined with lifting and thrusting slightly for 1–2 min to make the needling sensation radiate to the homolateral temporalis part, and twirling and rotating once again for 1–2 min. *Hegu* (LI 4) and *taichong* (LR 3) are punctured perpendicularly to induce *qi*, with the needles retained. The needles are retained in each point for 30 min, during which manipulation is applied once every 10 min. Acupoints of the head are selected from the affected side, and points of the four limbs from both sides and the opposite side. The operation is performed once daily, 10 times as a course.

Bloodletting

Selection of points: Commonly used point — *taiyang* (EX-HN5). Supplementary points — *taichong* (LR 3) and *yintang* (EX-HN3).

Manipulation: The commonly used point is taken as the main point and one supplementary point is added according to symptoms. *Taiyang* (EX-HN5) and *yintang* (EX-HN3) are given pricking needling with sterilized three-edged needles shortly before cupping for 2–3 min. When one is puncturing *taichong* (LR 3), with the patient in the supine posture, a filiform 1.5 *cun* long is inserted to a depth of 1.2 *cun* till the arrival of *qi*, followed by twirling, rotating, lifting and thrusting the needle at a high frequency for 3–5 min, with a retention of 15–30 min. The manipulation is applied once every other day, 10 times as a course, at an interval of 5 days between courses.

Ear acupuncture

Selection of points: Commonly used points — temple and *shenmen*. Supplementary points — heart, liver, ear apex and central rim.

Manipulation: Commonly used points are employed, and supplementary points are added according to symptoms, four or five points at each session. At an acute episode, select two or three points; they are pricked for bloodletting with thin three-edged needles, and the others with filiform needles. At catabasis, electroacupuncture is applied by connecting to the electroacupuncture apparatus with an irregular wave and an intensity tolerable to the patient for 15–20 min on switch, with unilateral points taken each time, and the two ears alternately. The manipulation is applied once every day or every other day, 10–15 times as a course.

Remarks

Headache may be an initial manifestation or obvious symptom of some severe diseases, so a systemic examination must be made prior to acupuncture treatment. Among the three therapies above, the first is the most common one but a little difficult for beginners. What is more, *taiyang* (EX-HN5) may be punctured perpendicularly or given penetrating needling at short distances. Bloodletting therapy focuses on cupping following bloodletting, and the cupping glass should be small-sized since the area selected is small. If there are no such glasses or jars, bloodletting may be performed by pressing. Ear acupuncture can relieve pain, and pressing therapy with *Vaccaria segetalis* seeds is also available at catabasis.

QUESTIONS

(1) Which acupoint or acupoints do you prefer in treatment of trigeminal neuralgia? How to manipulate?
(2) Briefly introduce the methods of point selection and manipulation in the three therapies of point stimulation in treatment of vascular migraine.

SCIATICA

Overview

Sciatica refers to pain in the pathway of the sciatic nerve and its areal area. It is marked by burning pain or tingling pain radiating from the lower back and upper buttock down the back of the thigh to the back of the leg. Obvious tenderness may be felt along the path, with positive response to the straight leg rising test and changes in the ankle reflex. Depending on different areas affected, sciatica is of two types: root and trunk. It pertains to the concept of *tong bi* (pain arthralgia) in TCM. Acupuncture treatment in modern times has accumulated a great deal of experience since the 1950s, and developed analgesia principles researches on acupuncture treatment of sciatica. At present, an effective rate above 90% has been achieved, and more than half of the patients may clinically recover.

Treatment

Body acupuncture

Selection of points: Commonly used points — *huantiao* (GB 30) and *yanglingquan* (GB 34). Supplementary points — *weizhong* (BL 40), *yinmen* (BL 37), *shenshu* (Bl 23), *ciliao* (BL 32), *kunlun* (BL 60) and *qiuxu* (GB 40).

Manipulation: Commonly used points are employed at each session, and supplementary points may be added according to symptoms. The root type (pain aggravated by coughing or sneezing) requires *shenshu* (BL 23) and *ciliao* (BL 32); the trunk type (obvious tenderness along the path of the sciatica nerve), points of the lower limbs. *Huantiao* (GB 30) is punctured deeply, with twirling and rotating combined with lifting and thrusting to make the needling sensation radiate to the sole or toes; *yanglingquan* (GB 34) is given the same manipulation to make the sensation reach the dorsum of the foot. The other points also require the needling sensation radiating to the extremities. On the arrival of *qi*, retain the needles. The retention varies from 20 to 60 min, depending on the degree of pain, and it may be prolonged to 2 h or more if the pain is not eased. Twirl and rotate the needle once every 5–10 min. Electroacupuncture is also available, with an intermittent wave, a frequency (240 cpm) and an intensity tolerable to the patient. The manipulation is applied once every day or every other day, at 10 sessions as a course.

Acupoint injection

Selection of points: Commonly used points — *huantiao* (GB 30), *yinmen* (BL 37), *yanglingquan* (GB 34) and *chengfu* (BL 36). Supplementary points — *dachangshu* (BL 25), *shenshu* (BL 23), *weizhong* (BL 40) and *kunlun* (BL 60).

Manipulation: Select one of the following injections: a 10% glucose injection (5–10 ml for each point); vitamin B1 2 ml (100 mg) with a 0.5% procaine hydrochloride injection 10 ml (4–6 ml for each point). Commonly used points are taken as the main points, and one or two supplementary points may be added for a better effect, all from the affected side. For the first session, only *huantiao* (GB 30) is punctured deeply with a long needle, slightly lifting and thrusting until the sensation of an electric shock arises (be sure not to insert the needle forcefully or aimlessly, in case of injuring the nerve). Then withdraw the needle 1–2 *fen*, before injecting the liquor. The points are alternately selected, according to the most obvious tenderness. *Huantiao* (GB 30) must be employed for the first three or four sessions. The operation is applied once every day or every other day, at 10–15 sessions as a course.

Remarks

Besides the acupuncture therapies for sciatica introduced above, there are other methods, such as needle-embedding, bloodletting, ear acupuncture, acupoint irradiation with microwave, and moxibustion which are all effective, to different degrees. The two methods here are the most common and confirmed ones in the clinic. Body acupuncture has been applied to 599 cases and an effective rate of 88.75%–99% achieved after 10 times of treatment on the average, and it is applicable to different types of sciatica; acupoint injection is applicable to the trunk type of sciatica with obvious tenderness along the path, but the procaine allergy test is to be conducted before injection.

LATERAL FEMORAL CUTANEOUS NEUROPATHY

Overview

This is a commonly seen peripheral nerve disease, clinically manifested by formication, numbness or pain in the lateral skin of unilateral or bilateral thighs, which may be aggravated by prolonged sitting or walking; and hypesthesia or allergy of local skin without amyotrophy or movement disorder. Modern reports about acupuncture treatment were rare in the 1950s–1960s, but many cases observed have proven acupoint injection to be effective since the 1970s. Now, acupuncture therapies, including electroacupuncture, tapping with a skin needle, moxibustion, cupping and elongated needles, have a similar curative effect. Electroacupuncture was once compared with elongated needles by researchers, and the latter proved superior, but clinically bloodletting–cupping is the most commonly used technique.

Treatment

Cupping

Selection of points: *Ashi* point. Location: focal zone (same as below).

Manipulation: Following routine sterilization of the point area, flicking manipulation is applied to the affected area from left to right with a skin needle, until there is a little bleeding in the local area. Then, apply cupping to the focal area with one or several jars; or plaster a layer of liquid paraffin before cupping with a medium-size or small-size jar, moving the jar about on the affected area until the skin becomes red. Generally, the jars are retained for 10–15 min, moving for 3–5 min. The cupping is applied once every other day, at five sessions as a course, at an interval of one week between courses.

Moxibustion

Selection of points: *Ashi* point.

Manipulation: With the patient in the lateral recumbent posture with the affected side upward, revolving moxibustion is applied with a moxa roll over the selected area, at a distance of 0.5–1 *cun* from the skin, until the skin becomes reddish. Massage the affected area rhythmically from gently to forcefully with the hypothenar, and the warmness by moxibustion disappears; repeat the moxibustion and massage the same way several times, until the patient feels the warmness reach the deep muscles and feels relaxed and comfortable. In the early stage, the moxibustion is applied once daily and changed to once every 2–3 days with improvement of the symptoms, at 10 sessions as a course.

Elongated needles

Selection of point: *Ashi* point.

Manipulation: Elongated needles 5 *cun* in length are inserted downward or along the skin into the superior and inferior borders of the affected area, penetrating to the contralateral boders, and 1 *cun* between the needles. Connect to the electroacupuncture apparatus with a frequency (100 cpm), a continuous wave and an intensity tolerable to patients. The stimulation lasts for 15–20 min. Elongated needling is applied once daily, five times as a course, with an interval of one week between courses.

Remarks

In the three therapies, the *ashi* point is employed and the manipulations except for elongated needling are easy to perform. Cupping is applicable to cases regardless of the area of the focus; moxibustion, to cases with a small focal area and a short course of disease; elongated needles, to cases with a large focal area and a long course. For those stubborn cases with a long course, combine three or two therapies together. The former is applied in the sequence of elongated needling, bloodletting–cupping and moxibustion for the local area; the latter is applied by combining moxibustion with cupping. It is necessary to note that elongated needling requires a certain experience and is inapplicable to beginners.

QUESTIONS

(1) Describe how to manipulate body acupuncture and point injection for treatment of sciatica.

(2) Do you think that it is workable to combine cupping with moxibustion for treatment of lateral femoral cutaneous neuropathy? How to operate that?

NEURASTHENIA

Overview

Neurasthenia is a frequent psychological disorder. It is characterized by fatigue and weakness, tonic pain in the head and neck, insomnia, loss of memory, agitation, irritability, etc., but there are no organic lesiohs. It belongs to *yu zheng* (melancholia), *bai he bing* (lily disease), *bu mei* (insomnia), *jian wang* (forgetfulness) and *xin ji* (palpitations) in TCM. Modern reports about acupuncture treatment for neurasthenia were first seen in 1955. Besides acupuncture, various point stimulation therapies have been introduced into the treatment, with good effect, and the total effective rate is 85%.

Treatment

Acupuncture with a skin needle

Selection of points: Commonly used points — bilateral to the vertebral column. Supplementary points — points of the head and hind neck, and *yuji* (LU 10) of both hands.

Manipulation: Commonly used points are taken as the main points for tapping needling. The manipulation begins with tapping the cervical vertebrae three times from above to below, then the thoracic vertebrae three times from No. 8 to No. 12, and finally the sacral vertebrae three or four times. The head is given netlike tapping, and the bilateral hind neck and *yuji* (LU 10) are tapped twice. Tapping needling requires strength of the wrist, lifting steadily and thrusting quickly with medium stimulation until the skin flushes without bleeding. The manipulation is applied once daily, 12 times as a course, with an interval of 3–5 days between courses.

Ear acupuncture

Selection of points: Commonly used points — heart, central rim and *shenmen*. Supplementary points — liver, kidney, spleen, subcortex and endocrine.

Manipulation: Commonly used points are employed at each session, and supplementary points are added according to different symptoms, such as liver for impatience and irritability, kidney and endocrine for menoxenia, spleen for poor appetite, and subcortec for insomnia. Choose one of the following: *Vaccaria segetalis* seeds (preferable), mung beans (halved and attached to the points with the flat), or borneol (prepared as grains of rice) to press points with adhesive plaster on one ear alternately for 1 min, until the auricle becomes hot. The patient is asked to press the points by himself or herself 3–5 times daily, and the pressing before bedtime is necessary. The plaster is changed once every other day at 5 sessions as a course, with an interval of 3 days between courses.

Bloodletting

Selection of points: Commonly used points — *ashi* point (tenderness of the upper half of both ear roots). Supplementary points — *neizhongkui* (on the middle line of the palmaris of the middle finger, one point at the middle of the second transverse crease, and two points at 1 *fen* anterior and posterior to it — in total six points on both hands).

Manipulation: Commonly used points are employed at each session. Detect the tenderness carefully at the ear root, mark it before routine sterilization, followed by pricking swiftly with a three-edged needle, with blood out like a mung bean. One side is inserted into each time, once daily or every other day, with the two ears alternately employed. It is better to apply manipulation in the morning or afternoon. If there is no obvious effect, the inner *zhongkui* of the opposite side may be punctured in the same way. One course needs 5–7 sessions, and the next course begins after a 7-day interval.

Remarks

Filiform needling is traditionally regarded as the main therapy in the treatment of neurasthenia, while other acupoint stimulations in recent years have proven to be effective as well as convenient. The three therapies introduced here have all been applied to more than 200 cases and confirmed the effectiveness. Patients may choose one of them according to their own condition and knowledge. Neurasthenia is so intractable that patients need not only perseverance but also psychological directions for the purpose of enhancing the curative effect.

RESTLESS LEGS SYNDROME

Overview

Restless legs syndrome (RLS) is a neurological disorder characterized by an irresistible urge to move one's body to stop uncomfortable or odd sensations like pins and needles, or creeping ants. It may affect anyone. The patient experiences no symptoms in the daytime but onset from dusk to bedtime, and insomnia, anxiety and tension accordingly. The cause remains unknown and modern medicine has no specific therapeutics for RLS except symptomatic treatments.

In TCM, RLS belongs to *bi zheng* (arthralgia *zheng*), caused either by damage to yang *qi* and blood due to affection of exogenous wind–cold and invasion of pathogens, or by stagnation of *qi*, blood stasis and atresia of arteries and veins due to deficiency of yin blood and failure to promote *qi*. So a good effect has been achieved by warming yang to dispell cold, and nourishing yin to benefit *qi*.

Acupuncture and moxibustion for RLS began in 1985, and three patients were cured by Chinese medication combined with acupuncture. In the following 20 years, many clinical reports have been published. Experience has shown that the main therapy is to combine acupuncture with other treatments (e.g. or medication, or exposure to a specific electromagnetic wave), or to integrate two or more acupoint stimulus methods (e.g. point injection, moxibustion, pricking therapy, scalp acupuncture, etc.). Comparing pure warm needling to the combination of scalp acupuncture and warm needling showed that the latter was more effective than the former (P < 0.05), indicating that the synthetic method is superior to the single method. Besides, quite a lot of authors emphasize warm reinforcing, which is consistent with the pathogenesis of RLS. It has been found from the material that the short-term effective rate for acupuncture treatment is above 90%, but few reports aim at long-term followup.

Treatment

Body acupuncture

Selection of points: Commonly used points — two groups, namely (1) *bizhong* (location: inside the forearm, the middle of the wrist and elbow transverse striations, between tendons) and (2) *xuehai* (SP 10), *yanglingquan* (GB 34), *sanyinjiao* (SP 6) and *taixi* (KI 3). Supplementary points — *zusanli* (ST 36), *weizhong* (BL 40) and *chengshan* (BL 57).

Manipulation: One group is employed, and supplementary points may be added if there is no obvious curative effect. *Bizhong* is punctured

2.5–4.0 *cun* deep and, on the arrival of *qi*, reinforcing manipulation is applied by twirling and rotating the needle for 3 min. *Zusanli* (ST 36), *yanglingquan* (GB 34), *chengshan* (BL 57), *xuehai* (SP 10) and *weizhong* (BL 40) are all punctured perpendicularly to a depth of 1–1.5 *cun*, making the needling sensation transmit upward or downward; *taixi* (KI 3) is punctured obliquely upward to 0.5–1 *cun*, with the sensation upward. Those points above are all given reinforcing manipulation by twirling and rotating on the arrival of *qi* with the needles retained for 10 min. The operation is performed once every day or every other day, at 7 sessions as a course, at an interval of 3–5 days between courses.

Warm needling

Selection of points: Commonly used points — *zusanli* (ST 36), *fenglong* (ST 40), *sanyinjiao* (SP 6), *xuehai* (SP 10), *weizhong* (Bl 40) and *yanglingquan* (GB 34). Supplementary points — foot-kinesthetic sensory area, and sensory area (upper one-fifth).

Manipulation: Only commonly used points or both are employed at each session. Commonly used points are given warm needling with No. 28 filiform needles inserted, and reinforcing or uniform reinforcing–reducing manipulation is applied by twirling, rotating, lifting and thrusting. A moxa stick 1.5–2 *cun* long or a moxa cone is put on the needle handle and ignited from the end point, and one stick or two or three cones are needed. Withdraw the needle after the burnout. Supplementary points are punctured with the same needle to a depth of 3 cm at an angle of 15°–30° with the scalp, swiftly twirling and rotating the needle at a frequency of 200 cpm, with the needle rotated two or three circles backward and forward, respectively. The needles are retained in each point for 3–5 min. Apply the manipulation once every other day, at 7 sessions as a course, at an interval of 3–5 days between courses.

Acupuncture and moxibustion

Selection of points: Commonly used points — three groups, namely (1) *zusanli* (ST 36), *chengshan* (BL 57) and *juegu* (GB 39); (2)

yanglingquan (GB 34), *jiexi* (ST 41) and *sanyinjiao* (SP 6); (3) *waiqiu* (GB 36), *weizhong* (BL 40) and *bafeng* (EX-LE10).

Manipulation: One group is employed at each session, bilaterally. A No. 28 filiform needle is inserted to induce soreness, numbness, heaviness or a slightly radiating sensation in the local area or legs, followed by uniform reinforcing–reducing manipulation with a retention of 30 min. After the acupuncture, select one or two points for warm moxibustion for 5 min, until the skin becomes red. The manipulation is applied every day or every other day, at 10 sessions as a course.

Remarks

Among the three therapies, the first is the most commonly used in the clinic, with the most-confirmed effect. It requires a needling sensation to be induced and is a little difficult for beginners. Warm needling is also effective and can be combined with scalp acupuncture for patients who respond badly to warm needling, and if swift twirling and rotating is hard to apply, impulse electrical stimulation is available, with a frequency of 300–500 cpm. Acupuncture and moxibustion is applicable to beginners, because of its convenience and steady long-term effect.

HYSTERIA

Overview

Hysteria is believed to be a psychoneurosis induced by psychological factors. It is divided into two groups in the clinic: (1) physical obstacles characterized by hysterical paralysis, loss of the voice, amaurosis, deafness and globus hystericus; (2) psychic seizures with sentiment disorder, crying, or even faintness. Acupuncture treatment for the disease was recorded in *Bei Ji Qian Jin Yao Fang (Important Formulas Worth a Thousand Gold Pieces for Emergencies)* in the Tang Dynasty. Modern reports appeared in the 1950s. The methods of acupoint stimulation tend to be fewer and more necessary, which is one of the features in treatment of hysteria with acupuncture and moxibustion. At present, an effective rate above 90% has been achieved.

Treatment

Body acupuncture

Selection of points: Commonly used points — Supplementary points — *neiguan* (PC 6) and *lianquan* (RN 23) added for loss of the voice; *jingming* (BL 1) and *qiuhou* (EX-HN7) for amaurosis; *zusanli* (ST 36) and *tiantu* (RN 22) for globus hystericus; *ermen* (SJ 21) and *yifeng* (SJ 17) for deafness; *shuigou* (DU 26) for spasm; *yanglingquan* (GB 34) and *quchi* (LI 11) for hysterical paralysis.

Manipulation: At the beginning, the method of multiple needles and strong stimulation is employed, and commonly used points are used at each session and supplementary points are added according to symptoms. On the arrival of *qi*, twirl, rotate, lift and thrust the needles at great amplitude with medium or larger stimulations, with the needles retained in each point for 15–20 min. When the symptoms are relieved, manipulation is changed into stimulations with fewer needles, i.e. only one commonly used point and one supplementary point employed are punctured by twirling, rotating, lifting, thrusting and scraping the needles with medium stimulations, with the needles retained for 20–30 min. This is applied 1–3 times a day in acute episodes and once every day or every other day after stabilization.

Electroacupuncture

Selection of points: Commonly used points — *shuigou* (DU 26), *baihui* (DU 20) and *neiguan* (PC 6). Supplementary points — *hegu* (LI 4), *zusanli* (ST 36), *shaoshang* (LU 11) and fenglong (ST 40).

Manipulation: Commonly used points are taken as the main points, and one or two pairs of supplementary points may be added if a better effect is not achieved. On the arrival of *qi*, connect to the electroacupuncture apparatus with high frequency and heavy current stimulation for 10–20 s. If the symptoms cannot be controlled, repeat the operation three times. After that, there is a change to low frequency and weak current stimulation for 15 min. For cases with restlessness or spasm, assistance from others is required in case of accidents. The treatment is applied once or twice every day.

Remarks

Various therapies are available for treating hysteria, but only two have been introduced here, as they have been proven to be effective. Body acupuncture has been applied to 1313 cases, with an effective rate of 92%; electroacupuncture to 725 cases, with an effective rate of 93.6%– 96%. The former is applicable to both types of hysteria; the latter, to psychic seizures. Treatment of hysteria requires quiet surroundings and the patient's trust and cooperation, combined with psychological suggestion by words.

QUESTIONS

(1) Which acupoint stimulation method do you prefer if a patient with neurasthenia goes to see a doctor? How to manipulate?

(2) Describe how to manipulate body acupuncture in treatment of restless legs syndrome.

(3) Describe how to select points and manipulate in treatment of hysteria by applying body acupuncture.

EPILEPSY

Overview

Epilepsy is a paroxysmal transitory brain disorder, classified into primary and secondary types. Acupuncture treatment is applicable to the former type. Epilepsy is clinically manifested by transitory unconsciousness, limb convulsions, sensation and mental disturbance, and behavior disorders, involving grand seizures, minor seizures, localized seizures and psychomotor seizures. This disease is similar to *xian zheng* (epileptic syndrome) in TCM, and its treatment with acupuncture and moxibustion was recorded in *nei jing* (*The Inner Classic*). Modern reports about the treatment appeared in the early 1950s. Clinical observations and experimental studies in the past 50 years have proven that acupuncture and moxibustion is effective in controlling the duration of the seizure and prolonging the paralysis time. At present, a total effective rate of 80% has been achieved.

Treatment

Body acupuncture

Selection of points: Commonly used points — *dazhui* (DU 14), *yaoqi* (EX-B9), *shuigou* (DU 26) and *houxi* (SI 3). Supplementary points — *baihui* (DU 20), *neiguan* (PC 6), *shenmen* (HT 7), *fenglong* (ST 40) and *weizhong* (BL 40).

Manipulation: Commonly used points are taken as the main points, and two or three supplementary points are added according to symptoms. *Dazhui* (DU 14) is punctured with a No. 28 filiform needle obliquely upward at an angle of 30° to a depth of 1.5 *cun*, with the needle inserted slowly. When the patient complains of a needling sensation (soreness and distension, or radiating downward), lift the needle a little, with retention. *Yaoqi* (EX-B9) is punctured perpendicularly 1.0–1.2 *cun* by twirling and rotating the needle with strong stimulation. *Shuigou* (DU 26) and *houxi* (SI 3) are punctured deeply, also twirling and rotating the needle with strong stimulation. The needles are retained for 15 min. After withdrawal of the needles, *dazhui* (DU 14) and *yaoqi* (EX-B9) may be given cupping. Supplementary points are applied to with routine acupuncture without retention on the arrival of *qi*. The manipulation is performed once every day or every other day, at 10 sessions as a course, at an interval of 5–7 days between courses.

Acupoint injection

Selection of points: Commonly used points — two groups, namely (1) *jianshi* (PC 5) and *waiguan* (SJ 5); (2) *shenmen* (HT 7) and *houxi* (SI 3). Supplementary points — two groups corresponding to the above — (1) *baihui* (DU 20), *zhangmen* (LR 13) and *daling* (PC 7); (2) *yuji* (LU 10), *zusanli* (ST 36) and *fenglong* (ST 40).

Manipulation: Prepare injections: 0.5% procaine marmal saline solution, and vitamin B1 injection (100 mg/2 ml); choose either of them. One group (commonly used points and one or two supplementary points) is employed at each session. Prior to the injection, a No. 4 or No. 5 needle for dentistry is inserted to induce *qi* or make the needling sensation radiate. Procaine 5 ml (a hypersensitive test is necessary) is injected into each point [*jianshi* (PC 5) and *zusanli* (ST 36) need 10 ml], and vitamin B1 0.3–0.5 ml into each point. Employ one group a day, and the two groups alternately. A course comprises 10 sessions.

Scalp needling

Selection of points: Commonly used points — motor area, and corresponding area to the focus (according to the electroencephalogram, locate the focus before selecting points in the corresponding areas in the scalp, usually divided into forehead, top of head, occiput and temples). Supplementary points — sensory area, vertigo and aural area, and choreiform tremor area.

Manipulation: One area is employed at each session, and one or two supplementary areas are added according to symptoms or curative effect. A No. 28 filiform needle is inserted to the depth required before swiftly twirling and rotating the needle for 1 min at a frequency of 200 cpm, with the needle retained for 30 min, and repeat the manipulation every 10 min. A G6805 electroacupuncture apparatus is also available. It takes 10–30 min on switch, with a frequency (240–360 cpm) and an intensity tolerable to the patient. The manipulaiton is applied once daily, at 10 sessions as a course.

Remarks

Among the three therapies above, the first is the most commonly used in the clinic, but more attention should be paid to the depth and maneuver while inserting into *dazhui* (DU 14) and *yaoqi* (EX-B9), especially *dazhui* (DU 14), to which accidents may happen. So it is applicable to practitioners with a certain experience. Scalp acupuncture has become popular in recent years in treatment of epilepsy, and is especially effective by needling in the corresponding area to the focus, with not only short-term but also obvious long-term effect. While acupoint injection is being applied, *daling* (PC 7) and *shenmen* (HT 7) need a smaller dosage, owing to their thinner muscles.

SCHIZOPHRENIA

Overview

Schizophrenia is the most commonly seen psychosis and is characterized by various psychoactivity disorders. It most commonly manifests itself as dyssynchrony between thoughts, emotions, behavior and surroundings (the so-called split personality). There are four types of schizophrenia, namely simple, young, catatonic and delusional. In acute onset, it presents as sudden excitation, restlessness, abnormal behavior and paraphasia. In TCM it belongs to *dian kuang zheng* (mania), and treatment with acupuncture and moxibustion was recorded in *Neijing*. Great importance has been attached to modern acupuncture treatment since the early 1950s. It has been proven that various methods of point stimulation are not only applicable to all types of schizophrenia, but also adjuvant to the three traditional therapies for psychiatry (electric shock, insulin shock and chlorpromazine medications). At present, the effective rate averages about 80%.

Treatment

Body acupuncture

Selection of points: Commonly used points — for mania, *dazhui* (DU 14) and *dingshen* (junction of one-third and two-thirds below the philtrum); for depression, *daling* (PC 7), *laogong* (PC 8) and *yongquan* (KI 1); delusion, *zhongwan* (RN 20) and *shenmen* (HT 7). Supplementary points — mania, *hegu* (LI 4) penetrating toward *houxi* (SI 3), and *taixi* (KI 3) toward *yongquan* CKI 1); for depression, *neiguan* (PC 6) toward *waiguan* (SJ 5), and *hegu* (LI 4) toward *laogong* (PC 8); for delusion, *jianshi* (PC 5) toward *zhigou* (SI 6).

Manipulation: Commonly used points are employed according to symptoms, and one pair of supplementary points may be added if the effect is not significant. *Dazhui* (DU 14) is punctured deeply to 1.2–1.5 *cun* (the same way as in the treatment of epilepsy). On the arrival of *qi*, lift the needle a little instantly, before repeating the manipulation. *Dingshen* is punctured obliquely upward to a depth of 1.5 *cun*. The remaining points are given routine acupuncture. For cases with mania, reducing manipulation is applied by lifting and thrusting of the needle combined with twirling and rotating with strong stimulation; for depression, reinforcing manipulation is applied with medium stimulation; for delusion, reinforcing with mild stimulation. At the beginning, the treatment is performed once daily, at 20 sessions as a course, and the second course may begin after a 1-week interval, with once-every-other-day manipulation if the symptoms are improved.

Acupoint laser Irradiation

Selection of points: *Yamen* (DU 15) [5 *fen* below *fengfu* (DU 16)].

Manipulation: Helium–neon laser is employed for irradiation with wavelength 632.8 nm and power 5.9–25 milliwatts for 10 min at each session, once daily, at 30 sessions as a course. There are many methods of point stimulation in treatment of schizophrenia, such as catgut embedding, point injection, big needles, electroacupuncture and five-person needles, some of which are omitted owing to their high requirements and risks. Body acupuncture is commonly used in the clinic; there was a good response in 88.4% of more than 500 cases. The maneuver should be focused upon while insertion into *dazhui* (DU 14) is performed. Acupoint laser irradiation is applied to fewer cases but its effectiveness has been confirmed with a similar curative effect to chlorpropham. It is easy and reliable in performance, and so is an alternative in treatment of schizophrenia.

SENILE DEMENTIA

Overview

Senile dementia is a chronic progressive mental deterioration. Symptoms occurring at the initial stage are manifested as loss of memory and changes in personality (like stubbornness or selfishness), then progress to decline in intellectual activities, or even inability to provide self-care. The most common forms of senile dementia are Alzheimer's disease (50%), vascular dementia (VD, or multi-infarct dementia; 15%), overlapping of the two (25%), and others (10%). In some major cities of the West and China (like Shanghai), senile dementia has become the fourth leading cause of death. Modern medicine has no effective therapies for it, so it is of great significance to prevent the disease. In TCM, senile dementia belongs to *dian ji* (depressive psychosis), *shan wang* (loss of memory), *dai chi* (dementia) and *shen yi bing* (hypochondriasis), and is believed to be caused by kidney deficiency as the root and stagnation of phlegm and blood stasis as the branch.

Acupuncture treatment for the disease was recorded in *Bian Que Xin Shu* (*The Teachings of Bian Que*) by Dou Caizhi in the Song Dynasty, but it did not draw much attention until early 1990. According to statistics, tens of articles about acupuncture treatment have been published since 1991 — mainly Chinese but also foreigners' clinical research. Body acupunture is often employed in treatment; it takes points of the face and head as commonly used points. Acupoint injection is also effective. Many practitioners apply acupuncture combined with Chinese medicine to enhance the curative effect. It has been confirmed that acupuncture is highly effective for vascular dementia (VD), but it needs further clinical and mechanism research because of its short-term practice, incomplete techniques, different evaluation criteria in different regions, and discrepancy in effective rates in different clinical documents.

Treatment

Electroacupuncture

Selection of points: Commonly used points — *sishenxue* (1.5 *cun* left, right, anterior and posterior to *bhaihui* (DU 20)) and *shenting* (DU 24). Supplementary points — *zusanli* (ST 36) and *dazhui* (DU 14).

Manipulation: Generally, commonly used points are employed at each session, and supplementary points are added according to symptoms. Filiform needles 1.5 *cun* long are inserted horizontally into *sishenxue* and *shenting* (DU 24) in the direction of *baihui* (DU 20), to a depth of

0.8–1 *cun*. Twirl and rotate the needles till the arrival of *qi*, and then connect to the G6805 electroacupuncture apparatus with a continuous wave, a frequency (45 cpm) and an intensity tolerable to the patient. The needles are retained for 45 min. *Zushanli* (ST 36) are punctured perpendicularly, and *dazhui* (DU 14) obliquely downward with manipulations applied once every 15 min by lifting, thrusting, twirling and rotating the needles. The operation is performed once a week, at 12 sessions as a course. Generally, 1–3 courses are carried out in half a year.

Acupuncture and moxibustion

Selection of points: Commonly used points — *baihui* (DU 20) and *sishencong* (EX-HN1). Supplementary points — *zusanli* (ST 36) and *mingmen* (DU 4).

Manipulation: Commonly used points are employed at each session, and one supplementary point is added. With a filiform needle 1.5–2 *cun* long, penetrating needling is applied. *Sishencong* (EX-HN1) is first punctured horizontally toward *baihui* (DU 20), with four tips at *baihui* (DU 20), and the needles are retained for 30 min. Manipulate the needles once every 10 min and, at the same time, *baihui* (DU 20) and the supplementary point are given pecking moxibustion with moxa sticks, for 15 min at each session. The manipulation is applied once a week, at 25 sessions as a course, one course a year.

Body acupuncture

Selection of points: Commonly used points — *baihui* (DU 20), *fengfu* (DU 16) and *shuigou* (DU 26). Supplementary points — *quchi* (LI 11), *shenmen* (HT 7), *sanyinjiao* (SP 6), *taixi* (KI 3) and *taichong* (LR 3).

Manipulation: Commonly used points are taken as the main points, and supplementary points as adjuvant. On the arrival of *qi*, *baihui* (DU 20) is punctured anterior, posterior, left and right respectively along the skin to make the sensation radiate around; *fengfu* (DU 16) is punctured slowly toward the lower mandible with reducing manipulation by twirling and rotating the needle to make the sensation reach the top; *shuigou* is punctured deep obliquely upward by lifting and thrusting repeatedly to enhance the sensation; *quchi* (LI 11) is punctured by lifting, thrusting, twirling and rotating combined with reducing manipulation; *shenmen* (HT 7) and *taichong* (LR 3) are given uniform reinforcing–reducing manipulation; and *sanyinjiao* (SP 6) and *taixi* (KI 3) are given lifting, thrusting, twirling and rotating combined with reinforcing manipulation; the needles are retained in each point for 30 min, twirling them once every 5–10 min. Acupuncture is performed once daily, 10 times as a course, two or three times a week from the second course. Four courses are needed for the treatment of senile dementia.

Remarks

There are many therapies for senile dementia with acupuncture and moxibustion, and the three above are convenient and commonly used. Electroacupuncture is mainly applied for control and prevention of senile VD with symptoms of the early stage, manifested as reduction in interest and work efficiency, loss of memory of recent things, inhibition of thought, and difficulty in concentration. Acupuncture and moxibustion is applicable to prevention of VD, and requires the patient's persistence because of its long process of prevention. Body acupuncture is highly effective in improving the intelligence of patients with VD. Generally speaking, the shorter the course is, and the younger the patient is, the better the curative effect will be.

QUESTIONS

(1) Describe how to manipulate the commonly used therapies in treatment of epilepsy.
(2) Describe in detail the body acupuncture treatment for schizophrenia.
(3) Which type of senile dementia is acupuncture applicable to? What methods of acupuncture and moxibustion are there for treatment?

CHAPTER 24

Acupuncture and Moxibustion for Diseases of the Urinary and Reproductive Systems

CHRONIC PROSTATITIS

Overview

Chronic prostatitis is quite common in men and is clinically manifested by frequent urination, urination difficulty and dropping urination, usually with white cloudy urine, a dragging and distending sensation at the perineum, or nocturnal emission, premature ejaculation, and impotence, accompanied by dizziness, fatigue and other symptoms. It belongs to the disease or syndrome categories of *niao jing* (尿精, seminal fluid) and *bai zhuo* (白浊, cloudy urine) in TCM, and was first recorded in *The Systematic Classic of Acupuncture and Moxibustion*, while the modern research on the treatment drew attention from the 1970s and made some worthwhile explorations of point selection and acupuncture techniques. At present, the effective rate for the treatment with acupuncture and moxibustion averages about 80%.

Treatment

Body acupuncture

Selection of points: Commonly used points — two groups, namely (1) *qianliexian* [the middle point between *huiyinxue* (RN 1) and the anus] and (2) *huiyin* (RN 1) (on the perineum, the middle point between the root of the scrotum and the anus) and *shenshu* (BL 23). Supplementary points — *qihai* (RN 6), *zhongji* (RN 3), *guanyuan* (RN 4) and *zhibian* (BL 54).

Manipulation: One group is employed at each treatment session, and two groups may be employed alone or alternately, adding two or three supplementary points. *Qianliexian* is punctured with a No. 28–30 filiform needle, 3 *cun* in length, by perpendicularly inserting to a depth of 1.5–2.5 *cun*, with the needle retained for 20 min, during which the sensation is strengthened by thrusting, lifting, twirling and rotating the needle. *Huiyin* (RN 1) is punctured with a filiform needle 3 *cun* long by perpendicularly inserting the needle to a depth of 2–3 *cun*, till soreness and distension occur. Manipulation is given by thrusting and lifting coupled with slight twirling and rotating 3–5 times, before withdrawing the needle. For *shenshu* (BL 23), a No. 28 filiform needle 2 *cun* in length is inserted obliquely toward the spine, to a depth of 1–1.5 *cun*, until local soreness and distension are felt, before withdrawing the needle. *Qihai* (RN 6), *guanyuan* (RN 4) and *zhongji* (RN 3) are perpendicularly punctured to a depth of 1.2–1.5 *cun*, until the sensation reaches the urethra. Withdraw the needle after thrusting, lifting, twirling and rotating for 1–2 min. *Zhibian* (BL 54) is punctured obliquely toward the inside with a filiform needle 3.5–4 *cun* long, to a depth of 3–3.5 *cun*, until the needling sensation radiates to the perineum and the urethra. Withdraw the needle immediately after thrusting, lifting, twirling and rotating for 1 min. The manipulation is given once every day or every other day, at 10 sessions as a course, at an interval of 3–5 days between the courses.

Acupoint laser irradiation

Selection of points: Commonly used points — two groups, namely (1) prostate and *ciliao* (BL 32) and (2) *huiyin* (RN 1). Supplementary points — *shenshu* (BL 23), *sanyinjiao* (SP 6), *zhongji* (RN 3) and *guanyuan* (RN 4).

Manipulation: One group of commonly used points and one or two supplementary points are employed at each session (or employed alternately). A helium–neon laser acupuncture device is used to irradiate the laser beam with specially made optical fiber, wavelength 632.8 nm and output power 0.5–1.8 mW. The main points are sterilized. A specially made hollow needle is used with the optical fiber inside. The left index finger is inserted into the anus as guidance, and the needle is inserted into the prostate from *huiyin* (RN 1) with output power 1.8 mW for 20 min. The remaining points are punctured by connecting to the laser beam with output power 0.5 mW for 15–30 min. The irradiation is given once daily, at 4 sessions as a course; another may be needed 7 days later, for those unrecovered.

Remarks

The two methods above are the most widely used and effective in clinic at the present time, with fewer points selected. Body acupuncture was applied to 200 cases, with a total effective rate of 84%, and 70 patients (35%) recovered completely; and acupoint laser irradiation to 184 cases, with an effective rate of 98.4%, and 97 patients (52.7%) recovered completely. While body acupuncture is being given, make sure that the patient evacuates urine, for fear that the insertion will injure the bladder. As for acupoint laser irradiation, it is critical to insert the hollow needle into the prostate while puncturing *huiyin* (RN 1).

IMPOTENCE

Overview

Impotence is a common problem among men, where the patient has sexual desire but fails to sustain an erection sufficient for sexual intercourse. It is classified into functional impotence and organic impotence. The former is the subject discussed here, for it constitutes 85%–90% of all cases. This disease is also called *yangwei* in TCM or *yinwei* in early documents. Acupuncture and moxibustion for impotence was first seen in *The Systematic Classic of Acupuncture and Moxibustion*, while modern reports appeared in 1935, and a large number of clinical observations have been made since the 1950s. For one thing, many acupoints are involved in the treatment; for another, the effective points are screened. The success rate is 90% or more.

Treatment

Acupuncture and moxibustion

Selection of points: Commonly used points — *zhongji* (RN 1), *guanyuan* (RN 4) and *qugu* (CV 2). Supplementary points — *ciliao* (BL 32), *dadun* (LR 1), *shenque* (RN 8), *sanyinjiao* (SP 6) and *fuliu* (KI 7).

Manipulation: Two of the commonly used points and two or three supplementary points are employed at each treatment session. Prior to acupuncture on abdominal points, evacuate urine. A needle 1.5–2.5 *cun*, in length is perpendicularly inserted to a depth of 1.2–2 *cun*, by thrusting and lifting the needle to induce the sensation of an electric shock radiating to the root of the urethra. *Ciliao* (BL 32), *fuliu* (KI 7) and *sanyinjiao* (SP 6) are punctured with the routine needling technique. When the sensation of soreness and distension is achieved, thrust, lift, twirl and rotate the needle for 1–2 min, with a retention of 15–20 min. *Dadun* (LR 1) and *shenque* (RN 8) are given sparrow-pecking moxibustion for 10–15 min once every day or every other day, at 10 sessions as a course, at an interval of 3–5 days between courses.

Acupoint injection

Selection of points: Commonly used points — *yangweixue* [consisting of five points: one point at the upper one-third, middle one-third and lower one-third respectively; bilateral points 1 *cun* to the one-third of the middle along the line between *shenque* (RN 8) and *qugu* (RN 2)]. Supplementary points — three groups, namely (1) *sanyinjiao* (Sp 6) and *shenshu* (BL 23); (2) *changqiang* (DU 1); (3) *ciliao* (BL 32).

Manipulation: The injections are 0.5% procaine, strychnine nitrate (2 mgL/1 ml) or 5% glucose 30 ml mixed with strychnine 1 ml. Commonly used points and one group of supplementary points are employed at each session. Five needles 2.5 *cun* long are inserted into five points successively, with thrusting, lifting, twirling and rotating of the needles to induce a sensation radiating to the penis. The needles are retained for 20 min, with interrupted stimulations. Supplementary points are given point injection. The first group is given strychnine injection; one pair of points is employed, with the two points used alternately. A No. 5 dental needle is inserted till the arrival of a needle sensation and then 0.5 ml strychnine is injected, twice per week. The second group is given 0.5% procaine. After the skin anaphylactic test, a No. 7 needle is inserted along *changqiang* (DU 1) and along the tailbone upward to the ischial rectal fossa, and then 20 ml procaine is injected (be sure not to inject it into the rectum), also twice per week. The third group is given the mixed injection, which is better to be prepared temporarily. With the patient in the prone sitting posture, locate *ciliao* (BL 32), insert a No. 5 needle to a depth of 1 *cun*, and inject 4 ml liquid, also twice per week. The three groups may be applied in turn, once a day, six times as a course.

Remarks

Acupoint stimulation for impotence varies a lot and the two methods here are widely used in clinics. Take acupuncture and moxibustion, for instance. Among 355 patients treated with acupuncture and moxibustion, 219 recovered, and the effective rate of point injection was much higher. Observations show that a greater effect will be achieved when the needle is inserted into abdominal or sacrum points with the sensation radiating to the perineum or the glans penis, and it is better to induce a needling sensation radiating to the abdomen even if the distal points are punctured. Besides, in order to enhance the efficacy, acupuncture treatment should be accompanied by psychological counseling, guiding the intercourse methods and imparting sexual knowledge. During the treatment, sexual life must stop.

QUESTIONS

(1) What are the characteristics of point selection and manipulation in the treatment of chronic prostatitis?
(2) What are the requirements for the needling sensation in the treatment of impotence with point stimulation?

SPERM ABNORMALITIES

Overview

Sperm abnormalities, the main cause of male infertility, include low sperm counts, slow sperm motility and abnormally shaped sperm, and other syndromes which may affect sperm mobility and survival, such as semen significantly higher or lower, overstickiness, semen without lique-faction, or an abnormal pH value. Sperm abnormalities belong to *jing bu zu* (sperm shortage) or *jing leng* (cold sperm) in TCM. Acupuncture treatment first appeared in *The Systematic Classic of Acupuncture and Moxibustion*, and modern application was reported in 1958, and great progress has been made in the past 30 years. The effective rate of acupuncture therapy is about 90%, especially for cases of simple sperm abnormalities without any other symptoms.

Treatment

Acupuncture and moxibustion (I)

Selection of points: Commonly used points — two groups, namely (1) *qihai* (RN 6), *guanyuan* (RN 4) and *sanyinjiao* (SP 6); (2) *shenshu* (BL 23), *ciliao* (BL 32) and *taixi* (KI 3). Supplementary points — *zhongji* (RN 3), *zusanli* (ST 36), *zhaohai* (KI 6) and *mingmen* (DU 4).

Manipulation: One group is employed at each session, with the two groups employed alternately, and one or two supplementary points are added according to different conditions. Acupuncture is given to the abdominal points by perpendicularly inserting or repeatedly thrusting or lifting the needle with the tip slightly downward to induce a transmitting sensation. The points on the lower back are inserted into perpendicularly with reinforcing manipulation by twirling and rotating the needles, and moxa sticks 2 cm long are placed on the points with warming needle moxibustion. *Sanyinjiao* (SP 6), *taixi* (KI 3) and *zhaohai* (KI 6) are punctured till the arrival of *qi*, followed by twirling and rotating the needle for 1–2 min. The needles are retained at each point for 15–20 min. After withdrawal of the needles, points on the abdomen and the lower extremities are given sparrow-pecking moxibustion with moxa sticks alternately for about 15 min, till the local skin becomes reddish, once every day or every other day, 10 times as a treatment course.

Acupuncture and moxibustion (II)

Selection of points: Two groups — (1) *qugu* (RN 2), *sanyinjiao* (SP 6), *zhongji* (RN 3) and *guanyuan* (RN 4), and (2) *ciliao* (BL 32), *shenshu* (BL 23) and *mingmen* (DU 4).

Manipulation: One group is employed at each session, with the two groups employed alternately every other day. *Qugu* (CV 2) and *sanyinjiao* (SP 6) are punctured first with reinforcing manipulation by thrusting and lifting the needle with mild stimulation on the arrival of *qi*, and the needles are retained at each point. Then *guanyuan* (RN 4) and *zhongji* (RN 3) are given ginger moxibustion with three cones till there is a local erythema of the skin. For the second group, *ciliao* (BL 32) is punctured first. On the arrival of *qi*, ginger moxibustion is given to *shenshu* (BL 23) and *mingmen* (DU 4) with three cones. The needle is retained for 15–20 min, during which it is manipulated once every 5–10 min, 15 times as a course, at an interval of 5–7 days between courses.

Remarks

Acupuncture and moxibustion for sperm abnormalities has a few methods, but it has been applied to many cases. The two methods above were respectively applied to 256 cases and 160 cases, among which 155 patients (60.5%) and 125 patients (78.3%) completely recovered, which showed that a higher cure rate had been achieved. In addition, followup visits proved that those who completely recovered had a higher fertility rate. The methods above are a combination of acupuncture and moxibustion, so it is important to employ a comprehensive way since sperm abnormalities are difficult to cure. Acupuncture on abdominal points should avoid inserting too deep, which is a rule beginners must observe.

EJACULATION DISORDER

Overview

Ejaculation disorder, belonging to *yang qiang* (阳强, excessive yang) in TCM, is a medical condition in which there is no semen from the penis at the time of climax, similar to phallodynia treated with acupuncture and moxibustion, mentioned in *Important Formulas Worth a Thousand Gold Pieces for Emergencies* in the Tang Dynasty. Acupuncture treatment for ejaculation disorder in modern times was first reported in the 1970s, and clinical cases have been increasing in recent years, with the rise of ontology with TCM. Acupuncture is the main method in point stimulations, with an effective rate of about 90%. Electroacupuncture and moxibustion are also applicable.

Treatment

Body acupuncture

Selection of points: Commonly used points — *qugu* (RN 2) or *guanyuan* (RN 4), and *dadun* (LR 1). Supplementary points — *zusanli* (ST 36) and *shenshu* (BL 23) for a weak constitution; *sanyinjiao* (SP 6) and *baihui* (DU 20) for insomnia.

Manipulation: Commonly used points are all employed, *qugu* (CV 2) and *guanyuan* (RN 4) alternately. The abdominal points are given deep acupuncture with exploration manipulation by thrusting and lifting the needles to induce a sensation radiating to the glans penis, with the needles retained for 30 min. *Dadun* (LR 1) is given sparrow-pecking moxibustion with a moxa stick for 5 min. Supplementary points are selected according to different symptoms. Insert the needle swiftly till the arrival of *qi*, followed by twirling and rotating it for 1–2 min. If the needling sensation is weak, twist the needle slowly to strengthen the sensation, with a retention of 15–20 min, once a day, 10–15 times as a course. The next course begins after 3–5 days.

Electroacupuncture

Selection of points: Two groups — (1) *sanyinjiao* (SP 6), *guanyuan* (RN 4), *zhongji* (NR 3) and *qugu* (RN 2); (2) *huiyin* (RN 1), *ciliao* (BL 32), *shenshu* (BL 23) and *zhibian* (BL 54).

Manipulation: One group is employed at each session, with the two groups employed alternately. Points of the first group are punctured with filiform needles 2 *cun* in length by inserting to a depth of 1.5–1.8 *cun*. Slightly thrusting, lifting, twirling and rotating the needles induces a sensation of soreness and numbness radiating downward. Then *sanyinjiao* (SP 6) is inserted to a depth of 1.5 *cun*, with the needle retained on the arrival of *qi*. Connect the points to an electric acupuncture device with irregular wave for 20 min. After withdrawal of the needles, *zhibian* (BL 32) is obliquely inserted inward with a filiform needle 4 *cun* long, to a depth of 3–3.5 cun, with a sensation radiating to the abdomen and the perineum. Manipulate the needle for 1–2 min by mildly thrusting and lifting without retention. For those with a long course of disease, the points mentioned above may be given moxibustion with moxa sticks until the local skin becomes reddish. The manipulation is applied once every other day, at 6 sessions as a course, at an interval of 5 days between courses.

Acupuncture and moxibustion

Selection of points: (1) *zhongji* (RN 3), *taixi* (KI 3) and *guanyuan* (RN 4); (2) *shenshu* (BL 23), *ciliao* (BL 32) and *mingmen* (DU 4).

Manipulation: One group is employed at each session, and the two groups are employed alternately. *Zhongji* (RN 3), *taixi* (KI 3) and *guanyuan* (RN 4) are punctured first with reinforcing manipulation by softly inserting and swiftly twirling and rotating the needles until the patient feels soreness, distension and numbness. Then apply ginger moxibustion to *guanyuan* (RN 4) or *mingmen* (DU 4). Withdraw the needles three cones later. The manipulation is given once daily, at 15 sessions as a course. Another course may be applied after 3–5 days if the effect is not obvious.

Remarks

Ejaculation disorder is classified into two types: organic and functional. Acupuncture and moxibustion mainly aims at the latter. The methods above, except for electroacupuncture, have proven effective in more than 150 cases. However, the following three points should be noted during the acupuncture treatment: (1) while needling the abdominal points, be careful to achieve a needling sensation that reaches the glans penis or urethral orifice; if not, a poor effect will be obtained; (2) the disease is stubborn and chronic, requiring two or three courses for treatment; (3) the disease is usually caused by psychological factors, especially lack of sexual knowledge, so normal treatment in combination with psychotherapy, and trust from the patient, will lead to a better curative effect.

QUESTIONS

(1) What are the similarities and differences between the two acupuncture and moxibustion methods in treating sperm abnormalities?

(2) Describe how to manipulate the two point stimulations in treating ejaculation disorder.

CHAPTER 25

Acupuncture and Moxibustion
for Diseases of Surgery

ACUTE INFLAMMATION

Overview

Acute inflammation is a commonly seen and important pathologic process, characterized by histic deterioration, hyperemia, increased permeability and histiocytic hyperplasia. Acute inflammation on the body surface manifests itself clinically with red swelling, thermalgia and dysfunction.

Treatment of various inflammatory diseases with acupuncture and moxibustion is well known, and infective inflammation is introduced here. Reports about anti-inflammation with acupuncture by electroacupuncture and point injection were published in the late 1950s; research documents about its anti-inflammatory mechanism through animal experiments appeared in the 1960s; and studies on the anti-inflammation of acupuncture made great progress from the late 1970s to the turn of the century. And methods vary a lot, including moxibustion, ear acupuncture, point laser irradiation, electroacupuncture and point injection, as well as body acupuncture. Thousands of cases with surgical infective inflammation have confirmed the effectiveness of acupuncture, with a total effective rate of 92.6%–100%. And researches have shown that acupuncture and moxibustion is able to inhibit the three main pathologic processes of inflammation and is highly effective for permeability.

The anti-inflammatory mechanism of acupuncture is believed to lie in its benign accommodation, which cannot only enhance defense response but also inhibit excessive defense response. That is to say, acupuncture is able to reinforce the immunological function of the body, restrain overincrease in the inflammatory vascular permeability and emigration and infiltration of leucocytes, ameliorate capillary and lymph circulation, and promote the absorption of inflammatory effusion so as to control the necrosis area of the focus and relieve the inflammation.

Treatment

Acupuncture and moxibustion

Selection of points: Commonly used points — points of the upper limbs: *quchi* (LI 11) and *hegu* (LI 4); lower limbs: *zusanli* (ST 36) and *yanglingquan* (GB 34) and *sanyinjiao* (SP 6); trunk: vertebral point, *weizhong* (BL 40); hands: *lingtai* (DU 10); feet: *xingjian* (LR 2). Supplementary points — upper limbs: *shousanli* (LI 10) and *neiguan* (PC 6); lower limbs: *biguan* (ST 31), *fengshi* (GB 31) and *ashi* point; trunk: *huantiao* (GB 30), *zhibian* (BL 54) and *ashi* point; hands: *hegu* (LI 4) and *ashi* point; feet: *sanyinjiao* (SP 6) and *ashi* point; fever: *dazhui* (DU 14) and *quchi* (LI 11). Location of the vertebral point: 0.2 *cun* directly posterior to *houxi* (SI 13). Location of the *ashi* point: focal zone (the same as below).

Manipulation: Commonly used points are taken as the main points and supplementary points as adjuvant. No. 26–30 filiform needles are inserted with the tips toward the focal zone by lifting, thrusting, twirling and rotating the needles repeatedly to transmit the sensation to the affected area, and then reducing manipulation is applied with strong stimulation for 0.5–1 min, with the needles retained for 20 min before withdrawing them. The *ashi* point is pricked to bleed with a sterilized three-edged needle or cupped to draw pus out according to symptoms. After that, 20 g pure moxa (or a moxa roll) is put into the warming moxibustion apparatus and ignited to apply revolving moxibustion for 20 min. The treatment is performed once or twice a day, or once every 6 h for severe cases, until the inflammation disappears completely.

Body acupuncture

Selection of points: Baliao, Quchi (LI 11) and *zusanli* (ST 36).

Manipulation: Commonly used points are employed at each session and only bilateral *quchi* (LI 11) is employed for cases with nonsurgical infection. No. 28 filiform needles, 2–3.5 *cun* long, are inserted deeply to the sacrum, into points from *xiaoliao* (BL 34) to shangliao (BL 31) via *zhongliao* (BL 33) and *ciliao* (BL 32), by twirling and rotating at great amplitude combined with slight lifting and thrusting of the needle for 1 min with strong stimulation, before withdrawing the needle. *Quchi* (LI 11) and *zusanli* (ST 36) are punctured deeply, to about 1.5 *cun*. Manipulation of three insertions and one lifting is applied, which is to needle the point three times, with twirling and rotating of the needles combined with slightly lifting and thrusting repeatedly every time when the needle is inserted to a depth of 0.5 *cun*, and lift the needle from the deep to the superficial layer all at one time. Do this repeatedly and withdraw the needle, with the pinholes pressed. Following the operation, only *quchi* (LI 11) is punctured the next day, once in the morning and once in the afternoon, for 3–7 days on end, and the course may be prolonged if the symptoms are not ameliorated.

Cupping

Selection of points: Dachui (DU 14), interscapular region, *shangliao* (BL 31) and corresponding area. Location of the interscapular region: the region between the medial border of the scapula and the 4th–6th thoracic vertebrae. Location of the corresponding area: the area in the back and the lower back corresponding to the inflammatory focus in the chest and the abdomen.

Manipulation: Select the point area according to the focus location. *Dazhui* (DU 14) indicates infections in the head, the face or the neck; the interscapular region, in the fingers or upper limbs; *shangliao* (BL 31), in the toes, lower limbs, buttocks or perineal region; the corresponding area, in the soft tissues of the chest or the abdomen. Different affected areas require different postures. The sitting position is taken for infections above the abdomen; the prone or lateral recumbent posture, for infections below the buttocks or perineal region. The point is located and sterilized as a routine, and is given cotton fire cupping or cupping with a vacuum jar shortly after being pricked lightly with a three-edged needle three times (no matter whether there is bleeding or not). Be sure that the three pinholes are included in the jar, which is retained for 10–15 min, until the local skin becomes scarlet. The cupping period should not be shortened for a better curative effect. The manipulation is applied once daily and the cupping area may be changed a little for the second session.

Moxibustion

Selection of points: *Ashi* point.

Manipulation: 20 g of moxa wool is put into the fumigating moxibustion apparatus, with the hole directly toward the *ashi* point (focal zone), 3–5 cm to the focus until the patient feels warm, for 20–50 min at each session. Generally, infections of *Staphylococcus aureus* or beta streptococcus need moxibustion of 20 min, *Escherichia coli* infections 30 min, and *Pseudomonas aeruginosa* infections 50 min. The moxibustion is applied once daily, at 10 sessions as a course.

Remarks

Among the four therapies, acupuncture and moxibustion is applicable to various surgical infections, and is more commonly used and effective in the clinic; body acupuncture, to postoperative infections or inflammatory infections of gynecology and obstetrics; cupping, to surgical infections, with easy manipulation and a short course of treatment which may be combined with acupuncture; moxibustion, i.e. fumigating moxibustion, for various superficial bacterial infections, is also convenient and effective. If there is no fumigating moxibustion apparatus, fumigating with moxa sticks is available. Acute inflammation is treated in one course, and other therapies may be alternative if acupuncture and moxibustion achieves no effect.

ERYSIPELAS

Overview

Erysipelas is an acute streptococcus bacterial infection of the deep epidermis with lymphatic spread that occurs in the face and lower extremities. It is characterized by sudden onset, erythematous skin lesions with a sharply demarcated raised edge, very red but fading if pressed. The skin is stretching and burning hot, enlarging rapidly, accompanied by fever, chills and headaches. Modern reports about acupuncture treatment for erysipelas appeared in the 1950s, and were small in number and remained restricted access material. In the past 30 years, more and more documents have proven the effectiveness of acupuncture therapy. Effect analysis of various soft tissue inflammations finds that acupuncture is highly effective for cellulitis and erysipelas, and that the bloodletting method is the most widely used in the clinic.

Treatment

Bloodletting

Selection of points: Commonly used points — *ashi* and *weizhong* (BL 40). Supplementary points — two groups, namely (1) *huantiao* (GB 30), *yanglingquan* (GB 34) and *sanyinjiao* (SP 6), and (2) *zusanli* (ST 36) and *yinlingquan* (SP 9). *Ashi* location: focal zone (the same as below).

Manipulation: Commonly used points are the main points. First, a violet engorged small vessel is found (if there is no clearly engorged small vessel, obvious veins around are available) and sterilized, followed by a round sharp needle (a No. 28 filiform needle is an alternative) inserted rapidly into the vessel, shaking and withdrawing it slowly. When bleeding occurs, press the pores with sterilized cotton balls. Four or five punctures are performed at each session. *Weizhong* (BL 40) is selected from the affected side and punctured for three or four drops of blood. Either of the supplementary groups is employed, and punctured perpendicularly 1–1.5 *cun* deep with a No. 28 filiform needle. On the arrival of *qi*, reducing manipulation is applied by lifting and thrusting combined with twirling and rotating, without retention of the needles. At the beginning, the treatment is performed once daily, and once every other day from the third session until total recovery, which will generally take 3–6 times.

Body acupuncture

Selection of points: Commonly used points — *diji* (SP 8), *xuehai* (SP 10), *sanyinjiao* (SP 6), *fenglong* (ST 40), *taichong* (LR 3), *ashi* and *sifeng*

(EX-UE10). Supplementary points — for the lower limbs, *yanglingquan* (GB 34), *zusanli* (ST 36) and *ligou* (LR 5); for the head and face, *yifeng* (SJ 17), *touwei* (ST 8), *sibai* (ST 2) and *hegu* (LI 4).

Manipulation: Commonly used points are taken as the main points, and supplementary points as adjuvant. On the arrival of *qi*, reducing manipulation (rapid insertion and slow withdrawal, first deep and then slow), from the slow–rapid reinforcing–reducing method, is applied by lifting, thrusting, twirling and rotating the needle for 1–2 min with strong stimulation, with the needles retained for 20–30 min, manipulating the needles once every 10 min. The *ashi* point is tapped forcefully with a three-edged needle or a dermal needle till blood is out, and this is combined with cupping if necessary. *Sifeng* (EX-UE10) is given pricking needling till mucus is out with a thick filiform needle or a three-edged needle. Acupuncture is performed once daily; other methods, once every other day.

Cupping

Selection of points: *Ashi* point.

Manipulation: After local sterilization, a small-sized three-edged needle is taken for rapid scattered needling from upper to lower to let beadlike blood out within the border of the skin lesion, followed by flash-fire cupping with a glass cup in a size depending on the area of the skin lesion, with the cup retained for about 1 min. Wipe off the blood stains after the cup is removed. The cupping is applied once every other day.

Remarks

The three methods introduced above all involve bloodletting therapy, which is the most widely used and highly effective, but other methods may be alternatives if there is no response to bloodletting two or three times. Body acupuncture combines needling with bloodletting, and it has a good short-term effect but the long-term effect remains unsatisfactory. Cupping, which involves bloodletting, is applicable to erysipelas in the early stage. In short, different conditions require different therapies.

CHOLELITHIASIS

Overview

Cholelithiasis refers to the presence or formation of gallstones in the biliary tract, usually in the gallbladder, and is clinically characterized by biliary colic (sweating and a pale face due to extreme pain), nausea, vomiting, icterus to different degrees, fever at acute episodes; loss of appetite, epigastric distension and pain, belching, pantothenic acid, constipation or diarrhea at intermission. The first report about acupuncture treatment appeared in 1959, and in the past 40 years various kinds of acupoint stimulations have been in practice and confirmed effective in treatment of cholelithiasis. Now it is believed to be applicable to cases with calculus of the common bile duct 1 cm or less in diameter and nonorganic stenosis in the inferior extremity of the bile duct; and cases with cholecystolithiasis less than 1 cm in diameter and good discharge function of the gallbladder.

Treatment

Electroacupuncture

Selection of points: Commonly used points — *riyue* (GB 24) (on the upper abdomen, directly below the nipple, in the seventh intercostal space, 4 *cun* lateral to the anterior midline) and *qimen* (LR 14). Supplementary points — *ashi* (2 *cun* lateral to the midline above the nipple from the right) and *danshu* (BL 19).

Manipulation: Commonly used points are taken as the main points, and supplementary points are added for severe pain and gallbladder enlargement, all from the right side. Perpendicular needling is applied [to *danshu* (LR 14) with the needle obliquely a little toward the vertebral column, and to the *ashi* point with a 6-*cun*-long filiform needle inserted horizontally into the center of the gallbladder enlargement to the oblique externus abdominis muscle]; on the arrival of *qi*, connect to the G6805 electroacupuncture apparatus with an irregular wave and an intensity tolerable to patients, for 60 min. After the needles are withdrawn, 50 ml of 33% magnesium sulfate is taken once daily, at 10 sessions as a course.

Ear acupuncture

Selection of points: Commonly used points — liver, pancreas and gallbladder, duodenum, sympathetic and shoulders. Supplementary points — spleen, stomach, *shenmen*, root of ear tragus, large intestine and endocrine.

Manipulation: Commonly used points are employed at each session, combined with two or three supplementary points. Press the ear acupoints with *Vaccaria segetalis* seeds or magnetic beads (380 G), one ear each time, the two ears alternately; and the patient is advised to repeat that by himself or herself after meals for 10–20 min, three or four times daily. The plaster is changed two or three times every week, at 20 sessions as a course, at an interval of 5 days between courses.

Acupoint laser irradiation

Selection of points: *Danshu* (BL 19) and *ashi* point (on the right upper quadrant, the most obvious tenderness).

Manipulation: *Ashi* point and *danshu* (BL 19) on the right are irradiated with a helium–neon laser irradiation apparatus with wavelength 632.8 nm, 30–60 cm between the pipe mouth and the skin, output 2 mW and facula diameter 2 mm. The irradiation is applied for 10 min at each point, once or twice daily, and 33% magnesium sulfate taken simultaneously, 10–20 ml each time, three times a day.

Remarks

Among the three therapies, ear acupuncture is the most widely used. It is mainly applicable to cholelithiasis in its intermission, and effective in discharging calculus and easing the symptoms for prevention of acute attacks. Point laser irradiation and electroacupuncture are often employed in the acute stage. The total lithagogue rate of electroacupuncture is 78.4%, obviously higher than that of 33% magnesium sulfate medication. Laser irradiation is also effective, but needs further verification since it is applied to relatively few cases.

QUESTIONS

(1) Which types of acute inflammation are the four acupuncture therapies applicable to respectively?

(2) The three acupuncture therapies for erysipelas involve bloodletting. State the features of the manipulations.

(3) Which therapy of point stimulations do you prefer in treatment of cholelithiasis?

TRANSFUSION REACTIONS

Overview

The most common and severe transfusion reactions are the pyrogenetic reaction and the allergic reaction. The former occurs 1–2 h after liquor and blood transfusion, with sudden rigors, high fever (up to 39°C–40°C) accompanied by flushing, headache, nausea, vomiting, or even delirium and coma; the latter presents as pruritus, localized or extensive hives, or angioneurotic edema, bronchial spasm, or even anaphylactic shock in more serious situations.

Reports about acupuncture and moxibustion for prevention of transfusion reactions were first seen in early 1970, in which ear acupuncture as the main treatment method was more applicable to clinical practice, and most of which focused on prevention of pyrogenetic reactions. A great number of clinical observations have shown that acupuncture and moxibustion is highly effective for prevention and cure of transfusion reactions. Clinical comparisons have shown that there are many more cases of pyrogenetic reactions and allergic reactions by preventive therapies without acupuncture, while ear acupuncture treatment may obviously lessen the extent of reactions and shorten the length of reactions.

Prevention and Treatment

Ear acupuncture

Selection of points: Commonly used points — shenmen, adrenal gland and lung. Supplementary points — for fever reactions, sympathetic and subcortex; for allergic reactions, endocrine and wind stream; *quchi* (LI 11) and *xuehai* (SP 10) (body acupoint).

Manipulation: Commonly used points are employed at each session, and one or two supplementary points may be added according to the extent of the reaction, ear points for prevention and body points for treatment. In treatment, a filiform needle is used with strong stimulation by continuous twirling and rotating until the reaction is relieved. The needle is retained for 30 min, during which twirling is applied interruptedly. Body acupuncture is applied with reducing manipulation, with the needles retained for 30 min. In prevention, prior to liquor or blood transfusion, press the ear points with *Vaccaria segetalis* seeds or magnetic beads for 5–10 min, until the patient complains of soreness, numbness, heaviness and distension on one side of the head, and the auricle of the ear becomes red and hot.

Body acupuncture

Selection of points: Commonly used points — two groups, namely (1) *zhongchong* (PC 9) and *hegu* (LI 4), and (2) *dazhui* (DU 4). Supplementary points — *shaoshang* (LU 11) and *shangyang* (LI 1) added for fever; *yintang* (EX-HN3) for head and forehead pain; *lieque* (LU 7) for head and neck pain; *neiguan* (PC 6) and *zusanli* (ST 36) for chest stuffiness and nausea.

Manipulation: One group of commonly used points is employed at each session, and supplementary points may be added according to symptoms. A 0.5-*cun*-long filiform needle is inserted into *zhongchong* (PC 9), with the needle retained for 2–15 min, for mild disease. For severe cases, one or two drops of blood are pricked out with a 2-*cun*-long filiform needle inserted perpendicularly into *hegu* (LI 4) with uniform reinforcing–reducing manipulation by strong stimulation, with the needle retained for 5–10 min. *Shaoshang* (LU 11), *shangyang* (LI 1) and *yintang* (EX-HN3) are pricked for bloodletting. The other points are punctured with uniform reinforcing–reducing manipulation, with the needles retained for 2–10 min. *Dazhui* (DU 4) is punctured obliquely upward with a 1-*cun*-long filiform needle to a depth of 0.5 *cun*, twirling and rotating the needle with strong stimulation, with the needles retained for 10 min. A better effect can be achieved if the acupuncture is applied as soon as a rigor and fever appear.

Moxibustion

Selection of points: Mingmen (DU 4).

Manipulation: When the patient complains of chills, rigors or fever, moxibustion is applied immediately to *mingmen* (DU 4). The practitioner holds the moxa roll and moves it around the acupoint horizontally so as to cause a burning sensation but no scalding of the local skin, for 2–3 min, and at most 10 min. At the same time, slow down the transfusion speed to 70–40 drops a minute. Stop the transfusion if the severe reaction occurs to the whole body.

Remarks

Among the three methods introduced above, ear acupuncture is the most widely applied, not only for operations in various postures, but also for prevention as well as treatment. Body acupuncture is applicable to diverse adverse reactions in the course of transfusion, and it can be combined with ear acupuncture if necessary. Moxibustion aims mainly to cure pyrogenetic reactions. Generally, 5-min moxibustion is enough. Otherwise, change to another therapy.

RADIATION REACTIONS

Overview

Radiation reactions are adverse reactions during the course of radiotherapy for malignant neoplastic diseases, including general reactions like anorexia, nausea, vomiting, headache and fatigue; hemogram reactions like leukopenia and thrombocytopenia; and local reactions. Absence of timely handling and treatment may lead to obvious postradiation. There is no specific therapeutics for radiation reactions except for adjusting the treatment protocols and dosages, or stopping treatment.

Acupuncture treatment for radiation reactions began in the 1950s and observations of many cases found that acupuncture and moxibustion could obviously ease the systemic symptoms, and be effective for leuko-penia, factitial proctitis and cutaneous ulcers. In the 1970s, ear acupuncture was applied to leukopenia induced by radiotherapy or chemotherapy and achieved a certain curative effect. There has been great development in methods of acupoint stimulation and observation of curative effect in recent 40 years. For example, helium–neon laser irradiation is applied to various types of radiation reactions, and its indications and practical effect have been observed and compared.

Much work has been done on the mechanism of treatment of radiation with acupuncture and moxibustion. It has been proven through empirical study that acupuncture and moxibustion is able to resist the inhibition to immune function caused by radiotherapy, to protect the hemogram, and to enhance marrow-blood-producing function so as to improve the human tolerance to radiotherapy. And it has been further confirmed in recent times that the major mechanism for increasing leukocytes by acupuncture and moxibustion lies in enhancing CSF (colony-stimulating factors) content and activity in blood serum, and promoting the division growth of bone marrow hematopoietic stem cells, so as to increase the leukocytic clono-genicity, and immature and mature granular leukocytes in bone marrow.

Treatment

Body acupuncture

Selection of points: Commonly used points — *quchi* (LI 11), *neiguan* (PC 6) and *zusanli* (ST 36). Supplementary points — *dazhui* (DU 14) added for leukopenia; *zhongwan* (RN 20) and *sanyinjiao* (SP 6) for poor appetite; *baihui* (DU 20) and *shenmen* (HT 7) for dizziness and insomnia; *tianshu* (ST 25) and *shangjuxu* (ST 37) for proctitis. Location of the *lei-yuan* point: 5 *fen* below the intersection point of the medioclavicular line and costal margin.

Manipulation: One or two commonly used points are employed at each session, and supplementary points may be added according to symptoms. On the arrival of *qi*, uniform reinforcing–reducing manipulation is applied by lifting, thrusting, twirling and rotating the needle with medium and strong stimulation, with the needles retained for 15–30 min. *Leiyuan, guanyuan* (RN 4) and *tianshu* (ST 25) are given moxibustion with moxa sticks for 15 min after acupuncture, until the local skin becomes red. The treatment is applied once daily, at 10 sessions as a course, and the next course begins after a pause of 3–5 days.

Acupoint laser irradiation

Selection of points: Commonly used points — two groups, namely (1) *ashi* point; (2) for dizziness and weariness, *mingmen* (DU 4), *gaohuang* (BL 43) and *zusanli* (ST 36); for poor appetite and nausea, *neiguan* (PC 6), *diji* (SP 8), *pishu* (BL 20) and *zhongwan* (RN 20); for reactions in the oral cavity and throat, *zhaohai* (Ki 6), *shaoshang* (LU 11) and *lianquan* (RN 23); for reactions in the rectum and bladder, *guanyuan* (RN 4), *tianshu* (ST 25), *dachangshu* (BL 25) and *zhongji* (RN 3). Location of the *ashi* point: focus of the radiative cutaneous ulcer.

Manipulation: Irradiation is performed with the helium–neon laser therapeutic apparatus at low power. The first group is punctured for treatment of radiation reactions of the skin. During irradiation, the power is 2–4 mW, the facula diameter 1.5–2.0 mm and the irradiating length 50 mm. If the area for direct radiation is larger than 10 cm, irradiation should be divided into different zones for 20–30 min at each session. The treatment is performed 6 times a week, at 10–12 sessions as a course, at an interval of 3–5 days between courses. The second group is for treatment of various clinical symptoms. Three or four points are selected according to symptoms at each session. Irradiation power varies according to symptoms — generally 3–5 mW, or 8 mW at individual points. Mark the point with gentian violet before irradiating perpendicularly 100 cm above the skin, for 3 min and no more than 15 times for each point. The treatment is applied once daily, at 10 sessions as a course, and the next course begins after an interval of 3–5 days.

Moxibustion

Selection of points: *Dazhui* (DU 14), *hegu* (LI 4), *zusanli* (ST 36) and *sanyinjiao* (SP 6).

Manipulation: Commonly used points are employed at each session. The patient sits up straight, with the acupoints exposed completely. Warm moxibustion is applied with moxa sticks, 1.5 cm above the skin, until the patient feels warmth but not burning pain. Each point requires 10–15 min of moxibustion, till the local skin becomes red, followed by massage for 3–5 min, respectively. The treatment is applied once daily, at 10 sessions as a course.

Acupoint injection

Selection of points: *zusanli* (ST 36).

Manipulation: A fluorodexamethasone injection is given as physic liquor, and bilateral points are employed at each session. 5–10 mg of fluorodexamethasone (5 mg/ml) is sucked into a 5 ml injector with a No. 5 pinhead for dentistry, which is inserted perpendicularly till the arrival of *qi*, and 2.5–5 mg is injected into each point. The treatment is performed once daily, at three sessions as a course.

Remarks

Among the four therapies above, body acupuncture is applicable to various types of radiation reactions, and is the most commonly employed in the clinic. Point laser irradiation is very useful, especially for injuries to the skin due to radiotherapy. Moxibustion and point injection aim to improve leukopenia caused by radiotherapy, and moxibustion can increase the leukocytes in cases with cancer after chemotherapy.

ACUTE APPENDICITIS

Overview

Acute appendicitis is the most common acute surgical condition of the abdomen, characterized by pain in the lower right abdomen that gets progressively more sharp and intense, nausea and vomiting, leukocyte and leukocyte neutrophil counts heightened in most cases, and tenderness in the lower right abdomen (called McBurney's point), which is the main symptom of the disease. Acute appendicitis is classified into four types: acute simple appendicitis, acute suppurative appendicitis, gangrene perforating appendicitis, and periappendiceal abscess. Acupuncture treatment is mainly applied to acute simple appendicitis, similar to *chang yong* (intestinal abscess) in TCM, which was recorded in *Bei Ji Qian Jin Yao Fang* (*Important Formulas Worth a Thousand Gold Pieces for Emergencies*) in the Tang Dynasty. Modern reports about acupuncture treatment began in the early period of the founding of China, and large-scale clinical observations were conducted in the 1950s. It has been shown that acupuncture and moxibustion are the main therapies in treatment of acute simple appendicitis and mild purulent appendicitis.

Treatment

Body acupuncture

Selection of points: Commonly used points — *lanweixue* (EX-LE7), *zusanli* (ST 36), *ashi* point (the most obvious tenderness in the lower right abdomen, i.e. McBurney's point). Supplementary points — *zhongwan* (RN 20) and *neiguan* (PC 6) added for nausea and vomiting; *quchi* (LI 11) and *chize* (LU 5) for fever; *dachangshu* (BL 25) and *ciliao* (BL 32) for abdominal distension.

Manipulation: Two or three commonly used points are employed at each session, and one or two supplementary points are added for obvious symptoms. *Chize* (LU 5) is pricked for drops of blood with a sterilized three-edged needle, and the others are punctured till the arrival of *qi* with reducing manipulation by twirling and rotating combined with lifting and thrusting, with strong stimulation for 1–2 min. The needles are retained in each point for 30–60 min, during which they are manipulated once every 5–10 min, or are connected to the G6805 electroacupuncture apparatus with an irregular wave and an intensity tolerable to patients. The treatment is applied once or twice every day.

Ear acupuncture

Selection of points: Commonly used points — *lanwei* (EX-LE7) [above the crista helicis, the middle of the anterior and central parts, i.e. below *dachang* (BL 25)], the middle part of the fassa helicis. Supplementary points — large intestine, shoulder, subcortex and ear apex for fever; root of the ear vagus for vomiting.

Manipulation: Commonly used points are employed at each session, and one or two supplementary points are added according to symptoms. The ear apex is pricked to bleed with a three-edged needle and the other points are punctured with a No. 28 filiform needle, which is inserted into the tenderness by rapid twirling and rotating for 2–3 min with strong stimulation, with the needles retained for 30–60 min, during which interrupted stimulation is performed on one ear at each session and the two ears alternately. The treatment is applied 1–3 times a day, and pricking the ear apex is applied once daily.

Acupoint injection

Selection of points: Lanweixue (EX-LE7).

Manipulation: Water for injection is taken as physic liquor, 10–20 ml at each session. Bilateral *lanwei* points (EX-LE7) are employed, with the tenderness punctured with a No. 5 needle for dentistry. For patients with strong constitutions and dull to needling, the needle points are inserted obliquely upward (at an angle of 45° with the skin) with slow injection of 10 ml for each point within 5 min; for patients with weak constitutions and sensitive to needling, the needle points are inserted perpendicularly downward or obliquely downward with slow injection of 5 ml for each point. The treatment is applied once daily.

Remarks

Body acupuncture is the major therapy in acupuncture and moxibustion treatment for acute appendicitis, and is effective for acute simple appendicitis and mild purulent appendicitis, with an effective rate of 85%–90%. It is preferable for the treatment because of its confirmed long-term curative effect. Ear acupuncture is also recommended; it was applied to 600 cases, with a recovery rate of 85%, and was able to relieve or remove other symptoms except headaches, to put the hemogram back. Point injection is effective for acute simple appendicitis.

QUESTIONS

(1) What characteristics does acupuncture manipulation have in treatment of transfusion reactions and radiation reactions?
(2) Describe in detail the body acupuncture in treatment of acute appendicitis.

ACUTE MASTITIS

Overview

Acute mastitis refers to inflammation of breast tissue caused by bacterial infections. It is clinically manifested by swelling and pain of the affected breast, a stiffened local area, skin redness, breast tenderness, and swelling of armpit lymph developing into suppuration in several days, accompanied by high fever, chills, fatigue and poor appetite. It is called *ru yong* (deep-rooted breast carbuncles) in TCM, and was recorded in *Zhen Jiu Jia Yi Jing* (*The Systematic Classic of Acupuncture and Moxibustion*), as well as its treatment with acupuncture and moxibustion. Modern reports were first seen in the early 1950s, and so far a great deal of material has been accumulated. It is generally believed that the shorter the course, the better the effect, and much better if the inflammation is treated within 24 h of the onset. According to statistics, the effective rate of acupuncture treatment is above 95%.

Treatment

Body acupuncture

Selection of points: Commonly used points — *jianjing* (GB 21) and *tianzong* (SI 11). Supplementary points — *zusanli* (ST 36), *quchi* (LI 11), *danzhong* (RN 17) and *zhongwan* (RN 20).

Manipulation: Either or both of the commonly used points are employed at each session, and two supplementary points according to symptoms. *Jianjing* (GB 21) on the affected side is punctured perpendicularly with a filiform needle 1.5 *cun* long to a depth of 0.8–1.0 *cun* (the depth depends on the patient's figure, whether lean or fat; not too deep, in case of injuring the apex of the lung), by twirling and rotating combined with lifting and thrusting slightly with strong stimulation which is tolerable to the patient, with the needle retained. *Tianzong* points (SI 11) on both sides are perpendicularly punctured to the periosteum by lifting, thrusting, twirling and rotating to make the sensation radiate to the shoulders and the breasts. The other points are given routine acupuncture with reducing manipulation by lifting and thrusting on the arrival of *qi*, with the needles retained for 20–30 min, during which fumigation and moxibustion with moxa sticks may be applied to the focal zone in the breast. The treatment is applied once daily, at six sessions as a course.

Cupping

Selection of points: Ashi point (the point on the affected side of the back corresponding to the focus of the breast).

Manipulation: The patient bestrides a chair, facing its back, with his or her back exposed completely. Smear some Vaseline or grease around the *ashi* point, before putting a cup 2 *cun* in diameter directly on the point. Then, push the cup upward, downward, to the right and the left four times respectively, till the local area becomes red or ecchymosis appears. Alternatively, the point may be pricked with a three-edged needle to let blood out before cupping. The treatment is applied once daily, at six sessions as a course.

Acupoint laser irradiation

Selection of points: Commonly used points — *danzhong* (RN 17), *zusanli* (ST 36) and *ashi* (the most obvious engorgement and sclerosis in the affected breast). Supplementary points — two groups, namely (1) *jianjing* (GB 21) and *shaoze* (SI 1), and (2) *liangqiu* (ST 34) and *hegu* (LI 4).

Manipulation: Commonly used points are employed at each session, and either of the supplementary groups is employed or the two alternately. The helium–neon laser therapeutic apparatus is used with wavelength 632.8 nm, output 7 mW and facula diameter 4 mm, with irradiation for 5 min at each point. The treatment is applied two or three times a day.

Remarks

Acute mastitis is one of the indications of acupuncture treatment, and applicable to all the needling techniques. Body acupuncture has been applied to 603 cases, with an effective rate of 95%–100%. *Jianjing* (GB 21) and *tianzong* (SI 11) are effective points in treatment of acute mastitis, but accidents may happen to *jianjing* (GB 21), which should avoid deep insertion. Cupping is relatively easy, and applicable to cases within a four-day course and without local suppuration. Acupoint laser irradiation is acceptable to patients as it is painless and safe, but it is limited to cases in the early stage of disease.

ACUTE LYMPHANGITIS

Overview

Acute lymphangitis refers to acute inflammation in the lymphatic vessels and around them caused by morbigenous bacteria spreading into the vicinal lymphatic vessels from the injured skin and infected focus, commonly affecting the extremities. The characteristic symptom is wide, red streaks near the site of infection. The affected areas are hard with pressing pain, accompanied by fever, chills and fatigue. The condition is called *hong si ding* (red-streaked infection) in TCM, whose treatment with the bloodletting method was recorded in some medical literature in the Ming and Qing Dynasties. Reports in modern times began in the early 1960s. At present, the recovery rate is above 95% and most patients recover in four or five days.

Treatment

Acupuncture and moxibustion

Selection of points: Commonly used points — *ashi* point (the beginning and the end point of the red line), 3–5 acupoints near or bilateral to the red line. Supplementary points — points which the red streak passes by, or *xi*-cleft points of the meridians it belongs to.

Manipulation: Commonly used points are preferable, and if there is no obvious effect supplementary points may be added or substituted. First, puncture the meridian points, and on the arrival of *qi* twirl, rotate, lift and thrust the needle with medium or strong stimulation, with the needles retained. Then the *ashi* point is given moxibustion with ignited moxa rolls, which are moved slowly from the beginning of the red line to the end point, 3 cm above the skin, until the patient feels warm and comfortable. The moxibustion is applied for 15–30 min, till the thin red line becomes wide and red. Supplementary points are given bloodletting therapy, i.e. press the area 1 *cun* to both ends of the *xi*-cleft points with the thumb and the index finger of the left hand to produce venous engorgement. A three-edged needle held by the right hand is rapidly inserted into the point to a depth of 2–3 mm, before being rapidly withdrawn. Repeat the manipulation by pricking right, left, up and down in the form of a plum flower, 1–2 mm above the point, until the blood drops like beads. The insertion should be light and swift, and not too deep; press a little for smooth bleeding. Sterilize the area with iodine tincture after the operation, before bandaging it with gauze. The operation is performed once daily, and needling and pricking points may be reduced with relief of the symptoms.

Hot needling

Selection of points: *Ashi* point (the primary focus and the red line).

Manipulation: Furunculosis of the primary focus employed is punctured rapidly to a depth of 0.3–0.5 mm with a needle burned red using an alcohol lamp. Withdraw the needle before the patient feels pain. Three-to-five needles are punctured at one session, until the patient no longer feels pain or itch. Cases with the red line thick and hard, and obvious tenderness, are punctured with fire needling along the red streak, one needle in each point, no more than three needles. Lastly, perform local sterilization with 75% alcohol, apply dephlogisticating paste, cover it with an aseptic dressing and fix it with an adhesive plaster. The treatment is generally applied only once.

Remarks

Bloodletting and moxibustion are the main therapies in treatment of acute lymphangitis with acupuncture and moxibustion, and have been influenced by traditional methods. *Ashi* and meridian points nearby are used as the main points. The first therapy is an extraction and colligation of various common methods, and was once applied to 139 patients with a total effective rate of 97.1%, out of whom 109 recovered after one treatment. The second is fire needling, which can cure the disease with one performance if applied correctly. In this therapy, the needle point must be burned red, and the needle is inserted into the point neither too deeply nor too shallowly. Beginners are advised to choose the first therapy.

QUESTIONS

(1) Which manipulation is preferred in treatment of acute mastitis with acupuncture?
(2) Describe in detail the acupuncture and moxibustion therapies in treatment of acute lymphangitis.

ACUTE URINARY RETENTION

Overview

Acute urinary retention refers to a sudden onset of filling and distension of the bladder due to difficulty in urination. It is clinically manifested by distension and pain in the lower abdomen, stillicidium urinae, jactation, etc. Depending on the causes, acute urinary retention is classified into mechanical obstruction and dynamic obstruction, and acupuncture therapy is applicable to the latter. It belongs to the category of *long bi* (uroschesis) in TCM, and treatment with moxibustion was recorded in the pre-Qin work *Jing Mai* (*Channels*). Modern reports about the acupuncture treatment began in the early 1950s. A great amount of clinical practice has proven that acupuncture and moxibustion is highly effective in treatment of acute urinary retention of various causes, and more effective in postoperative urinary retention. The effective rate is above 90% on the average.

Treatment

Selection of points: Commonly used points — *qugu* (RN 2), *guanyuan* (RN 4) and *sanyinjiao* (SP 6). Supplementary points — *zhongji* (RN 3), *yinlingquan* (SP 9), *zhaohai* (KI 6), *qihai* (RN 6), *dazhui* (DU 14) and *baihui* (DU 20).

Manipulation: Commonly used points are taken as the main points, and supplementary points as adjuvant for better effectiveness. Points of the lower abdomen are punctured with slow insertion, with the left hand holding the needle shaft to avoid injuring the inflated bladder. On the arrival of *qi*, lift and thrust the needles swiftly to make the sensation radiate to the perineal region. Alternatively, *guanyuan* (RN 4) is given transverse insertion (at an angle of 10° with the skin) penetrating to *qugu* (RN 2), twirling and rotating rapidly for 1 min. *Sanyinjiao* (SP 6) is punctured with the tip upward, with lifting and thrusting of the needle to transmit the sensation upward. The other points are all punctured by lifting, thrusting, twirling and rotating the needles on the arrival of *qi*, with the needles retained for 20–30 min, during which manipulate the needles once every 5 min with short-time and strong stimulation. Digital compression is also applied to *guanyuan* (RN 4) as adjuvant, with the palm of the right hand toward the umbilicus, the middle finger pressing *guanyuan* (RN 4), the thumb of the left hand pressing the first dactylopodite of the middle finger of the right hand, both hands strengthened gradually, and the patient is asked to urinate until evacuation. The treatment is applied once or twice a day.

Electroacupuncture

Selection of points: *Qihai* (RN 6), *guanyuan* (RN 4) and *zhongji* (RN 3). Supplementary points — *shuidao* (ST 28) (on the lower abdomen, 3 *cun* below the umbilicus, 2 *cun* lateral to the midline) and *sanyinjiao* (SP 6).

Manipulation: Commonly used points are taken as the main points, and supplementary points are added according to symptoms. *Qihai* (RN 6) is punctured with transverse insertion penetrating to *guanyuan* (RN 4), or from *guanyuan* (RN 4) to *zhongji* (RN 3), or from *shuidao* (ST 28) to *zhongji* (RN 3); *sanyinjiao* (SP 6) is punctured perpendicularly to a depth of 1.5 *cun*. On the arrival of *qi* in each point, connect to the electroacupuncture apparatus with medium or strong stimulation, with a frequency of 120–240 cpm and a continuous wave, for 15–30 min. The treatment is applied once or twice a day.

Wrist–ankle acupuncture

Selection of points: Lower 1 and Lower 2.

Manipulation: The needle tip, pointing to the abdomen, is inserted at an angle of 30° between the needle and the skin, and then inserted to a depth of 1.5 *cun* along the superficial layer under the skin, with the needle retained for 20–40 min.

Remarks

Acupuncture therapies for acute urinary retention involve needling, moxibustion, electroacupuncture, ear acupuncture, point injection, point application, electrotherapy with low frequency, and wrist–ankle acupuncture, among which body acupuncture is the most commonly used one because of its confirmed curative effect. During the operation, urination occurs instantly after the needle is removed if the needling sensation is induced to radiate to the abdomen or perineal region until the patient feels micturition desire or constriction in the abdomen. Electroacupuncture is in fact another effective therapy which is a stimulating factor in addition to body acupuncture. Wrist–ankle acupuncture is easy to perform but the practical value needs further verification.

URINARY CALCULI

Overview

Urinary calculi (UC) is one of the most common diseases in the urinary system. It may occur in any part the (kidney, ureter or bladder), but originally in the kidney. The clinical manifestions involve sudden onset, severe lower back pain that is continuous or intermittent, radiating to the fossa iliaca, perineum and scrotum along the ureter, as well as other symptoms like hematuria or pyuria, difficulty in urination and interrupted urination. It is similar to *shi lin* (urinary stone) in TCM. In modern times, acupuncture treatment for UC was reported in the late 1950s, and it has been found in the past 50 years that acupuncture and moxibustion not only relieve the colic caused by calculi but also promote the discharge of small-sized stones. According to statistics on more than 1000 cases, the total effective rate is 72.93%–95%, and the lithagogue rate 50%–65.3%.

Treatment

Acupoint injection

Selection of points: Commonly used points — *shenshu* (BL 23), *guanyuan* (RN 4) and *yinlingquan* (SP 9). Supplementary points — *zusanli* (ST 36), *sanyinjiao* (SP 6), *yanglingquan* (GB 34), *daheng* (SP 15), *zhongji* (RN 3) and *huantiao* (GB 30).

Manipulation: A 10% glucose injection is taken as the physic liquor. Commonly used points are employed at each session, according to symptoms, *Yanglingquan* (SP 9) and *Huantiao* (GB 30) are added for colic onset; *sanyinjiao* (SP 6), for dysuria and hematuria; *zhongji* (RN 3), for distension in the lower abdomen and interrupted urination; *zusanli* (ST 36), for dry vomiting and abdominal distension; and *dasheng* (SP 15), for abdominal pain around the umbilicus. Needle the points with slight lifting, thrusting, twirling and rotating till the arrival of *qi*, followed by injecting 2–8 ml of the liquor into each point. The treatment is applied once every day or every other day, at 30 sessions as a course.

Electroacupuncture

Selection of points: Commonly used points — three groups, namely (1) renal calculi: *shenshu* (BL 23), *guanyuan* (RN 4) and *yinlingquan* (SP 9); (2) ureteral calculi: *shenshu* (BL 23), *pangguangshu* (BL 28) and *shuidao* (ST 28); (3) bladder and urethral calculi: *guanyuan* (RN 4), *zhongji* (RN 3), *shuidao* (ST 28) and *sanyinjiao* (SP 6). Supplementary points — three groups, namely (1) renal calculi: *pangguangshu* (BL 28), *zhaohai* (KI 6) and *tianshu* (ST 25); (2) ureteral calculi: *qihai* (RN 6), *sanjiaoshu* (BL 22), *ciliao* (BL 32) and *zhongji* (RN 3); (3) bladder and urethral calculi: *neiguan* (PC 6) and *yinlingquan* (SP 9).

Manipulation: Points of the back and the abdomen on the affected side are employed, two or three points at each session, with supplementary points added according to symptoms. Common points are stimulated with electroacupuncture to induce *qi* by lifting, thrusting, twirling and rotating, with lifting and thrusting as the main manipulations, to make the sensation radiate to the affected kidney area or lower abdomen. Then connect to the G6805 electroacupuncture apparatus with an interrupted wave and irregular wave alternately, with the current strength tolerable to the patient. Supplementary points are punctured with filiform needles by lifting and thrusting combined with twirling and rotating, with the needles retained for 40 min. For cases with obvious onset of pain, the retention can be prolonged to 1 h. During the retention, manipulate the needles two or three times. The treatment is performed once daily, at 10 sessions as a course.

Remarks

It has been indicated by experiments in recent years that acupuncture is able to enlarge the amplitude of the ureteral peristalsis wave, and increase the urinary flow so as to move the stones downward, which confirms the function of acupuncture and has been proven by both methods introduced above. Acupoint injection was applied to 805 cases, with a total effective rate of 72.92%, and was found applicable to stones less than 1.7 cm in diameter and 1 cm in transverse diameter. The effective rate of electroacupuncture is 73.0%. Acupuncture treatment for UC will attain superior effectiveness under the condition that the stones exist in the middle and inferior segment of the ureter, less than 1 cm in transverse diameter, smooth and glossy outside, with no deformity of the urethra, and the kidney on the affected side functions well, with the stones in the active phase.

QUESTIONS

(1) Which therapy is preferable in treatment of acute urinary retention? Describe how to manipulate it.
(2) Describe briefly two methods of point stimulation in treatment of urinary calculi.

STIFF NECK

Overview

Stiff neck is a disease with muscular soreness in the back and limitation of activity. It is clinically characterized by neck rigidity, difficulty in turning the neck right and left, soreness in the local area with tenderness but no red swelling, and is commonly found in the morning. In ancient medical literature it was named *xiang qiang* ("stiff neck") and recorded in *Bei Ji Qian Jin Yao Fang* (*Important Formulas Worth a Thousand Gold Pieces for Emergencies*) by Sun Si-miao in the Tang Dynasty. In modern times, especially in the past dozens of years, lots of reports about acupuncture and moxibustion for treatment of stiff neck have been published. Acupuncture stimulation methods include needling, cupping, digital pressing, ear acupoint pressing, eye acupuncture, magnetic needling and electron excitation, all of which are highly effective.

Treatment

Body acupuncture

Selection of points: xuanzhong (GB 39), yanglao (SI 6) and houxi (SI 3). Supplementary points — waiguan (SJ 5), zhongzhu (SJ 3) and yanglingquan (GB 34).

Manipulation: Commonly used points are taken as the main points one point at each session, and supplementary points may be added or altered if a satisfactory result is not achieved. *Xuanzhong* (GB 39) is punctured perpendicularly to a depth of 1.5–1.8 *cun*, with strong or medium strength, with the needle retained for 15–20 min after the arrival of *qi*; *yanglao*

(SI 6) is punctured obliquely upward to a depth of 1.5 *cun*, transmitting the sensation to the shoulder; and *houxi* (SI 3) perpendicularly 0.5–0.8 *cun*, twirling and rotating the needle for 1–3 min after the arrival of *qi*, or combined with electro acupuncture with a frequency of 40–50 cpm and a continuous wave. Supplementary points are given routine acupuncture; insert deeply to induce a strong needling sensation. During the course of manipulation, the patient is asked to move the neck by himself or herself gradually. All the needles are retained for 15 min and the treatment is performed once daily.

Cupping

Selection of points: *Ashi* point. Supplementary points — *fengmen* (BL 12) and *jianjing* (GB 21). Location of the *ashi* point: the most obvious tenderness spot in the neck (the same as below).

Manipulation: The *ashi* point is kneaded and pressed for a moment and sterilized before being given rapid pricking needling 3–5 times with a three-edged needle, or tapping at medium strength with a dermal needle on an area in the caliber size of the cup, followed by being sucked with an appropriate jar or cup. One or two supplementary points are punctured till the arrival of *qi*, with the needles retained, before cupping on the needles. Sucking lasts for 10–15 min. After the cups are removed, revolving moxibustion is applied with moxa rolls to the *ashi* point for 5–7 min. The treatment is performed once daily.

Digital pressing

Selection of points: Waiguan (SJ 5), *neiguan* (PC 6) and *ashi* point. Supplementary points — *fengchi* (Gb 20), *jianjing* (GB 21), *jianzhen* (SI 9), *yanglao* (SI 6), *tianzhu* (Bl 10), *fengfu* (DU 16) and *dazhui* (DU 14).

Manipulation: Commonly used points are taken as the main points, and supplementary points may be added if there is no satisfactory result. Gently tap at or press the *ashi* point with fingers for 1 min. The practitioner pinches and presses *neiguan* (PC 6) of the patient with the thumb, with the middle finger or the index finger reaching *waiguan* (SJ 5), 2–3 min at each session, with the strength from light to strong to make the pressure reach *waiguan* (SJ 5) from *neiguan* (PC 6) while the patient feels soreness, numbness, distension and heat, or a sensation of *qi* transmitting upward. During the pressing, asked the patient to move the neck from left to right. For supplementary points, *fengchi* (GB 20) is massaged with a single hand 20 times, *jianjing* (GB 21) with both hands 20 times, and the rest are pressed with fingers or pushed and pressed up and down, right and left, for 1–2 min at each point. The treatment is applied once daily, 3 times as a course.

Otopoint pill pressing

Selection of points: Neck and *shenmen* (HT 7).

Manipulation: Bilateral commonly used points are employed at each session. One or two mung beans are put on a piece of Huoxue Zhitong emplastrum (activating blood for relieving pain) or Shangshi Zhitong emplastrum (dissolving dampness for relieving pain), sold in the market with an area of 1 × 1 cm², which is pasted to the ear acupoints selected, with the borders impacted. Then, press the ear point for 0.5–1 min gradually, until the patient feels distension and pain, and ask the patient to move the neck for 2–3 min. The patient presses the points by himself or herself 3 times every day, and the paster cannot be removed until complete recovery.

Acupuncture and moxibustion

Selection of points: Commonly used point — *dazhui* (DU 14). Supplementary point — *jianjing* (GB 21).

Manipulation: The patient sits up straight, with the head inclining forward. Insert the needle into the commonly used point with the tip deviating to the affected side to a depth of 0.5–1 *cun*, making the sensation transmit to the affected area of the neck and the shoulder. On the arrival of *qi*, the practitioner presses *jianjing* (GB 21) on the affected side with one hand, asking the patient to turn the neck left and right maximally, and at the same time twirling the needle with the other hand for 3–4 min. If a satisfactory result is not achieved, a moxa stick about 5 cm long is pierced into the needle handle and ignited, for moxibustion, after which cupping is added to the point area. The treatment is performed once a day.

Remarks

The five therapies introduced here are all easy to perform. The first one is the most commonly used and is applicable to cases with acute onset and a short course of disease. It needs only one point, but manipulation must fit the requirements. Cupping is often applied to cases with obvious symptoms and a longer course, and is in fact combined with acupuncture, but *jianjing* (GB 21) should avoid deep insertion. Digital pressing is for cases with puncture phobia, and requires a certain force of the fingers, but it has its flaws — more points are selected and a longer period of time is needed in treatment. Otopoint pressing is for cases with mild symptoms and is combined with other methods. Acupuncture is actually a comprehensive therapy and requires a certain experience in manipulation.

ACUTE LUMBAR SPRAIN

Overview

An acute lumbar sprain is usually caused by muscular exertion disturbance in the lower back due to turning the body forcefully. It is clinically manifested by sudden pain in the lower back after a sudden and rapid activity, limitation of motions, aggravated cough and deep breathing. It belongs to *yao tong zheng* (lower back pain) in TCM, and treatment with acupuncture and moxibustion was recorded in *Nei Jing* (*The Inner Classic*) for special description. An acute lumbar sprain is one of the indications responding well to acupuncture therapy, and modern reports appeared in the mid-1920s, with abundant experience accumulated till now. The effective rates for the various acupuncture therapies are all above 95%.

Treatment

Body acupuncture

Selection of points: Commonly used points — *shuigou* (DU 26), *houxi* (SI 3) and *yaotongdian* (EX-UE7). Supplementary points — *weizhong* (BL 40), *mingmen* (DU 4), *yaoyangguan* (DU 3) and *dachangshu* (BL 25).

Manipulation: Commonly used points are generally employed and supplementary points may be added if no satisfactory effect is achieved, with the points selected according to the affected regions. For injuries in the middle part of lumbar vertebrae, *shuigou* (DU 26) is punctured obliquely upward to a depth of 0.2–0.3 *cun* twirling and rotating repeatedly for 2 min or, at 1 cm lateral to *shuigou* (DU 26), pinch the upper lip of the patient with the left thumb and index finger, and insert a 2-*cun*-long filiform needle with the right hand from the left to the right side, pulling the needle back and forth with strong stimulation for 5–10 s; meanwhile, the patient is asked to move the lower back, like bowing forward and leaning backward, or revolving left and right 20 times. For cases with mild soft tissue injuries, *houxi* (ST 3) on the opposite or pain-affected side is punctured toward *hegu* (LI 4) to a depth of 1–1.5 *cun*, twirling, rotating, lifting and thrusting the needle at macroamplitude with strong stimulation for 2 min; meanwhile, the patient moves the body as said above. For cases with a larger area of soft tissue injury in the lower back, *yaotongdian* (EX-UE7) on the opposite side is punctured obliquely toward the palm to a depth of 0.8–1 *cun* till the arrival of *qi*, twirling, rotating, lifting and thrusting the needle at macroamplitude with strong stimulation for 2 min; meanwhile, the patient moves the body as said above. All the needles in the treatment are retained for 15–20 min at each point, during which the manipulation is applied once or twice. If there remains pain or pain is not relieved significantly, supplementary points are available. *Weizhong* (BL 40) is pricked for blood; *dachangshu* (BL 25) on the affected side is given deep insertion for lower back pain on one side, making the needling sensation radiate to the heel; or puncture the tenderness spot in the lower back; for pain in the middle part of lumbar vertebrae, puncture *mingmen* (DU 4) or *yangguan* (DU 3). Cupping should be applied after acupuncture to the points of the lower back. The treatment is performed once or twice a day.

Electroacupuncture

Selection of points: Commonly used points — *ashi* (the most obvious tenderness spot) and *weizhong* (BL 40). Supplementary point — *jiajixue* (EX-B2).

Manipulation: The patient is in the prone position on a slat bed, with the hands above the head. The practitioner presses the psoas muscles bilateral to lumbosacral vertebrae one by one with the thumb and index finger of the right hand, finding the tenderness spot, i.e. the *ashi* point. *Weizhong* (BL 40) is first punctured to a depth of 1.5 *cun*, twirling, rotating, lifting and thrusting the needle to transmit the sensation to the feet, followed by puncturing the *ashi* point. If the injury occurs in the middle of the lumbar vertebrae, *jiajixue* (EX-B2) bilateral to the tenderness spot may be added to make the senfsation radiate downward. Connect to the electroacupuncture apparatus with a continuous wave, a frequency (200–300 cpm) and a current strength tolerable to the patient, for 20 min at each session, once daily.

Remarks

Point stimulation methods for acute lumbar sprains vary a lot, but the two introduced above are the most commonly used according to practical experience. Body acupuncture was reported to have been applied to 1300 cases, which responded well to the treatment, with a recovery rate for one time of 59.4%. Electroacupuncture applied to 800 cases has achieved a total effective rate of 95%–100%. The key point of acupuncture treatment lies in strong stimulation while needling the main points, as well as the patient bending from the waist repeatedly to provoke pains. Body acupuncture, applicable to acute lumbar sprains, is ineffective for chronic lumbar muscle strains, while electroacupuncture is effective for chronic injuries.

CERVICAL SPONDYLOSIS

Overview

Cervical spondylosis is a common degenerative condition of orthopedics and traumatology, commonly seen in adult men. Clinically it is classified into cervical spondylotic radiculopathy, cervical spondylotic myelopathy (CSM), the vertebral artery type of cervical spondylosis, and the sympathetic type of cervical spondylosis. The first is the most frequent type and manifests itself as neck and shoulder pain radiating to the arm and fingers, limitation of neck activity, or even numbness and weakness in fingers, tinnitus and dizziness in severe cases; it is the main object of acupuncture treatment. It belongs to *jing xiang tong* (neck pain) or *gu bi* (bone impediment) in TCM, and the treatment with acupuncture and moxibustion was recorded in *Nei Jing*. There were not many articles about modern treatment until after the 1970s. With the development of geriatric medicine, cervical spondylosis has drawn enough attention from the field of acupuncture and moxibustion. Thousands of cases have been reported and an effective rate of 90% has been achieved.

Treatment

Body acupuncture

Selection of points: Commonly used points — *jiaji* points (C4–C7). Supplementary points — *jianjing* (GB 21), *quchi* (LI 11), *hegu* (LI 4), *houxi* (SI 3) and *yanglao* (SI 6) added for the nerve root type; *baihui* (DU 20), *taiyang* (EX-HN5), *sanyinjiao* (SP 6), *taixi* (KI 3) and *xingjian* (LR 2) for the vertebral artery type; *baihui* (DU 20), *xinshu* (BL 15), *ganshu* (BL 18), *danshu* (BL 19) and *taichong* (LR 3) for the sympathetic type; *zusanli* (ST 36), *taiyang* (EX-HN5), *waiguan* (SJ 5), *weizhong* (BL 40) and *yanglingquan* (GB 34) for the spinal type.

Manipulation: Generally, *jiaji* points C5–C6 are employed, and two or three supplementary points according to different types. No. 28–30 filiform needls are inserted toward the vertebral column at an angle of 75° or inserted 0.5 *cun* lateral to *jiaji* at an angle of 45° until the needle point reaches something hard; then withdraw the needle 0.5 *cun*, with lifting and thrusting combined with twirling and rotating to transmit the sensation. Cases of severe pain are given swift lifting and slow insertion, while cases of body numbness and coldness are given swift insertion and slow lifting. Supplementary points are punctured for the arrival of *qi*, followed by lifting, thrusting, twirling and rotating. All the needles are retained for 20 min, during which they are manipulated once every 5 min. The treatment is applied once every day or every other day, at 10–12 sessions as a course.

Pricking

Selection of points: Ashi point.

Manipulation: The *ashi* point refers to the reactive site, commonly seen in the neck and the back with a skin injury like *dangshen* flowers (*Codonopsis pilosula*), which is usually round or oval, beanlike or peanut-kernel-sized, with neat borders, slightly darker than normal skin with weak reflection, and more often in big vertebrae or cervical hyperplasia. Two or three points are employed at each session. After routine sterilization and local anesthesia with 2% procaine, a thin three-edged needle is used to prick the epedermis and then the superficial skin cellosilk with the needle point inserted transversely along the skin, first sliding forward and then raising the needle slightly, pricking cellosilk broken. Cut off the cellosilk ends exposed outside the skin before the next pricking. The treatment is applied once every 5 days, at 5 sessions as a course. But make sure that at least one of the pricking spots is on the cervical vertebrae.

Remarks

The first method, body acupuncture, is the most common in the clinic. It is easy to perform and applicable to all types, and has been applied to 700 cases with a total effective rate of 95% — most effective for cervical spondylotic radiculopathy and least for cervical spondylotic myelopathy. While applying body acupuncture, what is most important is to induce the needling sensation in puncturing *jiaji* points; however, this is not necessary for beginners. The second method, pricking is one of the bloodletting therapies. It was applied to 560 patients, among whom 504 recovered completely, and the total effective rate was 100%.

QUESTIONS

(1) Describe how to manipulate body acupuncture and cupping in treatment of stiff neck
(2) What are the characteristics of body acupuncture and electroacupuncture in treatment of acute lumbar sprains?
(3) Illustrate the concrete operation procedures in treatment of cervical spondylosis with pricking therapy.

SCAPULOHUMERAL PERIARTHRITIS

Overview

Scapulohumeral periarthritis refers to a recessive and inflammatory lesion of the capsula articularis humeri and the surrounding soft tissues, commonly seen among people over 45. It is clinically manifested by pain in the early stage, light in the day and heavy at night; and dysfunction in the late stage due to adhesions, and limitation of activities like adduction, external rotation and backward extension. It is called *lou jian feng* and *jian ning* (frozen shoulder) in TCM, and its treatment with acupuncture and moxibustion was recorded in *Zhen Jiu Jia Yi Jing* (*The Systematic Classic of Acupuncture and Moxibustion*). The first modern aritcle about the acupuncture treatment of scapulohumeral periarthritis was published in 1954. Traditional needling methods have given way to various point therapies in recent years. At present, an effective rate of 85% has been achieved.

Treatment

Body acupuncture

Selection of points: Commonly used points — *jianyu* (LI 15) penetrating to *jiquan* (HT 1); *tianzong* (SI 11) and *tiaokou* (ST 38) [2 *cun* below *shangjuxu* (ST 37)] penetrating to *chengshan* (BL 57). Supplementary points — *quchi* (LI 11), *chize* (LU 5), *jianjing* (GB 21), *hegu* (LI 4) and *yanglingquan* (GB 34).

Manipulation: Commonly used points are employed at each session, and supplementary points added according to symptoms. The patient keeps the hands down and the elbows bent. A No. 28 filiform needle is inserted into *jianyu* (LI 15) penetrating to *jiquan* (HT 1) to make a sensation of soreness and distension radiate to the whole articular cavity. *Tianzong* (SI 11) is punctured to the bone. *Tiaokou* (St 38) is punctured to *chengshan* (Bl 57) on the healthy side until the arrival of *qi*, lifting, thrusting, twirling and rotating the needle as well as asking the patient to move his or her affected shoulder like rotating or extending forward and backward for

3–5 min, followed by manipulation on other points, which are given lifting and thrusting after the arrival of *qi* to induce a strong needling sensation. The treatment is applied once every day or every other day, at 10 sessions as a course, at an interval of 5 days between courses.

Cupping

Selection of points: *Ashi* point (tenderness spot).

Manipulation: Press the affected shoulder to find the tenderness spot, and apply pricking needling to the most obvious spot with a three-edged needle to a depth of 0.1–0.2 *cun*, followed by pricking the spots above, below, right and left of the tenderness, with the whole area slightly larger than the mouth of the cupping jar, and bloodletting like beads. If the tenderness spots are scattered, two or three spots are employed for pricking. Then flash-fire cupping or vacuum cupping is applied for cupping and sucking for 10–15 min, until 1–3 ml of static blood is sucked. Remove the jar and press the pinholes with sterilized cotton balls; and passive activity is performed for 5–10 min. Do cupping and sucking once every 3 or 4 times, at 3 sessions as a course, at an interval of a week between courses.

Ear acupuncture

Selection of points: Commonly used points — shoulder, clavicle (below the shoulder points, the fifth quinquesection of the scapha zone) and *shenmen* (HT 7). Supplementary points — liver, spleen and subcortex.

Manipulation: Commonly used points are employed, and one or two supplementary points may be added according to symptoms. The tenderness spot found, a No. 28 filiform needle is rapidly inserted for the arrival of *qi*, twirling and rotating the needle with medium and strong stimulation for 0.5–1 min, during which the patient is asked to move the affected shoulder. For cases with severe pain, shoulder points are given pricking needling with three-edged needles till drops of blood are let out. One ear each time and the two ears alternately, the treatment is applied once every day or every other day, at six sessions as a course.

Remarks

Among the three therapies above, the first is used in wider areas. It is more effective for cases in early or later stages, and was applied to 448 cases with a total effective rate of 97.5%. Cupping is applicable to the cases in later stages, and ear acupuncture to cases of pain in early stages. In practice, the three therapies may be combined together to enhance the curative effect. It is necessary to point out that the patients must do some function exercises during the treatment, like climbing a fence, otherwise the effectiveness may be greatly affected.

EXTERNAL HUMERAL EPICONDYLITIS

Overview

External humeral epicondylitis, also called tennis elbow, is clinically manifested by pain in the lateral elbow joint, aggravation in a forcefully clenched fist or pronation stretching of the forearm (like twirling a towel or sweeping the floor), and local tenderness (near the external humeral epicondyle), but no abnormality is seen on the appearance. It belongs to *zhou tong* (elbow pain), *shang jin* (consumption of fluid) in TCM, and the treatment with acupuncture and moxibustion was first recorded in *Zhen Jiu Jia Yi Jing* (*The Systematic Classic of Acupuncture and Moxibustion*). There was no much clinical data in the 1950s–1960s about the modern treatment, but more and more cases have been treated and reported in the past 40 years. At present, an effective rate of 90% or more has been achieved.

Treatment

Electroacupuncture

Selection of points: Commonly used points — *ashi* points. Supplementary points — *shousanli* (LI 10) and *chize* (LU 5).

Manipulation: *Ashi* has two points, one at the anterior border depression of the external humeral epicondyle, and the other at the posterior border depression; both are employed. The former is punctured perpendicularly with a 1-*cun*-long filiform, while the latter is punctured to the depression at an angle of 45° from the middle of the condyle toward the wrist back. *Shousanli* (LI 10) is added for pronation limitation of the forearm, and *chize* (LU 5) for supination limitation, both with routine acupuncture. On the arrival of *qi*, reducing manipulation is applied by lifting and thrusting the needle for 1 min; then connect to the electroacupuncture apparatus with a continuous wave, a frequency (300 cpm) and a strength tolerable to the patient. The treatment is performed once every other day, at 10 sessions as a course, at an interval of 5–7 days between courses.

Moxibustion

Selection of points: Commonly used points — *ashi* point (the most obvious tenderness, and the same as below). Supplementary point — *taixi* (KI 3).

Manipulation: Commonly used points are given moxibustion; supplementary points, acupuncture. Moxibustion is performed by drug-separated moxibustion, with the same amount of Gong Dingxiang (*Flos caryophylli*) and Rougui (*Cortex cinnamomi*) ground to powder and mixed even, which is Ding Gui San. Fresh ginger (cleaned) is cut into thin slices measuring 2 mm, and six or seven holes are pricked with a three-edged needle. A bit of Ding Gui San is spread evenly on the *ashi* point with a ginger slice on it, and a moxa cone in a peanut kernel size is put on the slice and ignited for moxibustion until the patient complains of scorching heat. Then change to another cone. Three to five cones are used at each session, till the local skin becomes reddish. *Taixi* (KI 3) is perpendicularly punctured with the point slightly upward. When a sensation of soreness and distension arises, manipulate the needle by twirling and rotating for 1–2 min, with a retention of 20 min. The treatment is applied once daily, at 7 sessions as a course, at an interval of 7 days between courses.

Skin needling

Selection of points: Commonly used point — *ashi* point. Supplementary points — *shousanli* (LI 10), *quchi* (LI 11) and *shaohai* (HT 3).

Manipulation: *Ashi* is employed at each session, combined with one supplementary point. Press for a moment the selected point with the thumb, and tap at it with a seven-star needle, first with mild stimulation and then more forcefully when the local area has a sensation of soreness and distension, until drops of blood come out, with the tapping area 1 cm in diameter. After wiping off the blood, apply revolving moxibustion with a moxa stick for about 15 min, until the local skin becomes reddish. The treatment is performed once daily, at 6 sessions as a course, at an interval of 3 days between courses.

Remarks

The three therapies introduced above are all common and effective in the clinic, since external humeral epicondylitis is so intractable. Generally, electroacupuncture is preferable, and if no satisfactory result can be achieved, moxibustion or skin needling is available. The key point of the treatment lies in the location of tenderness and the perseverance of treatment at the same time.

QUESTIONS

(1) Describe the three methods of point stimulation in treatment of scapulohumeral periarthritis.
(2) What are the acupuncture and moxibustion methods for external humeral epicondylitis?

CHAPTER 26

Acupuncture and Moxibustion for Obstetrics and Gynecology Diseases

DYSMENORRHEA

Overview

Dysmenorrhea refers to the aching pain in the lower abdomen and lower back before, after or during menstruation It is manifested by menstrual pain that gradually or quickly increases, and paroxysmal cramps in the lower abdomen and lower back. When cramps are severe, the symptoms may include a pale face, general fatigue, cold extremities, or even fainting. Dysmenorrhea can be classified as either primary or secondary, and acupuncture therapy is mainly applied to the former. The first report on acupuncture and moxibustion for dysmenorrhea was seen in 1951. In the 1950s–1960s, traditional point stimulation was taken as the main therapy, and acupuncture therapy for dysmenorrhea has made great progress since the 1980s. At present, a curative rate of 90% has been achieved.

Treatment

Body acupuncture

Selection of points: Commonly used points — (1) *chengjiang* (RN 24) and *dazhui* (DU 14); (2) *shiqizhuixia* (below the spinous process of L5) and *ashi* points (tender spots on the lower abdomen). Supplementary points — *chengshan* (BL 57) and *shenshu* (BL 23).

Manipulation: One group of commonly used points is employed at each session, with the two groups employed alternately, and supplementary points may be added or substituted when the effect is not satisfactory.

Chengjiangxue (RN 24) is punctured with a No. 28 needle 1 *cun* long by inserting obliquely downward to a depth of 5 *fen*. When the patient feels the needling sensation, swiftly thrust, lift, twirl and rotate the needle for 2 min, with a retention of 30 min, during which manipulation is applied once every 10 min. Insert a needle into *dazhui* (DU 14) and push it gently forward till the sensation spreads to the lower back, with a retention of 30 min. *Shiqizhuixia* is rapidly punctured with a No. 28 filiform needle, with the needle point directed to the spinous process of L5, obliquely downward by lifting, thrusting, twirling and rotating the needle to make the sensation radiate to the uterus and perineum. If the severe pain is relieved, manipulate the needle by lifting, thrusting, twirling and rotating for 5–10 min according to different conditions, with the needle retained for 30 min. The *ashi* point is given warm moxibustion with a moxa roll at a distance from the skin where the patient feels warmth but not burning heat. *Chengshan* points (BL 57) on both sides are rapidly punctured with 2-*cun*-long filiform needles, which are inserted by twirling them slowly until the sensation becomes strong, with a retention of 15–30 min. The other points are given manipulations by lifting, thrusting, twirling and rotating to make the sensation expand to the abdomen, with the needles retained for 15 min. The treatment is applied once daily until complete recovery is achieved.

Skin needling

Selection of points: Xingjian (LR 2), *gongsun* (SP 4), *yinbai* (SP 1), *taichong* (LR 3), *sanyinjiao* (SP 6) and *guanyuan* (RN 4).

Manipulation: All the points are employed. After routine sterilization, a seven-star needle is used for tapping needling with the wrist strength, during which the insertion has to be stable and precise, and the needle point is vertical to the skin. Tap the point 70–90 cpm, 1 min for each point, with medium stimulation until the local skin becomes red. The treatment is applied three days before the menstrual onset, once daily, three times as a course, and three courses are needed for observation (three months).

Remarks

Body acupuncture has a reliable curative effect, with both short-term and long-term efficacy, but for beginners it is advisable to choose skin needling since the manipulation of the former method is so complicated. Besides, the patient is required to ensure that there is menstrual hygiene and to avoid strenuous exercise, cold–dampness, mental stress, etc. during menstrual periods.

ACUTE DYSFUNCTIONAL UTERINE BLEEDING

Overview

Acute dysfunctional uterine bleeding (DUB) is a common disease in gynecology, caused by endocrinopathy and clinically manifested by menstrual blood increasing too much. The patients usually suffer from anemia to some degree, while organic pathological changes cannot be seen in general or gynecological examinations. This disease belongs to *xue beng* (血崩 metrorrhagia) in TCM. There were records about it with acupoint prescription in *The Systematic Classic of Acupuncture and Moxibustion* in the Jin Dynasty. Reports on modern acupuncture and moxibustion for acute DUB appeared in the early 1940s, and a large amount of clinical material has been accumulated over the past 60 years. At present a cure rate of 90% on average has been achieved.

Treatment

Body acupuncture

Selection of points: Commonly used points — *guanyuan* (RN 4) penetrating to *zhongji* (RN 3), *xuehai* (SP 10), *zigong* (EX-CA1) and *diji* (SP 8). Supplementary points — *sanyinjiao* (SP 6), *changqiang* (DU 1) and *dachangshu* (BL 25).

Manipulation: Commonly used points are taken as the principal points, with one or two supplementary points, at each session. A filiform needle 2 *cun* in length is inserted horizontally into *guanyuan* (RN 4) with penetration to *zhongji* (RN 3), while *diji* (SP 8) and *xuehai* (SP 10) are punctured to a depth of 1–1.5 *cun*, both of which are given manipulation by thrusting and lifting or twirling and rotating the needle for 1–2 min, with a retention of 10 min, followed by lifting the needle beneath the skin and inserting it along the spleen channel to a depth of 1 *cun* with retention. *Zigong* (EX-CA1) is inserted obliquely to a depth of 2–2.5 *cun*, till the needling sensation arises. Then connect the points to the G 6805 electric acupuncture device with an intermittent wave and a frequency of 120 cpm until the patient feels a rising sensation in the vagina and anus. At other points, the needles are retained at the arrival of *qi* for 15–30 min. The manipulation is given once or twice a day, seven times as a treatment course.

Ear acupuncture

Selection of points: Commonly used points — internal genitalia and ear center. Supplementary points — spleen, endocrine, subcortex, *shenmen* (HT 7) and liver.

Manipulation: Commonly used points and one or two supplementary points are employed at each session. Insert the filiform needles, then twirl and rotate them with strong stimulation, with a retention of 30–60 min; or inject each point on both sides with vitamin K 0.1 ml. The filiform needling is applied once or twice a day, and the otopoint injection once a day three times, successively.

Fibrous-tissue-broken pricking

Selection of points: Commonly used points — lumbosacral region. Supplementary points — internal genitalia, endocrine, spleen and liver.

Manipulation: Commonly used points are employed at each session, and supplementary may be added if necessary. In the lumbosacral region, select a pricking spot between *yaoyangguan* (DU 3) and the sacral hiatus (points of the lower back), better to be a brown papule (projecting on the skin surface and not disappearing by pressing), and use a three-edged needle to prick the skin and break many a white fibrous tissue. The spot pricked and broken is about 0.2–0.3 mm in diameter, 0.1–0.15 mm in depth. Then cover it with a sterilized dressing and bind it up. This method may be carried out on the second day after the menstruation, once per month for three months on end, with a different spot each time. Supplementary points are given pill pressing stimulation with *Semen vaccariae* seeds to both ears on the same day with pricking until the end of menstruation. The patient is advised to press the points by himself or herself three or four times a day.

Remarks

Acute DUB is an emergency condition in gynecology. The three methods above have all produced satisfactory effects in clinics, especially ear acupuncture, the easiest one, which was once applied to 110 patients with a total effective rate of 95%–97% and a marked improvement rate of 85.7%, and 70 of the patients completely recovered with otopoint injection. Fibrous-tissue-broken pricking is applicable since it is also effective, with a total effective rate of 89.6%–97.9% in 192 cases. If there is no obvious effect, it is advisable to combine with or change to other therapies, either modern or Chinese medicine, for fear of delaying treatment.

QUESTIONS

(1) Which point stimulation method or methods do you prefer in the treatment of dysmenorrhea? Describe the manipulation process.
(2) Restate the point selection and manipulation in the treatment of acute DUB with acupuncture and moxibustion.

HYPERPLASIA OF THE MAMMARY GLANDS

Overview

Hyperplasia of the mammary glands, also known as cystic hyperplasia of the breasts, is clinically manifested by multiple lumps without any abnormal condition seen from the appearance, as well as soreness and pain in the breasts. All of the symptoms will be aggravated before menstruation. This is a frequently occurring disease in women between 25 and 40 years of age. It was listed as one of the precancerous lesions, which drew the attention of the public. Hyperplasia of the mammary glands is included in TCM, in the category of *ru pi* (乳癖, nodule of the breast). There was no record of it in ancient books. Articles about treatment of hyperplasia of the mammary glands with acupuncture and moxibustion were first seen in the late 1950s, but it did not attract attention from the field of acupuncture and moxibustion until the late 1970s; then a great deal of further clinical and experimental research was conducted. An effective rate of 90% for the disease has been achieved.

Treatment

Body acupuncture

Selection of points: Commonly used points — (1) *wuyi* (ST 15) (on the chest, in the second intercostal space, 4 *cun* lateral to the anterior midline), *zusanli* (ST 36), *danzhong* (RN 17) and *hegu* (LI 4); (2) *tianzong* (SI 11), *jianjing* (GB 21), *ganshu* (BL 18) and *rugen* (ST 18) (directly below the nipple, on the lower border of the breast, in the fifth intercostal space). Supplementary points — *qimen* (LR 14) and *taichong* (LR 3) are added for liver constraint, and *pishu* (BL 20) and *sanyinjiao* (SP 6) for disharmony between the *chong* channel and the *ren* channel.

Manipulation: One group is employed at each session, and the two groups are employed alternately, with supplementary points added according to different conditions. *Wuyi* (ST 15) is punctured at an angle of 25° outward to a depth of 1.5 *cun, danzhong* (RN 17) horizontally downward to 1.5 *cun, jianjing* (GB 21) horizontally forward to 1 *cun*, and *tianzong* (SI 11) at an angle of 25° outward and downward to 1.5 *cun*, until the arrival of *qi*. Other points are given acupuncture with routine techniques. With the needling sensation present, reducing manipulation is applied by thrusting and lifting in combination with twirling and rotating the needle for those with liver constraint, and mild reinforcing–reducing manipulation for those with disorder of the *chong* and *ren* channels. The needle is retained for 20–30 min, during which the same manipulation is carried out twice. Apply the operation once every day or every other day, 10–14 times as a treatment course, at an interval of 3–5 days between courses. Stop needling after menstruation.

Acupuncture laser irradiation

Selection of points: Ashi (at the middle of the breast lump).

Manipulation: The patient is in the supine position with the affected area exposed, and gentian violet is used to label *ashi*. Irradiate the affected area with a helium–neon laser acupuncture device with a wave of 632.8 nm, an output power of 5–7 mW, a spot diameter of 1.5–10 mm and an irradiating length of 10–20 cm. If the lump is big, an astigmatism lens may be used for irradiation or zoning irradiation for 20 min each time. In zoning irradiation, each zone needs 5–10 min of irradiation. This manipulation is applied once a day, 10 times as a course, at an interval of 3–5 days between courses.

Ear acupuncture

Selection of points: Commonly used points — mammary gland (at the anti-helix, below the level parallel to the superior thyroid notch) and endocrine. Supplementary points — *shenmen* (HT 7) (otopoint) is added for lobular hyperplasia, and *rugen* (ST 18) (body point) for cystic hyperplasia.

Manipulation: Commonly used points are all employed and supplementary points are added according to syndromes. If the lesion occurs on one side, one needle is inserted in one ear, with the two ears applied to alternately; if the lesion occurs on both sides, puncture on both ears. With the sensitive spot of otopoints found, immediately puncture it till distension and pain are felt, with the needle retained for 2–3 h. *Rugen* (ST 18), parallel with the chest wall, is needled upward or outward and upward until the arrival of *qi*, followed by twirling and rotating the needle for 0.5–1 min, with a retention of 20–30 min. The manipulation is given once a day, 10 times as a course, at an interval of 3–5 days between courses.

Remarks

The first method, body acupuncture, is a summary of many years' experience. It was once applied to 622 patients, and 271 (43.6%) recovered, with a total effective rate of 94.1%. Compared to 80 cases without any treatment, for which the effective rate (self-cured and relieved) was only 10%, body acupuncture was proven to have a better curative effect. In addition, 152 cases were observed for 1–3-year effect with a effective rate of 81.4%–92.4%, which proved that acupuncture has a good long-term curative effect. Body acupuncture is the first choice in treating hyperplasia of the mammary glands, but point laser irradiation and ear acupuncture are also applicable since they are more convenient and safe with an obvious effect (though inferior to the first method), and so are more suitable for beginners.

UTERINE PROLAPSE

Overview

Uterine prolapse refers to descent of the uterus from its normal position in the vagina, and is clinically manifested by a sensation of distenstion and pulling in the perineum, and tissue protruding from the vagina, accompanied by low back pain, a sensation of heaviness or pulling in the abdomen, urinary difficulties, etc. It varies in severity, in three stages. It belongs to the disease or syndrome categories of *yin ting* (prolapse of the uterus) in TCM. The treatment of *yin ting* with acupuncture and moxibustion first appeared in *The Systematic Classic of Acupuncture and Moxibustion*. In modern times, the early documents about the acupuncture treatment were seen in the late 1950s. Previous experience has shown that acupuncture therapy is suitable for three cases in stage I (the uterus descends but is still in the vagina) and stage II (the cervix and part of the uterus slip outside of the vagina). At present, the average effective rate is about 90%.

Treatment

Body acupuncture

Selection of points: Commonly used points — *zigong* (EX-CA1), *qihai* (RN 6), *guanyuan* (RN 4) and *Baihui* (DU 20). Supplementary points — *zusanli* (ST 36), *shenshu* (BL 23), *taixi* (KI 3) and *pishu* (BL 20).

Manipulation: Commonly used points are all employed, and two of the supplementary points may be added according to different conditions. *Zigong* (EX-CA1) and *qihai* (RN 6) are punctured by inserting the needle obliquely toward the pubic symphysis to a depth of 2 *cun*, and *guanyuan* (RN 4) by inserting it perpendicularly to a depth of 1.5 *cun*. On the arrival of *qi*, twirl and rotate the needle till the patient feels the rising of the vagina or the uterus, then ask her to contract the abdomen and suck in a deep breath, and then push forward the thumb, manipulating the needle to enhance the sensation and boost the rising of the uterus. Insert the needle into *zusanli* (ST 36) and *taixi* (KI 3) with the tip slightly upward; for points on the back, insert it obliquely toward the backbone, till the arrival of *qi*. *Baihui* (DU 20) is given sparrow-pecking moxibustion for 15–20 min. The needles (except on the back) are retained at each point for 2–3 h, and 1–2 h for those with a mild condition and a short course. The manipulation is applied once every day or every other day, 10 times as a treatment course, at an interval of 7 days between courses.

Ear acupuncture

Selection of points: Commonly used points — lumbosacral vertebrae (at the upper two-fifths of the antihelix, below the bifurcating point between the superior and inferior antihelix cruses), internal genitalia, subcortex, liver and spleen. Supplementary points — sympathetic and mouth.

Manipulation: Two to four of the commonly used points are employed at each session, and supplementary points may be added if the effect is not obvious. The sensitive spot found, filiform needles 5 *fen* in length are inserted perpendicularly on both sides. When the sensation of distension and pain arrives, repeat the twirling and rotating of the needles for half a minute. Connect them to an electric acupuncture device with an intermittent wave and an intensity tolerable to the patient. The needles are retained at each point for 15–20 min. Apply the manipulation once a day, 7–10 times as a treatment course, at an interval of 3–5 days between courses.

Remarks

Body acupuncture is applied to those with uterine prolapse at stages I and II. While one is needling the points on the abdomen, the key technique is to induce the rising sensation in the vagina or the uterus by twirling and rotating manipulation. Ear acupuncture is applied only to cases at stage I, and may be replaced by body acupuncture if an obvious effect cannot be achieved. But if the uterine prolapse is complicated by infection, the infection should be controlled prior to the acupuncture; the acupuncture should not be applied to those with severe ascites, portal hypertension, or cancer in the hypogastric region.

QUESTIONS

(1) Describe in detail the point selection and manipulation in the treatment of hyperplasia of the mammary glands with body acupuncture.
(2) What are the key techniques and points for attention in the treatment of uterine prolapse with acupuncture?

INFERTILITY

Overview

Infertility is the inability of a couple to achieve pregnancy after two years of unprotected sexual intercourse. It comprises primary infertility (referring to a woman who has never had a successful birth) and secondary infertility (the inability to conceive after having a successful birth or abortion). The cause or causes can involve the male (sexual dysfunction, dyspermia, etc.) or the female, and the latter is associated with the main causes, such as ovulation disorders, or anovulation induced by ovary dysfunction caused by various factors, and is the main subject of acupuncture therapy. Infertility is called *jue zi* (绝子, "no offspring") in TCM, and the treatment of *jue zi* with acupuncture and moxibustion was first recorded in *The Systematic Classic of Acupuncture and Moxibustion*. Modern reports on the treatment appeared in the 1920s, but it did not draw attention until the 1980s. At present, a series of clinical and mechanism researches has been done with great effectiveness.

Treatment

Body (ear) acupuncture

Selection of points: Commonly used points — *guanyuan* (RN 4), *zigong* (EX-CA1), *zhibian* (BL 54), *baomen* [on the left, 2 *cun* lateral to *guanyuan* (RN 4)] and *zihu* [on the right, 2 *cun* lateral to guanyuan (RN 4)]. Supplementary points — endocrine, internal genitalia, adrenal gland and *yuanzhong* (central rim) (all are otopoints).

Manipulation: Commonly used points are taken as the principal points, and two or three points are employed at each session. On the arrival of *qi*, thrust, lift, twirl and rotate the needles for 1–2 min, with a retention of 30–40 min, during which manipulate the needle once every 5–10 min. Three or four supplementary points on one side are used, with the two sides employed alternately. After routine sterilization, embed a thumbtack-shaped needle, stick and fix it with a piece of adhesive tape, and ask the patient to press it by himself or herself two or three times per day. Body acupuncture is first carried out once a day for 3 days, and then changed to 2 or 3 times a week, 10–12 times as a course, at an interval of 5–7 days between courses. The embedment is replaced once every 3 days, 10 times as a course, at the same interval as for body acupuncture.

Electroacupuncture

Selection of points: Commonly used points — *sanyinjiao* (SP 6), *zhongji* (RN 3), *zigong* (EX-CA1) and *guanyuan* (RN 4). Supplementary points — *xuehai* (SP 10), *diji* (SP 8) and *zusanli* (ST 36).

Manipulation: Two or three commonly used points and one or two supplementary points are employed at each session. The acupuncture is applied at the middle of two menstruations for 3 days on end, or on the 12th–14th days of a menstrual cycle (for those with amenorrhea, the treatment begins one month after pneumoperitoneography and enterocoelic examination) once per day for 3 days on end. Insert the needle, followed by thrusting, lifting, twirling and rotating it with moderate strength for half a minute; then connect it to the electric acupuncture device with a continuous wave, a frequency (60–120 beats/min) and an intensity tolerable to the patient. The needle is retained for 1 h. Electroacupuncture is applied for 2–7 menstrual cycles as a course. Another course may be given if the effect is not obvious.

Remarks

Both the methods above are effective for infertility and so are applicable. Body (ear) acupuncture was once applied to 106 patients, among whom, 46 (43.3%) gave birth and 18 (17.1%) became pregnant, and the cure rate was 60.4%; electroacupuncture was applied to 106 patients, among whom, 76 (59 conceived) ovulated (79.2%) and 20 had no ovulation (20.8%), and the cure rate was 79.2%. In recent years, it has been found in mechanism research that ovulation with electroacupuncture has a relation to the temperature changes of the hand skin, i.e. if the temperature of the fingers and the palm is low and may rise after the electroacupuncture, the ovulation rate may rise significantly, which shows that electroacupuncture is able to boost ovulation.

MALPOSITION OF THE FETUS

Overview

Malposition of the fetus refers to the lying of the fetus in the uterus for 28 weeks after conception. It is usually seen in multiparas or those with a lax abdominal wall. No symptoms are found in most cases. It is only made known by prenatal examination. The commonly seen positions are the posterior, breech, transverse, oblique, etc. positions, which may cause difficult labor if not corrected in time. Correcting malposition is termed in TCM *zhuan tai* (转胎, "turn the fetus"). Acupuncture treatment for *zhuan tai* was recorded in ancient Chinese medical classics like *Pictorial Appendices to "The Classified Classic."* Modern reports on the treatment of malposition with acupuncture and moxibustion were seen in the 1950s, and in the 1960s the treatment was applied in quite a few hospitals. Comprehensive researches, from the clinical to the mechanism, have been conducted in the past 40 years, and acupuncture and moxibustion has been affirmed especially for correction of malposition. *Zhiyinxue* (BL 67) has been found to be the best point among the points employed.

Treatment

Moxibustion

Selection of points: Commonly used point — *Zhiyinxue* (BL 67). Supplementary points — *yinbai* (SP 1) and *sanyinjiao* (SP 6).

Manipulation: Bilateral *zhiyinxue* points (BL 67) are employed at each session, but one or two supplementary points may be added if the effect is not obvious. After two moxa rolls (30 cm in length and 1.2 cm in diameter) are ignited, the operator holds them with the hands and applies the mild-warming moxibustion to the bilateral points, 2–3 cm above them, until the pregnant woman feels obvious warmness instead of burning pain. The moxibustion is given for 10–15 min, once a day, 4 times as a course. During the manipulation, the woman may take the sitting position with her feet on a bench and her trouser belt unfastened, or the supine position with her legs stretching out. When the moxibustion is over, she is advised to unfasten her trouser belt while sleeping that night, and to attend the clinic every day; this stops as soon as the fetal position is corrected, but re-examinations are required.

Ear acupuncture

Selection of points: Commonly used points — internal genitalia, sympathetic and subcortex. Supplementary points — liver, spleen and kidney.

Manipulation: Commonly used points are all employed and supplementary points may be added according to different conditions. After finding sensitive spots with the needle tail and sterilizing them, paste and press the vaccaria seeds to the point, and ask the patient to press it by herself 3 times a day, once for 5 min; the paste is replaced once daily on one ear with the two ears employed alternately, for 4 days as a course, and the manipulation may last for 1–4 courses.

Acupoint laser irradiation

Selection of points: *zhiyin* (BL 67).

Manipulation: Bilateral *zhiyin* points (BL 67) are employed. They are directly irradiated by the he–neon laser device with optical fiber, with an output power of 7–8 mW, a wavelength of 632.8 nm, and a spot 3 mm in diameter, for 5 min at each point, once daily, for 3–5 days as a course.

Remarks

Of the three methods above, the first one is the most widely used. It was once applied to 3282 cases, and 2842 were corrected and 440 failed; the total successful rate was 86.6%, and it mostly gained success in one course. It was found that the correction of the transverse position was the most successful, the breech position took second place and the foot position had the lowest percentage. Acupoint laser irradiation has been rising in recent years and has been reported on a great deal. Painless and easy to operate, it is popular and acceptable to both patients and doctors. Pill pressing is also an easy and safe way to correct fetal malposition, and has a higher correction rate than the other methods.

QUESTIONS

(1) Introduce briefly the two methods of acupoint stimulation in the treatment of infertility.
(2) Which method do you prefer in the treatment of fetal malposition?

CHAPTER 27

Acupuncture and Moxibustion
for Pediatric Diseases

INFANTILE DIARRHEA

Overview

Infantile diarrhea, also termed "simple dyspepsia," is a common disease in infants below two years old. It comprises mild diarrhea and severe diarrhea. The former occurs several times in one day with loose, watery and unformed stools, sometimes with milk vomiting accompanied by light abdominal distension; while severe diarrhea occurs more than ten times in one day, or even tens of times, with watery stools, vomit, fever, agitation, or even coma and convulsions. This disease is included in TCM, in the category of *xiao er xie xie zheng* (小儿泄泻证, infantile diarrhea). In *The Teachings of Bian Que*, there were records about the treatment of critical infant diarrhea with acupuncture and moxibustion. In modern times, more and more reports on the treatment have appeared since the 1950s. It has been proven clinically that acupuncture and moxibustion is not only able to cure mild diarrhea, but is also significantly effective for severe diarrhea in combination with other modern and Chinese therapies.

Treatment

Body acupuncture

Selection of points: Commonly used points — *zusanli* (ST 36) and *sifeng* (EX-UE10). Supplementary points — *neiguan* (PC 6) is added for vomiting, *quchi* (LI 11) for fever, and *tianshu* (ST 25) and *Guanyuan* (RN 4) for severe diarrhea.

Manipulation: Commonly used points are employed for mild diarrhea, and supplementary points may be added according to syndromes. A No. 30 filiform needle 1 *cun* in length is inserted into *zusanli* (ST 36) or a supplementary point, to a depth of 5–6 *fen*, by swiftly twirling and rotating or thrusting and lifting the needle for 30 s or 1 min; then withdraw the needle. *Sifeng* (EX-UE 10) is punctured by swift pricking with a thicker filiform (No. 26) or a thin three-edged needle, with white–yellow grume squeezed out. In the case of high fever, *quchi* (LI 11) should be pricked to bleed.

Moxibustion

Selection of points: Commonly used points — *zhongwan* (RN 20), *tianshu* (ST 25), *shenque* (RN 8) and *zhixie* (at the midline of the abdomen, 2.5 *cun* below the center of the umbilicus). Supplementary points — *zusanli* (ST 36) and *shangjuxu* (ST 37); *neiguan* (PC 6) is added for vomiting, and *dazhui* (DU 14) or *quchi* (LI 11) for fever.

Manipulation: Three or four common points are employed at each session, and one or two supplementary points may be added according to different conditions. Commonly used points are given rounding moxibustion with moxa rolls, at the points above, below, left and right of *shenque* (RN 8) for 15–30 min, two or three times per day. The supplementary points are given acupuncture by slightly thrusting, lifting, twirling and rotating the needles after the arrival of *qi* before the needles are withdrawn without retention, once daily.

Acupoint laser irradiation

Selection of points: Commonly used points — *tianshu* (ST 25), *shenque* (RN 8) and *shangjuxu* (ST 37). Supplementary points — *zhixie* and *zusanli* (ST 36).

Manipulation: Two or three commonly used points are employed at each session, and supplementary points, at most three, may be added if the effect is not satisfactory. The points are irradiated by a he–neon laser therapeutic device with a wavelength of 632.8 nm, an output power of 1.5 mW and a spot 1–2 mm in diameter, 30 mm above the skin. The irradiation is given 3–5 min each time, once or twice per day.

Remarks

Point stimulations for infantile diarrhea vary a lot — the acupoint-mounting method, acupoint injection, ear acupuncture, etc. Presented here are only the commonly used ones, easy to use and acceptable to infants. Body acupuncture is the most widely used one, with a firm curative effect, and was once applied to more than 600 cases, with an average cure rate of 90%. As to moxibustion, it is easy to find the materials for treating. In particular, mild-warming moxibustion is acceptable for infants, and the curative effect will be boosted if it is combined with acupuncture. Acupoint laser irradiation is a method that has been rising and gaining increasing attention in recent years; without injury or pain, it is the most applicable to infants. Clinical observations have shown that it is worth promoting, with a total effective rate ranging from 92% to 95%.

PERTUSSIS

Overview

Pertussis is a highly contagious bacterial disease caused by *Bordetella pertussis*. The symptoms are initially mild, and then develop into severe coughing fits, which produce the high-pitched "whooping" sound (like the calling sound of a rooster) in infected babies and children when they inhale air after coughing, which is repeated many times until there is vomiting, accompanied by edema of the face, purpura, subconjunctival hemorrhage, etc. In TCM it is termed *dun ke* (顿咳), but there is not any record about acupuncture treatment for the disease in ancient books. Reports on the treatment of pertussis with acupuncture and moxibustion did not appear until 1958, and it was propagated in the 1960s. In recent years, acupuncture and moxibustion has improved a lot in clinics, with an effective rate of nearly 100%.

Treatment

Cupping

Selection of points: *Shenzhu* (on the back, at the depression below the spinous process of the third thoracic vertebra).

Manipulation: With the infected child in the sitting or prone position, the point is precisely located and inserted into perpendicularly with a filiform needle to a depth of 3–5 *fen*. Then slightly twirl and rotate or thrust and lift the needle till the arrival of *qi*, with a retention of 5 min. After the needle is withdrawn, attach a small glass jar on the point until the local skin becomes reddish, and take it off 10–15 min later. The infected child should lie still for 1 h after the manipulation is over.

Acupuncture with a skin needle

Selection of points: Commonly used points — neck and sacrum. Supplementary points — anterior neck, back and lower back, upper abdomen and lateral neck.

Manipulation: Stimulating spots on the neck, back, lower back and sacrum are all on the skin area 3–4 cm bilateral to the vertebral column, the anterior neck on both sides of the trachea, the lateral neck on the anterior and posterior crest of the sternocleidomastoid, and the upper abdomen on the area between the two horizontal lines from the xiphoid process and the costal arch to the umbilicus. Only commonly used points are employed for simple pertussis, but if it is complicated by tonsillitis, anterior neck is added, and other supplementary points may be added if it is complicated by pneumonia or dyspepsia. A seven-star needle is inserted top-down with moderate flicking manipulation, with the two spots 1–1.5 cm apart, until the local skin becomes reddish. The manipulation is given once or twice daily, for seven days as a course.

Bloodletting

Selection of points: Commonly used point — *sifeng* (EX-UE10). Supplementary points — *shaoshang* (LU 11) and *shangyang* (LI 1).

Manipulation: *Sifeng* (EX-UE10) is employed first and if the effect is unsatisfactory, add or replace the supplementary points. A three-edged needle (a No. 28 needle 5 *fen* long for infants) is inserted into *sifeng* (EX-UE10) with spot pricking till a little white–yellow grume is squeezed out. *Shaoshang* (LU 11) and *shangyang* (LI 1) are given spot pricking with thin three-edged needles to squeeze out blood of granule size. Lastly, press gently on the pinhole with dry medicinal cotton. The commonly used point is given the manipulation once or twice a day on one side each time with the two hands used alternately. Supplementary points are manipulated once every five days.

Remarks

The three methods introduced above are all widely used in clinics, especially cupping, which is safe and easy, and was once applied to 628 cases with a total effective rate of 99.2%. Skin needling has a better effect for those with complicated syndromes, though the area for tapping pricking is complicated. The pricking method, also effective, was applied to 112 cases with only spot pricking on *sifeng* (Extra 25), among which, 82 cases were completely recovered and 21 markedly effective, and the "cured and markedly effective" rate was 92.0%. There are other methods for pertussis, such as body acupuncture or point injection, but it is unnecessary to go into details.

MUMPS

Overview

Mumps is an acute infectious disease caused by the mumps virus. Commonly seen in children, it is clinically characterized by painful swelling of the salivary glands. Generally, it initially occurs on one side, and then the other side is attacked, but there are cases with only one side attacked. Mumps usually occurs suddenly and quickly, with the following symptoms: fever, mild discomfort, poor appetite, vomiting, etc. This disease is termed *zha sai* (痄腮) in TCM, and there were prescriptions for mumps with acupuncture and moxibustion in *The Classic of Nourishing Life with Acupuncture and Moxibustion* in the Song Dynasty. As for the modern acupuncture treatment, quite a few cases have been reported in the past 50 years. Acupuncture and moxibustion not only has remarkable curative effect, but is also able to prevent mumps as well.

Treatment

Body acupuncture

Selection of points: Commonly used points — *yifeng* (SJ 17), *jiache* (ST 6), *shaoshang* (LU 11) and *hegu* (LI 4). Supplementary points — *lieque* (LU 7), *fenglong* (ST 40), *jiexi* (ST 41) and *tinghui* (GB 2).

Manipulation: Commonly used points are employed as the principal points, and supplementary points may be added if the effect is unsatisfactory. *Shaoshang* (LU 11) is given spot pricking with a thin three-edged needle for bloodletting. The remaining points are given reinforcing and reducing manipulation by rapid and slow insertion and withdrawal of the needles on the arrival of *qi*, i.e. first insert the needles swiftly to a certain depth till the arrival of *qi*, then thrust, lift, twirl and rotate the needles slowly, and withdraw them layer by layer with strong stimulation; repeat the manipulation to induce a needling sensation on the facial points (only the affected side is selected) radiating to the swelling parotid gland, then retain the needles for 30–60 min, during which manipulate them two or three times, once or twice daily, till the disease is cured.

Electroacupuncture

Selection of points: Commonly used points — *ashi* point (posterior–inferior to the ear lobe of the affected side, or the upper border of the intumescent parotid), *hegu* (LI 4), *jiaosun* (SJ 20) and *shaoshang* (LU 11). Supplementary points — *quchi* (LI 11) and *neiguan* (PC 6).

Manipulation: Commonly used points are employed, and *quchi* (LI 11) is added for high fever and *neiguan* (PC 6) for vomiting. First, *ashixue* is punctured from the upper crest of the swelling parotid gland, at an angle of 45°, obliquely toward the center, to a depth of 1–1.5 *cun*; then *hegu* (LI 4) (affected side) is inserted into till the arrival of *qi*. Both points are connected to the electric acupuncture device with a continuous wave, a frequency (100–120 beats/min) and an intensity tolerable to the infected child. The needles are retained at each point for 10–15 min. Bilateral *shaoshang* points (LU 11) are selected and pricked with three-edged needles for bloodletting of 3–5 drops at each point. *Jiaosun* (SJ 20) is given strong stimulation without retention of the needle, and *quchi* (LI 11) and *neiguan* (PC 6) are punctured in the same way. The manipulation is applied once daily, and twice for severe cases.

Rush-burning moxibustion

Selection of points: Commonly used point — *jiaosun* (SJ 20). Supplementary points — *lieque* (LU 7).

Manipulation: *Jiaosun* (SJ 20) is usually employed, and *lieque* (LU 7) may be selected if the effect is not obvious. Both points are on the affected side. Cut off the hair around *Jiaosun* (SJ 20) in the size of a coin, ignite a rush of 7–10 cm long with a little rapeseed oil or soybean oil, press it directly over the point and move it away quickly. When the ignited end of the rush touches the skin, the sound "pa" is heard. The moxibustion may leave a blister of mung bean size on the skin, so tell the child not to scratch it and to let it subside by itself. Generally, the moxibustion is given once, and the same operation may be performed on to *lieque* (LU 7) if the effect is not obvious. Without a rush, a matchstick may be ignited and quickly pressed onto *jiaosun* (SJ 20) in the perpendicular direction. After the rush-burning moxibustion, the local skin becomes red or white, which should be ignored.

Remarks

There are many clinical methods in the treatment of mumps, and the three above are the main ones. Body acupuncture is the principal therapy, and was once applied to 1100 patients, with all of them cured. Electroacupuncture is suitable for those with complications. Rush-burning moxibustion is a traditional way which was highly recommended by physicians for children in the Qing Dynasty. In recent years, it has been found in clinics that rush-burning moxibustion is definitely effective for mumps, and therefore more and more reports on it have been appearing. And more than 1000 cases have proven it to be effective, most of the patients being cured with once-only moxibustion. What is more, the selection of points and the manipulation are very easy and suitable for propagation. It is better to explain to the infected child before the moxibustion, since the burning rush may frighten some.

QUESTIONS

(1) What are the characteristics of the point stimulation method in the treatment of infantile diarrhea?

(2) Describe how to treat pertussis with acupuncture and moxibustion.

(3) What are the differences between body acupuncture and electro-acupuncture in the treatment of mumps?

SEQUELAE OF PEDIATRIC BRAIN DISEASE

Overview

Pediatric brain disease refers to diseases caused by various encephalitis or other factors. Sequelae appear due to there being no prevention or timely treatment. They are clinically manifested by: (1) disturbance of intelligence; (2) limb paralysis, including central paralysis (spastic paralysis of one limb or limbs) and extrapyramidal paralysis (ataxia, unsteady steps, fast and slow actions that are unchangeable); (3) others, including aphasia, loss of sight or hearing. Modern treatment for sequelae of pediatric brain disease appeared between the 1950s and the 1960s, and the curative effect has been enhanced with increasingly more point stimulation methods since the 1970s. Currently, a cure rate of 80% has been achieved.

Treatment

Body acupuncture

Selection of points: Commonly used points — *sishenzhen* [four needles, anterior, posterior, left and right of *baihui* (DU 20)], *zhisanzhen* [three needles, *shenting* (DU 24) 0.5 *cun* above the hairline, and bilateral *benshen* (GB 13) 3 *cun* lateral to *shenting* (DU 24)]. Supplementary points — *taichong* (LR 3), *hegu* (LI 4), *neiguan* (PC 6) and *yongquan* (KI 1) added for the restless; *fengfu* (DU 16) and *tongli* (HT 5) for the quiet; *quchi* (LI 11), *jianyu* (LI 15), *waiguan* (SJ 5), *huantiao* (GB 30), *yanglingquan* (GB 34) and *xuanzhong* (GB 39) for movement disorder.

Manipulation: Commonly used points are all employed and supplementary points may be added according to syndromes. No. 30 filiform needles 1.5 *cun* long are inserted horizontally into the point on the head to a depth of 1 *cun*, and into the extremities to a routine depth, with the needles retained at each point for 30 min on the arrival of *qi*, during which manipulation by twirling and rotating the needles is given once every 10 min. For the first 20 days, this is applied once daily, followed by manipulating once every other day, for 4 months as a complete course.

Acupoint injection

Selection of points: Commonly used point — three groups, namely (1) *fengfu* (DU 16) and *shenshu* (BL 23); (2) *fengchi* (GB 20) and *zusanli* (ST 36); (3) *dazhui* (DU 14) and Neiguan (PC 6). Supplementary points — *jianyu* (LI 15), *jianliao* (SJ 14), *quchi* (LI 11), *waiguan* (SJ 5), *chize* (LU 5) and *hegu* (LI 4) added for upper limb paralysis; *huantiao* (GB 30), *Yinmen* (BL 37), *weizhong* (BL 40), *yanglingquan* (GB 34), *xuehai* (SP 10), *kunlun* (BL 60) and *jiexi* (ST 41) for lower limb paralysis; *shanglianquan* (RN 23), *hegu* (LI 4), *jiache* (ST 6) and *yifeng* (SJ 17) for dysphagia and dysmasesis; *lianquan* (RN 23) and *tongli* (HT 5) for speech disorder; *chengqi* (ST 1) and *qiuhou* (EX-HN7) for vision disorder; *ermen* (SJ 21) and *yifeng* (SJ 17) for hearing disorder.

Manipulation: Injections include aceglutamide, piracetam and vitamin B1; vitamin B12 (0.1 mg/ml) for the eyes. Select one of them. A 0.3–2 ml injection is given to the points, and the dose varies according to the condition, injection site, properties and concentration. A low dose is needed for points on the head, the face and thin muscles, and a high dose for points on the limbs, back and lower back. The manipulation is given once every other day, 10 times as a course, at an interval of 7–10 days between courses. Generally, three or more courses are necessary.

Remarks

The two methods above are typically effective in treating pediatric brain disease. The first one is mainly applicable to mentally handicapped children, and was applied to 558 cases with 127 markedly effective and 314 effective, and a total effective rate of 79.0%. The second one is for children with paralysis and other symptoms, and was once applied to 371 cases with the total effective rate ranging from 64.8% to 82.18%, being especially effective for postencephalitis. There are other therapies, like body acupuncture and head acupuncture, but here it is unnecessary to go into details.

SEQUELAE OF POLIOMYELITIS

Overview

Sequelae of poliomyelitis, also called postpolio syndrome (PPS), are caused by paralysis at the acute stage of polio not being positively managed. The main clinical manifestations are muscular atrophy, limb deformation, skeletal development constraint, etc. PPS is included in TCM in the category of *wei zheng* (痿证), and acupuncture and moxibustion for *wei zheng* was recorded in *The Inner Classic*, which made it clear to select *yangming* meridian only for the treatment of *wei zheng*. Modern treatment of polio with acupuncture and moxibustion, including PPS, was reported a great deal in the early 1950s, and from the late 1960s to the early 1970s acupuncture and moxibustion for PPS was booming. At present, an effective rate of 90% has been achieved, and the "completely recovered" rate is about 30%.

Treatment

Comprehensive method

Selection of points: Commonly used points — *jianyu* (LI 15), *quchi* (LI 11), *shousanli* (LI 10), *hegu* (LI 4), *huantiao* (GB 30), *siqiang* (4.5 *cun* directly above the middle of the upper border of the patella), *yanglingquan* (GB 34), *zusanli* (ST 36), *xuanzhong* (GB 39) and *biguan* (ST 31). Supplementary points — *ganshu* (BL 18), *pishu* (BL 20) and *shenshu* (BL 23).

Manipulation: The method includes acupuncture and acupoint injection. Acupuncture: two or three common points are employed at each session, depending on the paralyzed area. Short and strong stimulation is applied without retention. When the body begins to restore the function, moderate stimulation is employed, with the needles retained at each point for 15–20 min. The manipulation is given once every other day. Acupoint injection: one vitamin B1 100 mg/2 ml and one vitamin B12 100 mg/ml are mixed together. Two or three commonly used points and one supplementary point are employed at each treatment session. Short and swift stimulations by thrusting and rotating the needles are given to the points until the arrival of *qi*, and then the mixed liquid of 0.5–0.8 ml is injected into each point, twice a week. Rounding moxibustion with moxa sticks may be applied to four or five points for those with cold limbs and obvious paralysis, for 15 min till the local skin becomes reddish, once daily.

Electroacupuncture with needles in alignment

Selection of points: Commonly used points — (1) spleen and stomach channel lines and points: *biguan* (ST 31), *liangqiu* (ST 34), *zusanli* (ST 36), *fenglong* (ST 40), *jiexi* (St 41), *xuehai* (SP 10), *yinlingquan* (SP 9), *sanyinjiao* (SP 6), etc.; (2) gallbladder and bladder channel lines and points: *huantiao* (GB 30), *fengshi* (GB 31), *yanglingquan* (GB 34), *qiuxu* (GB 40), *zhibian* (BL 54), *yinmen* (BL 37), *weizhong* (BL 40), *chengshan* (BL 57), *kunlun* (BL 60), etc. Supplementary points — points on the *renmai* and *dumain* channels: *dazhui* (DU 14), *mingmen* (DU 4), *yangguan* (DU 3), *qihai* (RN 6), *zhongwan* (RN 20), *guanyuan* (RN 4), etc.

Manipulation: Two groups of commonly used points are employed alternately, combined with two or three supplementary points, at each treatment session. Selection of points should depend on the pathological area and the direction of the channels and collaterals, in combination with the distribution and the functioning condition of the paralyzed muscles. There is a better effect if the acupuncture is carried out between 7 and 11 o'clock in the morning. First, select the channels concerned, and insert the needles successively in rows at an interval of 3 cm from the top of the affected area into the points of two channels; then manipulate the needles in sequence to induce *qi*, followed by strengthening the force of fingers to thrust and lift the needles with thrusting as the main manipulation. Induce the needling sensation to transmit along the channels directly to the pathological area. Finally, each needle is connected to the electric acupuncture device with thin copper wires for electric stimulation, initially with a dense wave for 1 min, a sparse wave for 7 min, an irregular wave for 2 min, and lastly an intermittent wave for 10 min. The current intensity is increased with the wave changes. The treatment is carried out for 20 min, once daily 12 times as a treatment course, at an interval of 1 week between courses. One phase consists of 3 courses, and the next phase should begin after 6 months from the end of the last course.

Remarks

There are many point stimulation methods for sequelae of poliomyelitis, but here only two have been presented. The first is a comprehensive method combining body acupuncture and point injection for stubborn cases. It was once applied to about 700 cases with a total effective rate of 90%. The second, a new method that appeared in recent years, is specially for sequelae of poliomyelitis. It was applied to 1000 cases with a total effective rate of 96%, and is especially effective for young patients with a short course of disease (less than five years), with buttock muscles recovering quickly and thigh muscles recovering slowly. Both methods are easy to operate and either is applicable.

QUESTIONS

(1) What does either of the point stimulation methods place extra emphasis on in treating sequelae of pediatric brain disease?
(2) Restate in detail the electric row needling therapy for sequelae of poliomyelitis.

ENURESIS

Overview

Enuresis, commonly called bed-wetting, refers to involuntary discharge of the urine of a child over the age of three years, occurring during sleep. In severe cases, involuntary micturition occurs once or twice or even more times a night, characterized by evacuation once of the bladder. In TCM the condition is termed *yi ni* (遗溺, enuresis) or *niao chuang* (尿床, bed-wetting). The acupuncture prescription first appeared in *Important Formulas Worth a Thousand Gold Pieces for Emergencies* in the Tang Dynasty. In the early 1950s, clinical observations on the modern treatment of acupuncture and moxibustion were made. Articles on the treatment of enuresis have made up an important proportion of all the theses concerning acupuncture and moxibustion in the past 50 years. At present, an average effective rate of over 90% has been achieved.

Treatment

Body acupuncture

Selection of points: Commonly used points — *guanyuan* (RN 4) or *qugu* (RN 2), and *sanyinjiao* (SP 6). Supplementary points — *baihui* (DU 20), *jingming* (BL 1) and nocturia point (a hand acupoint, on the facies pal-maris, at the middle of the cross-grain of the second digital joint of the little finger).

Manipulation: *Guanyuan* (RN 4) and *qugu* (CV 2) are employed alter-nately, and supplementary points may be added or employed if the effect is not obvious, with at most three points at each treatment session. *Guanyuan* (RN 4) is inserted into perpendicularly to a depth of 0.5–1 *cun* by thrusting and rotating the needle repeatedly to induce a sensation of reaching the external genitals; *qugu* (CV 2) is inserted into obliquely at an angle of 15° with a No. 28 filiform needle till the arrival of *qi*, and then scraping manipulation (scrape the needle handle with the nail of the thumb) is applied 20–30 times, followed by lifting the needle just beneath the skin and then inserting it obliquely at an angle of 35° to the muscular layer to both left and right, and withdrawing the needle in the same way. *Sanyinjiao* (SP 6) is inserted into with the needle tip slightly upward till the arrival of *qi*, and then thrusting and lifting the needle in combination with twirling and rotating is performed to transmit the sensation to the knees; *baihui* (DU 20) is inserted into horizontally forward to a depth of 0.5–1 *cun*; the nocturia point is is given a perpendicular insertion to 0.2–0.3 *cun*; while puncturing *jingming* (BL 1), ask the child to close the eyes, and insert a No. 30–32 filiform needle into the point to a depth a 0.5–1 *cun*, with no thrusting, lifting, twirling or rotating of the needle. The needles are retained in each point for half an hour, during which they are manipulated once every 5 min. *Jingming* (BL 1) and the nocturia point are given the scraping method. The manipulation is applied once daily, 7–10 times as a course, at an interval of 3–5 days between courses.

Ear acupuncture

Selection of points: Commonly used points — kidney, bladder (in the middle of the kidney and the anterior upper angle of the cymba concha), spleen and central rim. Supplementary points — lung and *shenmen* (HT 7).

Manipulation: Commonly used points are taken as the principal points, and supplementary points may be added according to conditions, with 3–5 points employed at each session. No. 28 filiform needles, 5 *fen* in length, are inserted into otopoints without penetrating the ear cartilage. On the arrival of *qi*, the needles are retained for 30 min, once daily for the first five times. From the sixth time, place *Semen vaccariae* seeds on the point and press it with the hand for 1–2 min, until the affected child feels distension and pain. One side is employed each time, with the two sides employed alternately. Ask the child to press it by himself or herself twice a day (another one may be added before sleeping), for 5 min every time. Replace the plaster twice per week, for 5 times as a course.

Wrist–ankle acupuncture

Selection of points — Lower 6.

Manipulation: Insert a No. 30 filiform needle, 2 *cun* in length, obliquely at an angle of 30° into the selected point, then immediately lay the needle flat, parallel to the skin surface, followed by pushing the needle upward slowly to a depth of 1.5 *cun*; the affected child should feel no pain or needling sensation. Both sides are punctured with the needles retained for 30 min, once daily, 10 times as a course, at an interval of 5 days between courses.

Remarks

There are many treatment methods for enuresis with acupuncture and moxibustion, but only three have been presented here. Body acupuncture is the most important one, especially in point selection and needling techniques, and was applied to 1000 cases, with a total effective rate of 95%. Since it varies a lot between individuals, certain points should be selected according to the effectiveness. Ear acupuncture and wrist–ankle acupuncture are mainly applicable to beginners and those who are afraid of needling on the abdomen.

MINIMAL BRAIN DYSFUNCTION SYNDROME

Overview

Minimal brain dysfunction syndrome, also known as pediatric hyperactivity syndrome, is a marginal psychiatric disorder clinically manifested by hyperactivity, naughtiness, inattention, difficulty in drawing oneself up, mental retardation, learning handicaps, etc. It does not draw the attention of the parents until school age, and is commonly seen in children at the ages of 6–16. There are no corresponding names in TCM and not any records about the treatment with acupuncture and moxibusiton in ancient documents. It is only in the past 10 years that the disease has gained attention from the field of acupuncture and moxibustion. At present, an effective rate of 90% has been achieved.

Treatment

Comprehensive method

Selection of point: Commonly used points — *neiguan* (PC 6), *taichong* (LR 3), *dazhui* (DU 14), *quchi* (LI 11) and *shenshu* (BL 23). Supplementary points — *baihui* (DU 20), *sishencong* (EX-HN1) and *daling* (PC 7) added for inattention, and *Shenting* (DU 24) (on the head, 0.5 *cun* above the midpoint of the anterior hairline), danzhong (RN 17) and *zhaohai* (KI 6) for dysphoria.

Manipulation: Two or three commonly used points and one or two supplementary points are employed at each treatment session. Insert the needles till the arrival of *qi*, then give reducing manipulation by twirling and rotating or thrusting and lifting the needles for 0.5–1 min, with a retention of 10–15 min. No retention is given to those who do not cooperate. If the effect is not obvious, the points may be connected to the electric acupuncture device with an irregular wave and an intensity tolerable to the patient. The needles withdrawn, tapping acupuncture is given three times with a seven-star needle along the *du* channel and the two bladder channels on the back from top to bottom repeatedly with mild stimulation, till the local skin becomes reddish. The manipulation is applied once every day or every other day, 10 times as a course, at an interval of 3–5 days between courses.

Electroacupuncture and ear acupuncture

Selection of points: Two groups — (1) *shenmen* (HT 7), *neiguan* (PC 6), *zusanli* (ST 36), *sanyinjiao* (SP 6) and *xuanzhong* (GB 39); (2) adrenal gland, central rim, liver, subcortex and *shenmen* (HT 7) (all are otopoints).

Manipulation: Both groups are employed at each treatment session, including 4 or 5 of the body points and 3–5 of the otopoints. Needle the body points till the arrival of *qi*, then connect them to the electric acupuncture device with a continuous wave and a frequency of 60–200 beats/min, with the needles retained in each point for 5–10 min. After withdrawing the needles, stick *Semen vaccariae* seeds to the otopoints and press them. Ask the patient to press the points by himself or herself twice daily, 200 times for each pressing. One ear is employed at each session, with the two ears employed alternately. Replace the plaster twice per week. The acupuncture is applied 10–15 times as a course. No courses are counted for sticking and pressing the otopoints.

Remarks

Both of the methods above, strictly speaking, are not mature but effective in clinics. The first one was once applied to 48 cases, with 39 completely recovered, 5 effective and 4 invalid, and a total effective rate of 91.7% was achieved, which should be confirmed in practice. Combination with modern and Chinese medicine, as well as psychotherapy, will enhance the curative effect.

TICS (TOURETTE SYNDROME)

Overview

Tics (Tourette syndrome) are an inherited neuropsychiatric disorder with onset in childhood, at the age of 4–16. They are clinically characterized by multiple involuntary movements, and vocal cord twitches, as well as other symptom like, blinking, pouting, head-shaking, shrugging or fist-making, accompanied by vocal tics, barking, etc. All the symptoms emerge slowly. Acupuncture and moxibustion therapy has been gaining more and more attention and has become preferable because of the increased morbidity and the side effects of a nerve blockade. Reports about the treatment of tics (Tourette syndrome) with acupuncture and moxibustion first appeared in the early 1990s, and more than 1000 cases have proven its effectiveness through needling, otopoint pill pressing or a combination of the two. Some acupuncture practitioners compared the treatment with drug therapies, and found that acupuncture is superior to Western medicine in both short-term and long-term effects. It has been confirmed experimentally that those with an abnormal EEG will return to normal after acupuncture and moxibustion is given.

Treatment

Body acupuncture

Selection of point: Commonly used points — *neiting* (ST 44), *quchi* (LI 11), *lianquan* (RN 23), *shenmen* (HT 7) and *yintang* (EX-HN3). Supplementary points — *fuliu* (KI 7), *hegu* (LI 4), *zusanli* (ST 36), *shenshu* (BL 23), *dazhui* (DU 14) and *fengchi* (GB 20).

Manipulation: Generally, only three or four commonly used points are employed, and two or three supplementary points may be added if the curative effect is not obvious. *Neiting* (ST 44) and *quchi* (LI 11) are given reducing manipulation by thrusting and lifting the needles; *shen-men* (HT 7) is given reinforcing manipulation by twirling and rotating the needles; *lianquan* (RN 23) is given sparrow-pecking manipulation, and *yintang* (EX-HN3) is inserted into horizontally downward till local soreness and distension are felt. Supplementary points are given the uniform reinforcing–reducing manipulation by routine needling. All the points are punctured once every day or every other day, with the needles retained for 30 min, 10 times as a course, at an interval of 3 days between courses.

Otopoint pill pressing

Selection of points: Commonly used points — liver, heart, *shenmen*, brain point (central rim) and wind stream. Supplementary points — spleen, adrenal gland, subcortex, endocrine and kidney.

Manipulation: Commonly used points are all employed, and two or three supplementary points may be added according to conditions. *Semen vaccariae* seeds are used for sticking, with one or two granules on one piece of adhesive plaster. Both ears are applied to. Advise the parent to help rub and press until the auricle becomes hot and distended, but tolerable to the patient. The manipulation is applied three times per day, 3 min each time. Change to the other ear every week, five times as a course. More than two courses are needed for a treatment.

Electroacupuncture

Selection of points: Commonly used points — *baihui* (DU 20), *sishencong* (EX-HN1) and choreiform tremor area. Supplementary points — *zusanli* (ST 36), *fenglong* (ST 40), *fengchi* (GB 20) and *taixi* (KI 3).

Manipulation: Commonly used points are all employed, and one or two supplementary points may be added according to conditions. Swift insertion is performed. When the head points feel the arrival of *qi*, connect them to pulse electric current at a frequency of 300–400 beats/min, with the intensity tolerable to the affected child. The rest of the points are given the uniform reinforcing–reducing manipulation after the arrival of *qi*, with the needles retained in each point for 30 min, during which twirl and rotate the needles three times. The operation is applied once every day or every other day, seven times as a course. Another course should begin after three days.

Acupoint application therapy

Selection of points — shenque (RN 8).

Manipulation: Medicinals for mounting — *tianma* (*Rhizoma Gastrodiae*) 15 g, Gouteng (*Ramulus Uncariae cum Uncis*) 15 g, Dilong (*Peretima*) 15 g, Dannanxing (*Arisaema cum bile*) 15 g, Fangfeng (*Radix Saposhnikoviae*) 20 g, human nail 5 g and pearl powder 10 g. First, the six medicinals are ustulated in an earthenware pot, ground to powder, mixed with the pearl powder, and put into a bottle. Three days after the first treatment course with acupuncture, the second course begins, coupled with mounting therapy. Clean the navel with warm water, wipe it dry, fill the navel with the powder, and seal and fix it with adhesive plaster. Make a replacement once every three days. For those allergic to adhesive plaster, the powder is put into a gauze pocket fixed onto the navel with a bandage until complete recovery without a replacement.

Remarks

The four acupuncture methods are all widely used in clinics. Body acupuncture is the first choice, but is difficult for beginners since it requires more points, reinforcing and reducing manipulation, and cooperation from the affected child. Otopoint pill pressing is easy and acceptable to patients but the curative effect is inferior to that of body acupuncture, and it needs a longer period of treatment. Head electroacupuncture coupled with body acupuncture has a better effect with safe point selection and no high technique requirement, so it is applicable to beginners. Acupoint mounting therapy may be applied if the condition allows.

QUESTIONS

(1) What are the commonly used acupuncture and moxibustion methods in the treatment of enuresis?

(2) Find some new material about the treatment of minimal brain dysfunction syndrome with acupuncture and moxibustion.

(3) Among the four acupuncture and moxibustion methods for tics (Tourette syndrome), which one is applicable to beginners? How to operate it?

CHAPTER 28

Acupuncture and Moxibustion for ENT Diseases

ACUTE CONJUNCTIVITIS

Overview

Acute conjunctivitis, a common eye disease, refers to acute epidemic inflammation of the conjunctiva caused by viral or bacterial infection. It is clinically manifested by red eyes (hyperemia) relating to the palpebral conjunctiva and the fornix, a sensation of heat and irritation in the eye, sticky eyes with purulent discharge, or even puffiness of the eyes in severe cases. The disease is equivalent to *bao feng ke re* (暴风客热) in TCM, and the treatment with acupuncture and moxibustion was recorded in *The Inner Classic*. Quite a lot of clinical articles about the modern acupuncture therapy appeared in the late 1950s, especially about the otopoint pricking method, which is able to prevent the disease to some degree. At present, an effective rate of 90% has been achieved.

Treatment

Pricking for blood

Selection of points: Zhongchong (PC 9).

Manipulation: If one eye is affected, a point on one side is employed; for two eyes, two points. Grip the patient's middle finger with the thumb and index finger of the left hand to cause local congestion, followed by spot pricking with a three-edged needle, and then gently press it and squeeze out drops of blood, once daily, three times as a course. Another course may given if the patient is not completely cured.

Ear acupuncture

Selection of points: Commonly used points — tip of the ear, vena behind the ear, and tenderness spots (press evenly the ear lobes with the handle of a filiform needle or a match for symmetrical tenderness spots which are different from the skin around, with a darker skin color and grainlike nodes; if the point cannot be found, replace it with acupoints of the eye). Supplementary points — *shenmen* (HT 7), liver and eye.

Manipulation: One or two commonly used points and one supplementary point are employed. First, massage the ear tip repeatedly with fingers to cause congestion, fold the ear forward, and prick it to bleed with a three-edged needle; or prick the most obvious vessel on the ear upheaval or the tender spot on the ear lobe, and press it with the thumb to squeeze out 4 or 5 drops of blood, or 7–10 drops for severe cases. Eye, *shenmen* (HT 7) and liver are given shallow puncture with filiform needles (if the tender spot is selected, give up eye points) by twirling and rotating, with the needles retained in each point for 20–30 min. One ear is employed at each session, once or twice per day.

Body acupuncture

Selection of points: Commonly used points — *jingming* (BL 1), *taiyang* (EX-HN5), *fengchi* (GB 20) and *hegu* (LI 4). Supplementary points — *chengqi* (ST 1), *zanzhu* (BL 2), *tongziliao* (GB 1) and *sizhukong* (SJ 23).

Manipulation: Commonly used points are taken as the principal points, and supplementary points may be added if the effect is not obvious. A No. 28–30 filiform needle is inserted into *taiyang* (EX-HN5) perpendicularly to a depth of 0.5–1 *cun*; *fengchi* (GB 20) is inserted into toward the eyeball on the same side to a depth of 1.5 *cun*, slightly thrusting, lifting, twirling and rotating the needle to induce a sensation reaching the eye; *hegu* (LI 4) is inserted into with the needle tip upward to transmit the sensation upward; and *jingming* (BL 1) is given shallow puncture with a filiform needle

0.5 *cun* long. Supplementary points are given routine acupuncture. The needles are retained in each point for 15–20 min. Drops of blood are squeezed out after the needle is withdrawn from *taiyang* (EX-HN5). Body acupuncture is applied once daily, without the courses counted.

Remarks

Among the three methods above, pricking for blood is the easiest and the most effective. It was once applied to 250 cases, with a cure rate of 96% in three days. Ear acupuncture also takes pricking as the main technique, with a total effective rate of above 95% and the effect seen in 5–7 days. Body acupuncture has been applied to the most cases, with similar effects. Be cautious when needling *fengchi* (GB 20) or *jingming* (BL 1): for the former, avoid inserting too deep and the inserting direction must be precisely controlled; for the latter, one must not pierce the vessel, in order to avoid accidents.

ELECTRIC OPHTHALMIA

Overview

Electric ophthalmia is an acute inflammatory reaction in the conjunctiva and cornea caused by fairly long and intense exposure to ultraviolet light. It is manifested by a sudden onset, a foreign body sensation in the eyes, severe pain, photophobia, lacrimation, blepharoedema, mixed congestion in the conjunctiva, and so on. There was not any record about the treatment of electric ophthalmia with acupuncture and moxibustion in ancient documents. Many a report appeared in the 1950s–1960s. In recent years, methods of point stimulation have been improved and increased, and an effective rate of 95% has been achieved according to statistics.

Treatment

Body acupuncture

Selection of points: Commonly used points — *fengchi* (GB 20), *hegu* (LI 4) and *jingming* (BL 1). Supplementary points — *zanzhu* (BL 2), *yangbai* (GB 14), *sibai* (ST 2) and *taiyang* (EX-HN5).

Manipulation: Commonly used points are taken as the main points, and one or two supplementary points are employed if the effect is not satisfactory, with three or four points at each session, all with No. 30 filiform needles. *Fengchi* (GB 20) is punctured obliquely toward the tip of the nose; *hegu* (LI 4) is perpendicularly punctured deeply till the arrival of *qi*, and then reducing manipulation is applied by twirling and rotating the needle with strong stimulation. *Jingming* (BL 1) is punctured perpendicularly close to the orbital border to a depth of 0.5–1 *cun*, slightly twirling, rotating, lifting and thrusting till the arrival of *qi*. The rest of the points are all given reducing manipulation by forceful lifting and slight thrusting after the arrival of *qi*. The needles are retained for 15–20 min, with interrupted stimulations. *Taiyang* (EX-HN5) is pricked for bloodletting with a three-edged needle. The treatment is applied once daily until complete recovery is achieved.

Acupuncture with intradermal needles

Selection of points: *Zanzhu* (BL 2) and *hegu* (LI 4).

Manipulation: Four thumbtack intradermal needles, the round part gripped with forceps, are inserted into bilateral to both points respectively after thorough sterilization; then fix them with adhesive plasters. Press each point for 1 min, while *zanzhu* (BL 2) is pressed with both thumbs, or the single index finger or middle finger pulp, and *hegu* (LI 4) is pressed simultaneously with the two thumb pulps. The needles are retained for hours to a day and not withdrawn until the symptoms ease or disappear.

Ear acupuncture

Selection of points: Commonly used points — eye, ear apex and *shenmen*. Supplementary points — middle of the ear and adrenal gland.

Manipulation: Commonly used points are taken as the main points, and supplementary points added if there is no obvious effect, with both ears employed. Bloodletting therapy is applied to the ear apex in the same way as for acute conjunctivitis; the rest of the points are punctured with filiform needles till the arrival of *qi*, twirling and rotating the needles for 0.5–1 min, with a retention of 10–15 min. In withdrawing the needles, a bit of blood is squeezed out at each point. The treatment is applied once daily till total recovery.

Remarks

Among the three therapies introduced above, body acupuncture is preferable. It was applied to 776 cases, with a total effective rate of 88.1%–98.1%. Intradermal needling is also available, and it was applied to 100 cases, with 94 cases completely recovered in the shortest time of 2 h, and the longest of 38 h. Ear acupuncture may be combined with other therapies. In order to enhance the curative effect and shorten the treatment courses, cold compresses may be applied for decongestion, or drops of sterilized milk placed in the eyes.

QUESTIONS

(1) Restate briefly the manipulation and point selection in treatment of acute conjunctivitis with acupuncture and moxibustion.
(2) What are the similarities and differences of the two point stimulation therapies in treatment of electric ophthalmia?

JUVENILE MYOPIA

Overview

Myopia is a very frequent refractive error, clinically manifested by blurred distance vision, fatigability of the affected eye, or even fundus oculi changes in medium or severe myopia. It is called *jin shi* (near-sightedness) and *neng jin qie yuan* (blurred distance vision but good near vision) in TCM. In ancient documents, the acupuncture treatment was recorded as early as in *Zhen Jiu Jia Yi Jing* (*The Systematic Classic of Acupuncture and Moxibustion*). Modern reports began in the 1950s and various kinds of point stimulation therapies have been applied to the treatment, especially dermal acupuncture. Experience has shown that acupuncture therapy for juvenile myopia has been confirmed to be effective in the short-term period, but the long-term effect remains unsatisfactory and the mechanism of action needs further intensification.

Treatment

Acupuncture with skin needles

Selection of points: Commonly used points — two groups, namely (1) *zhengguan* 1 (at the junction of three-quarters exterior to the margo supraorbitalis and one-quarter interior) and *zhengguang* 2 (at the junction of one-quarter exterior to the margo supraorbitalis and three-quarters interior); (2) *jingming* (BL 1) and *chengqi* (ST 1). Supplementary points — *fengchi* (GB 20), *neiguan* (PC 6) and *dazhui* (DU 14).

Manipulation: The first group is taken as the main points, or the second group, or alternately. One to three supplementary points are employed according to symptoms. Dermal needles are used to tap the *zhengguan* 1 and *zhengguang* 2 area measuring 0.5–1.2 cm 20–50 times; *jingming* (BL 1) and *chengqi* (ST 1) are tapped for about 5 min; supplementary points are tapped the same way as for *zhengguang*. The treatment is applied once every day or every other day, at 10–15 sessions as a course, at an interval of half a month between courses.

Ear acupuncture

Selection of points: Commonly used points — eye, liver, kidney, short-sightedness (lateral to the cavity of the auricular concha). Supplementary points — eye 1 (on the ear lobe, anterior–inferior to the intertragic notch), eye 2 (on the ear lobe, posterior–inferior to the intertragic notch), *shenmen* and heart.

Manipulation: Three commonly used points and supplementary points are employed at each session. *Vaccaria segetalis* seeds or magnetic beads (380 G) are pressed with adhesive plaster onto the sensitive spot, the exterior and interior auricles for reinforcing stimulation. Ask the patient to press the points three or four times by himself or herself, 1 min for each point, and one ear at each session. If both ears are pressed, the number of auricular points should be reduced to three, for the purpose of taking turns. Change to another plaster once a week, at four sessions as a course, at an interval of one week between courses.

Acupoint laser irradiation

Selection of points: Commonly used points — *jingming* (BL 1), *chengqi* (ST 1) and *hegu* (LI 4). Supplementary points — *zuguangming* (GB 37) and *yanglao* (SI 6).

Manipulation: Commonly used points are taken as the main points, and supplementary points as adjuvant. The helium–neon laser is employed, with wavelength 632.8 nm, power 1.5–2 mW, current strength 6 mA, and beams irradiating perpendicularly. The patient is in the upright sitting position, eyes closed. Irradiate the points of the eyes for 2 min, and the others for 4 min, with the facula diameter less than 1.5 mm and the angle of emission less than 2 milliradians. Two or three points are selected at each session, once daily, at 10 sessions as a course, at an interval of 3–5 days between courses.

Body acupuncture

Selection of points: Commonly used points — *Chengqi* (ST 1), *jingming* (BL 1) and *qiuhou* (EX-HN7). Supplementary points — *yiming* (EX-HN14), *fengchi* (GB 20), *sibai* (ST 2), *hegu* (LI 4), *zanzhu* (BL 2) and *taiyang* (EX-HN5).

Manipulation: One or two commonly used points are employed at each session, combined with one or two supplementary points. *Chengqi* (ST 1) is punctured obliquely toward *jingming* (BL 1) at an angle of 30° to a depth of about 1 *cun*, with a No. 30 filiform needle, until a sensation of soreness and distension arises in the ocular region or tears drop, followed by continuously lifting-thrusting slightly 3–5 times, with the needle retained for 10 min. *Qiuhou* (EX-HN7) and *jingming* (BL 1) are perpendicularly punctured with filiform needles 2 *cun* long to a depth of 1.5 *cun*, inserting the needle slowly without twirling, rotating, lifting or thrusting.

The needle is retained for 10 min, after inducing the obvious sensation of soreness and distension in the eyeball, and the rest of the points are given routine acupuncture till the arrival of *qi*, twirling and rotating the needle with medium or strong stimulation, with a retention of 15 min. The treatment is applied once daily, at 10 sessions as a course, at an interval of 3–5 days between courses.

Remarks

Among the four acupuncture therapies for myopia, the first three are easy and safe to perform, acceptable for juvenile patients, and have been applied to more than 2000 eyes respectively except for point laser irradiation. Dermal needle acupuncture is the best in curative effect while ear acupuncture is inferior, and laser irradiation is similar to dermal needling and is advised to be the first choice in treatment. Body acupuncture has been applied to 6186 eyes and has achieved a total effective rate of 94.5% and a recovery rate of 38.2%; it is an alternative if the other three therapies have no satisfactory effect. The patients have to reinforce the protection of the eyes during treatment, otherwise long-term effectiveness will be affected.

STYE

Overview

Stye (or sty), also known as a hordeolum, is an acute purulent inflammation caused by staphylococcal infections of the meibomian glands or sebaceous glands around the eyelash follicle. Pricking therapy was mentioned in *Zhen Jiu Ju Ying* (*A Collection of Gems in Acupuncture and Moxibustion*) in the Ming Dynasty. In the late 1950s, there were a lot of clinical data about the treatment of styes with acupuncture and moxibustion, and it underwent great development in the late 1980s. It has been proven that acupuncture and moxibustion (including various kinds of stimulation methods) has a curative effect and is able to cause cases without pus to fade away, and to expel pus, with an effective rate of over 90% on the average.

Treatment

Ear acupuncture

Selection of points: Two groups — (1) ear apex; (2) cymba conchae auriculae and the cavity of the auricular concha.

Manipulation: Either group is employed — one only or the two alternately. Select the ear apex on the affected side, sterilize it, and pinch its skin with the left hand. Then a small-sized three-edged needle is inserted with the right hand to a depth of 5 *fen*, twirling and rotating it partly three times, with 8–10 drops of blood squeezed out. Sterilized cotton balls are used to stop the bleeding. For the second group, if the palpebra frontalis is affected, the cymba conchae auricula on the affected side is selected, while the cavity of the auricular concha is selected for lower lid affection. If the upper and lower lids are affected at the same time, give priority to the more serious affection, with both sides selected if both eyes are affected. After sterilization, a No. 26 filiform needle or a thin three-edged needle is used to prick the point area 3–5 times, and be sure not to pierce the cartilage. A bit of blood is let out; otherwise, squeeze out some. The treatment is applied once daily, and generally three sessions are needed.

Pricking for blood

Selection of points: Interscapular area.

Manipulation: A reactive site is found in the interscapular area. The patient is to bestride a chair, with his or her back exposed to the outside. The reactive site is usually the eminent papula, miliary or oval. If it cannot be found, *gaohuang* (BL 43) is employed. After routine sterilization, a three-edged needle is inserted 0.1–0.3 cm, with the skin pricked. Thrust rapidly and lift slowly till there is bleeding. Do not press or knead the pores, but slightly press the area around the pricking point to eliminate static blood, 0.2–0.3 ml. Wipe dry with sterilized cotton balls. Generally, prick the reactive site on the affected side, once daily, until complete recovery.

Remarks

Besides the therapies introduced above, there are many others in treatment of styes, such as acupoint laser irradiation, wrist–ankle acupuncture, point application, rush-fire cauterization and ear point needle embedding. The two therapies here are the most common and are both pricking for blood methods, one for ear points and the other for body points. The former was applied to 360 cases, with 317 completely recovered, and a total effective rate of 91.9%; the latter to 288 cases, with a total effective rate of 100%. Either is available in practice.

QUESTIONS

(1) Describe briefly the four commonly used therapies for treatment of juvenile myopia.
(2) Which method of point stimulation do you prefer for treatment of styes?

DYSCHROMATOPSIA

Overview

Dyschromatopsia is classified into color blindness and color amblyopia. Color blindness refers to inability or decreased ability to see color or perceive color differences, including anerythroblepsia (red blindness), deuteranopia (green blindness), tritanopia (blue blindness) and achromatopsia, but the last two are rare. Color amblyopia refers to deficiency in perceiving color differences, including amblyopia for red, green and blue, the first two being common in life. The condition is called *shi wu yi se* or *shi chi ru bai* in TCM. No record about treatment with acupuncture and moxibustion has been found in ancient medical literature, while the first modern report was seen in 1959. In the 1970s, a great amount of practice confirmed that acupuncture and moxibustion therapies are effective. Since then much work has been done at home and abroad, but ideal long-term effectiveness has not been achieved due to different curative effects in different places.

Treatment

Body acupuncture

Selection of points: Commonly used points — *tongziliao* (GB 1), *zanzhu* (BL 2), *jingming* (BL 1) and *sibai* (ST 2). Supplementary points — *fengchi* (GB 20), *sizhukong* (SJ 23), *yangbai* (GB 14), *hegu* (LI 4) and *zusanli* (ST 36).

Manipulation: Two or three commonly used points and one or two supplementary points are employed at each session, selected alternately. For eye points, No. 30 filiform needles are slowly inserted to a depth of 1–1.5 *cun*, till the eyeball has a strong sensation of distension, and the remaining points are punctured perpendicularly till the arrival of *qi*, followed by lifting and thrusting, or twirling and rotating, making the sensation radiate to the head and the eyes. The needles are retained for 15–20 min in each point, during which shake the needle handle 20 times in the eye points every 5 min and manipulate the other needles once respectively. The first therapeutic course needs 10 treatments, once daily. The second is given after an interval of 3–7 days, once every other day.

Ear acupuncture

Selection of points: Two groups — (1) eye, central rim and kidney; (2) eye 1, eye 2, adrenal gland and subcortex.

Manipulation: One group is employed at each session. White mustard seeds or *Vaccaria segetalis* seeds are used for application contralateral to the exterior and interior auricles to strengthen the stimulation. The patient is asked to press the points three times every day, for 5 min each time, with application twice a week, on either side alternately.

Scalp acupuncture

Selection of points: Commonly used points — visual area. Supplementary points — *zusanli* (ST 36) and *zuguangming* (GB 37).

Manipulation: Commonly used points are employed at each session, and one supplementary point is added according to symptoms. A 2-*cun*-long

No. 28 filiform needle is rapidly inserted into the selected point to the required depth, twirling the needle with the thumb and the index finger for 1 min with a frequency of 180–200 cpm, and a retention of 15 min, during which the same manipulation is applied once every 5 min. Alternatively, the electroacupuncture apparatus is connected with a continuous wave, a frequency (240 cpm for 15–30 min) and an intensity tolerable to the patient. Supplementary points are punctured till the arrival of *qi*, followed by lifting and thrusting the needles, with a retention of 15–30 min. The treatment is given once every day or every other day, at 10 sessions as a course, at an interval of 3–5 days between courses.

Remarks

Among the three therapies introduced above, body acupuncture has been applied to the most patients, namely 804, of whom 429 recovered in a short period (53.4%) with a total effective rate of 97.5%, and cases of dyserythrochloropsia were significantly more than those of anerythrochloropsia. Both pressing on ear points and scalp acupuncture are easy to perform, and are applied to cases similar in number, with an effective rate slightly lower than that of body acupuncture. Electroacupuncture, acupoint injection and laser irradiation are also available, with similar therapeutic effect as well as similar point selection; they are not introduced here.

ENDOLYMPHATIC HYDROPS

Overview

Endolymphatic hydrops, also known as Meniere's disease, is a disorder of the inner ear with symptoms such as a sudden onset of dizziness with a sensation of revolving or shaking of the body or the surroundings, generally accompanied by nausea, vomiting, a pale complexion, perspiration, tinnitus, hearing impairment and nystagmus. It belongs to the category of *xuan yun* (vertigo) in TCM, and treatment with acupuncture and moxibustion was recorded in *Zhen Jiu Jia Yi Jing* (*The Systematic Classic of Acupuncture and Moxibustion*). Modern reports were seen in the early 1960s. Electric scalp acupuncture and pressing moxibustion with moxa wool, developed in recent years, have an obvious effect in controlling an acute episode. At present, an effective rate of 90% on average has been achieved in treatment with acupuncture and moxibustion.

Treatment

Moxibustion

Selection of points: Commonly used points — *baihui* (DU 20). Supplementary points — *zusanli* (ST 36).

Manipulation: Moxa wool, a bamboo tongue spatula, a pair of curved scissors, incense thread, Vaseline, matches and gentian violet are employed. Select a spot 0.5 cm left of *baihui* (DU 20) for left tinnitus and 0.5 cm rigHT for rigHT tinnitus, marked with gentian violet, then cut the hair in an area of 1 cm × 1 cm with the acupoint exposed, and smear some Vaseline on it. The patient is asked to sit on a low chair, and the operator, sitting hehind him or her in a higher position, puts two moxa cones on baihui (DU 20), ignited using the incense thread. When half of the cones are burned out, or the patient complains of burning pain, put it out with the tongue spatula, with the moxa wool left, on which moxa cones are added one after another. Each cone is burned till no smoke appears, and then put it out. Repeat the manipulation with the pressure from ligHT to heavy, using 25–50 cones at each session; the patient may feel comfortable when the heat penetrates into the brain from the scalp. After moxibustion, needle *zusanli* (ST 36) with reducing manipulation by lifting and thrusting, with a retention of 15 min. The patient is required not to wash the head in half a month in order to form moxibustion sores, but to keep the sores clean. No special treatment is needed and generally there will be recoverey in about a month.

Body acupuncture

Selection of points: Commonly used points — *taichong* (LR 3), *hegu* (LI 4), *neiguan* (PC 6), *zusanli* (ST 36) and *sanyinjiao* (SP 6). Supplementary points — *baihui* (DU 20), *fenglong* (ST 40), *tinggong* (SI 19) and *lieque* (LU 7).

Manipulation: Three or four commonly used points are employed at each session, and supplementary points are added according to symptoms. All the points are deeply inserted into till the arrival of *qi*, with twirling and rotating combined with lifting and thrusting for 1–2 min. The needles are retained for 30 min and there may be continuation if dizziness cannot be controlled, during which manipulate the needles once every 5–10 min. The treatment is applied once or twice daily, at 10 sessions as a course.

Remarks

Of the two therapies introduced here, the first, i.e. moxibustion, is effective based on experience of many years. It was applied to 432 patients, among whom 357 recovered (82.6%) and 73 responded well (16.9%), and the short-term effective rate was 99.5%. A total of 88 patients were followed up for 3 months to 22 years, and 50% have never been affected again, which confirms the long-term effectiveness. So this therapy should be given priority despite its complex manipulation. Body acupuncture is also available, but it is applied to relatively few cases and needs further verification.

QUESTIONS

(1) Describe in detail how to treat dyschromatopsia with body acupuncture.
(2) Describe how to treat endolymphatic hydrops with moxibustion.

ACUTE SUPPURATIVE OTITIS MEDIA

Overview

Acute suppurative otitis media (ASOM) is an acute pyogenic infection caused by the presence of pathogenic bacteria in the middle ear. It is clinically manifested by distending pain, burning pain or stabbing pain in the early stage, radiating to the occiput and temples; fever, and decreased appetite prior to eardrum empyema or eardrum perforation; vomiting, or even convulsions in severe cases. Reports about the treatment of ASOM with acupuncture and moxibustion were first seen in the 1950s. Clinical practice of so many years has proven that both acupuncture and moxibustion have great effectiveness, not only in relieving severe pain in the ear but also in inhibiting inflammatory secretion in the tympanic cavity and enhancing absorption.

Treatment

Moxibustion

Selection of points: *Yifeng* (SJ 17).

Manipulation: Suspended moxibustion is applied with moxa sticks. Wipe clean the external acoustic meatus using sterilized q-tips with hydrogen peroxide, ignite the moxa stick, and suspend it 3 cm above *yifeng* (SJ 17) on the affected side with sparrow-pecking moxibustion until the local skin becomes flushed and has a sensation of ironing heat when pressed. Generally, it lasts 1 min, and a draining strip is used for drawing pus out after moxibustion. The treatment is applied once daily, at five sessions as a course.

Acupoint laser irradiation

Selection of points: Commonly used points — *tinghui* (GB 2), *yifeng* (SJ 17), *zusanli* (ST 36) and *qiuxu* (GB 40). Supplementary points — *ermen* (SJ 21), *quchi* (LI 11), *taixi* (KI 3) and the *ashi* point (hole of the affected ear).

Manipulation: Commonly used points are taken as the main points, and supplementary points are added according to symptoms. First, clean off the pus in the ear with 2% hydrogen peroxide and wipe it dry. The helium–neon laser apparatus is then employed with wavelength 632.8 nm, power output 10 mW, facula diameter 1.5 mm, and distance from the point 20 cm, irradiating for 5 min. The *ashi* point can be given optical fiber while being irradiated, also for 5 min. The treatment is applied once daily, at 10 sessions as a course, at an interval of 5–7 days between courses.

Body acupuncture

Selection of points: Commonly used points — *tinghui* (GB 2), *yifeng* (SJ 17), *qiuxu* (GB 40) and *waiguan* (SJ 5). Supplementary points — *quchi* (LI 11), *zusanli* (ST 36), *hegu* (LI 4), *ermen* (SJ 21) and *taixi* (KI 3).

Manipulation: Commonly used points are taken as the main points, and supplementary points are added if there is no control over fever and pain, three or four points at each session, among which local points are selected from the affected side, and distal points from the contralateral or bilateral points, all by twirling and rotating combined with lifting and thrusting, with medium or strong stimulation, and the needles are retained for 20–50 min, during which manipulate them two or three times. The treatment is applied once daily in the acute stage, and once every other day in the remission stage, at 7–10 sessions as a course, at an interval of 5 days between courses.

Remarks

These three methods are the most common in the clinic. Moxibustion is preferable, because of its easy manipulation and significant effect. It was applied to 402 cases of acute or chronic suppurative otitis media, for which the recovery rate was 99.0%, and it needs only 3.15 times of moxibustion on average. Acupoint laser irradiation is applicable to those fearing pain, and infants. Body acupuncture is also effective, and applicable to cases at the acute stage or with an acute onset of chronic otitis media. During treatment, patients should be offered a digestible diet, much water, and bed rest for high fever. Surgery is available if the symptoms are not relieved and headache is aggravated after acupuncture and moxibustion.

PERCEPTIVE DEAFNESS

Overview

Deafness refers to hearing impairment that is classified into conductive deafness and perceptive deafness. The latter is due to drug intoxication and is focused on here. It is similar to *xu long* (deficient deafness) and *jiu long* (chronic deafness) in TCM. The treatment of deafness with acupuncture and moxibustion was recorded as early as in *Jing Mai* (*Meridians*), in the Spring and Autumn Period and the Warring States Period. The first modern clinical report was published in 1927, and two upsurges occurred from the 1950s to the early 1970s in the treatment of deafness with acupuncture and moxibustion, including treatment of perceptive deafness. In the past 30 years, it has been getting more objective and more delicate, and the effective rate has risen to 80%, from 24%–65% in the 1970s.

Treatment

Body acupuncture

Selection of points: Commonly used point — *wangu* (SI 4). Supplementary points — *tinggong* (SI 19), *yifeng* (SJ 17), *ermen* (SJ 21), *baihui* (DU 20) and *jiaosun* (SJ 20).

Manipulation: *Wangu* (SI 4) is employed at each session, and two or three supplementary points may be added according to symptoms. The patient is sitting upright, with the head slightly forward. *Wangu* (SI 4) on the affected side is punctured with a No. 28–30 filiform needle, 2–2.5 *cun* long, at an angle of 60° with the neck, toward the exterior margin of the homolateral orbit, to a depth of 1.5–1.8 *cun*, until the arrival of *qi*, i.e. a sensation of numbness, distension, itching, heat or ringing, ventilation, etc. Then manipulate the needle by rapid twirling and rotating combined with sligHT lifting and thrusting for 0.5–1 min, and withdraw it when there is a strong needling sensation. *Yifeng* (SJ 17) is punctured with a 2-*cun*-long No. 30 filiform needle obliquely upward to a depth of 1.5 *cun* to induce a sensation of distension in the ear, as if winding through. *Baihui* (DU 20) is tapped with medium stimulation using a dermal needle for 5 min, and the rest of the points are given routine acupuncture, with the needles retained in each point for 30 min. Retention may be omitted if the infant sufferer is not cooperative. The treatment is applied once every day or every other day, at 10 sessions as a course. Another course begins after an interval of 3 days.

Electroacupuncture

Selection of points: Commonly used points — *tinggong* (SI 19) and *ermen* (SJ 21). Supplementary points — *yifeng* (SJ 17), *tinghui* (GB 2), *waiguan* (SJ 5), *zhongzhu* (SJ 3) and *hegu* (LI 4).

Manipulation: Commonly used points are employed at each session, and two supplementary points are added according to symptoms, one on the ear and one on the upper limb. The inserting depth varies in patients of different ages; 1–1.5 *cun* for those below 9, 1.3–1.5 *cun* for those 10–15, and 1.6–2 *cun* for those above 16. On the arrival of *qi*, connect to the electroacupuncture apparatus with a continuous wave, a frequency (100 cpm) and a strength tolerable to the patient, for 25–30 min. Supplementary points are given rapid needling till a sensation of soreness, numbness and distension arises and radiates around, with the needles retained for 25–30 min, during which manipulate them two or three times with medium stimulation. The treatment is applied once every other day, at 15 sessions as a course, at an interval of 7 days between courses.

Remarks

There are many therapies of point stimulation for perceptive deafness, such as promontory needling, embedding, acupoint injection and scalp acupuncture. In recent years, many a practitioner has performed great exploration of the point selection and manipulations. Deep insertion into *wangu* (SI 4) is highly effective, with a mild sensation, and was applied to 160 cases, with an excellence rate of 85%. It is hard for beginners to master the inserting technique, which requires further practice. Electroacupuncture is applicable to poisoning deafness by antibiotics as well as other forms of perceptive deafness. It was applied to 315 cases, with an effective rate of 73%–94%. The effective rate tends to rise as the course of treatment increases, so it is advisable for patients to adhere to the treatment.

QUESTIONS

(1) Describe briefly the three methods of point stimulation in the treatment of acute suppurative otitis media.

(2) What characteristics do the two methods of point stimulation have with regards to point selection and manipulation in the treatment of perceptive deafness?

CHRONIC SINUSITIS

Overview

Chronic sinusitis, also known as chronic suppurative sinusitis, is characterized by drainage of a mucous or purulent nasal discharge, nasal stuffiness, headache, and reduction in or loss of the sense of smell. The disease is named *bi yuan* (thick rhinorrhea) or *nao lou* (sinusitis) in TCM, and was recorded in *Zhen Jiu Jia Yi Jing* (*The Systematic Classic of Acupuncture and Moxibustion*). Reports about treatment of chronic sinusitis with acupuncture and moxibustion were first seen in 1954, and more and more articles have been published since the 1960s. Some patients who have responded poorly to antibiotics or physical treatment tend to achieve a good result by acupuncture and moxibustion, which is able not only to decrease or relieve symptoms like headache, but also to shrink the swelling of hyperemic mucous membrane so as to contribute to ventilation and drainage of the discharge. At present, an effective rate of 90% has been achieved.

Treatment

Body acupuncture

Selection of points: Commonly used points — *yingxiang* (LI 20), *yintang* (EX-HN3), *baihui* (DU 20) and *hegu* (LI 4). Supplementary points — *fengchi* (GB 20), *chize* (LU 5), *shangxing* (DU 23), *lieque* (LU 7) and *zanzhu* (BL 2).

Manipulation: Commonly used points are taken as the main points, and supplementary points are added if there is no obvious effect, three or four points at each session. *Yingxiang* (LI 20) is punctured with a 2-*cun*-long No. 28 filiform needle perpendicularly to a depth of 0.2–0.3 *cun*, followed by inserting the needle obliquely upward at an angle of 35°–40° until the anterosuperior extremity of the inferior concha, to a depth of 1.5 *cun*, during which drops of blood may come out of the nasal cavity but no hemostasis is needed, and much discharge and sneezing may occur at the same time. The needle is retained for 40 min without lifting, thrusting, twirling or rotating. For *yintang* (EX-HN3), the patient is sitting upright, with the forearms on a table or on the knees, and the practitioner pinches the nasal root upward slightly with the thumb and index finger of the left hand, and inserts the needle with the other hand into the point, obliquely downward along the nasal median line to a depth of 0.6–0.7 *cun*, with the tip toward the middle nasal concha, until the patient complains of soreness and distension. *Baihui* (DU 20) is given horizontal insertion till a sensation of distension and heaviness arises; *hegu* (LI 4) is punctured obliquely toward the index finger till there is a sensation of soreness and distension. Supplementary points are given routine acupuncture and reducing manipulation on the arrival of *qi* by lifting and thrusting, with the needles retained for 20–30 min. The treatment is applied once daily or every other day, at 10 sessions as a course, at an interval of 3–5 days between courses.

Electroacupuncture

Selection of points: Commonly used points — *hegu* (LI 4), *neiguan* (PC 6), *zusanli* (ST 36) and *neiting* (ST 44). Supplementary points — two groups, namely (1) *fengchi* (GB 20); (2) below the first and second cervical vertebrae.

Manipulation: Commonly used points and either group are employed at each session. Commonly used points are punctured with gentle manipulation and shallow insertion, regardless of the arrival of *qi*. Then electroacupuncture is applied. Prepare one cathode conductor jointed to the lead plate, wrapped with charpie backing and soaked in saline, and placed on the supplementary point; and four anode conductors jointed to points of the four limbs. The treatment is performed with a high frequency (280–320 cpm) and an output current tolerable to the patient, who will instantly feel numb at the points of the four limbs when the on switch is flipped, and 10 min later he or she may experience coolness of the extremities, sweating of the palms and soles, then flushing and heating of the head, dryness of the throat and lips, and reduced discharge in the nose. The duration of each electric stimulation is about 1–1.5 h. The treatment is applied once daily or every other day, at 10 sessions as a course, at an interval of 7–10 days between courses.

Remarks

Of the two methods introduced above, the first is effective, in spite of there being a little difficulty in manipulation. It was applied to 82 cases, with 40 recovered, 21 excellent and 17 effective, and the total effective rate was 95.1%. The second method is convenient to perform, and has a total effective rate of 97.6%. It is more effective in cases with a short course and superior in juveniles to adults, but it needs further verification as there are insufficient experimental cases.

ALLERGIC RHINITIS

Overview

Allergic rhinitis is an allergic disorder, clinically manifested by paroxysmal rhinocnesmus, nasal congestion, sneezing, watery nasal discharge, tunica mucosa nasi edema, a pale complexion and turbinate swelling. The first report about the treatment of allergic rhinitis with acupuncture and moxibustion was seen in 1957, and many clinical articles were published in the following years. Besides acupuncture and moxibustion, other therapies are available, like acupoint injection or acupoint application. In the past 20 years, there has been great development in the treatment of allergic rhinitis, and an effective rate of 95% has been achieved.

Treatment

Acupoint mounting

Selection of points: Three groups — (1) *dazhu* (BL 11) (1 *cun* lateral to the posterior midline, below the spinous process of the first thoracic vertebra) and *gaohuang* (BL 43); (2) *fengmen* (BL 12) and *pishu* (BL 20); (3) *feishu* (BL 13) and *shenshu* (BL 23).

Manipulation: Drugs for moxibustion — Bai Jie Zi (*Semen Sinapis*) 50%, Xi Xin (*Radix et Rhizoma Asari*) 30% and Gan Sui (*Radix Kansui*) 20% are ground to powder and attempered with fresh ginger juice, and made into pieces of therapeutic cake 1 cm in diameter. The treatment is applied in dog days every year. The application begins with a bit of *shexiang*

(*Moschus*) spread on the cake, which is stuck to an adhesive plaster measuring 4 cm², and it is applied to the point for 1–3 h. Remove the cake beforehand if the patient complains of intolerable scorching heat. Half an hour is needed for infants. Some patients may have blisters after application; then apply gentian violet and cover them with aseptic dressings. Three groups are employed alternately, at three sessions as a course, one course each year. This method is used with caution in pregnant women.

Acupuncture and moxibustion

Selection of points: Commonly used points — *yintang* (EX-HN3) and *bitong* (EX-HN8) (at the depression below the nasal bone, near the upper end of the nasolabial groove). Supplementary points — *baihui* (DU 20), *yingxiang* (LI 20), *hegu* (LI 4) and *fengchi* (GB 20).

Manipulation: Commonly used points are taken as the main points, and one or two supplementary points as adjuvant. *Yintang* (EX-HN3) is punctured with a 1.5-*cun*-long No. 30 filiform needle, inserted while pinching the skin, to a depth of 0.2 *cun*. On the arrival of *qi*, insert the needle slowly along the skin to a depth of 1 *cun*, with twirling and rotating combined with lifting and thrusting to make the sensation reach the apex nasi and nasal cavity. *Bitong* (EX-HN8) is punctured with a 1-*cun*-long No. 30 filiform needle, at first to a depth of 0.2 *cun*, followed by oblique insertion toward *yintang* (EX-HN3) along the skin on the arrival of *qi*, until there is a sensation of distension in the nasal cavity. The needles are retained for 20 min, during which manipulate them once every 5 min. *Baihui* (DU 20) is given sparrow-pecking moxibustion with moxa sticks for 15–20 min. Supplementary points are punctured for the arrival of *qi* with lifting and thrusting of the needles. Then the electroacupuncture apparatus is connected with a continuous wave and an intensity tolerable to the patient. The electric stimulation lasts 30 min. The treatment with acupuncture is applied once daily, and moxibustion twice daily, for 10 days as a course.

Remarks

Many therapies with acupoint stimulation for allergic rhinitis are available, including finger pressing, acupoint laser irradiation, moxibustion, acupoint application, ear point pressing, ear acupuncture and body acupuncture, all with a similar curative effect. The two methods introduced above are commonly used in the clinic. Acupoint application is convenient and safe to perform, and has been applied to 556 cases, with 58 recovered, 405 effective and 93 with no response, and the total effective rate was 83.2%. Acupuncture and moxubustion is more complicated to perform, and was applied to 160 cases, with 51 effective and 4 with no response, and the total effective rate was 97.5%. The two methods are alternatives, according to clinical conditions in practice.

ACUTE TONSILLITIS

Overview

Acute tonsillitis is an acute inflammation or infection of the pharyngeal lymphatic tissues, most obviously in the tonsils. The clinical manifestations are sudden and rapid onset, aversion to cold with fever (as high as 38°C–40°C), sore throat, red and enlarged tonsils with yellow and white effusion, accompanied by muscular stiffness, fatigue, headache and leukocyte increase. Acute tonsillitis is similar to *feng re ru e* (anemopyretic tonsillitis) in TCM, and its treatment with acupuncture and moxibustion was recorded in *Zhen Jiu Jia Yi Jing* (*The Systematic Classic of Acupuncture and Moxibustion*). Modern reports began in the early 1950s. Since then the clinical data and methods of point stimulation have increased and diversified. Repeated comparisons support the view that acupuncture and moxibustion, not inferior to benzylpenicillin medication in effectiveness, can relieve the general symptoms rapidly and is superior to medication. At present, the recovery rate is 90% on average.

Treatment

Body acupuncture

Selection of points: Commonly used points — *jiache* (ST 6), *hegu* (LI 4) and *shaoshang* (LU 11). Supplementary points — *tianzhu* (BL 10) and *yuji* (LU 10).

Manipulation: Commonly used points are taken as the main points, and supplementary points are added according to symptoms, three points at each session. Points of the head and face are selected from the affected side; those of the four limbs, from both sides. *Shaoshang* (LU 11) and *yuji* (LU 10) are given pricking needling with three-edged needles for blood to come out, and the rest of the points are punctured by lifting and thrusting combined with twirling and rotating with strong stimulation. The needles are retained for 15–20 min, and no retention is needed for infants. The treatment is applied once or twice a day, until total recovery is achieved.

Acupoint injection

Selection of points: Commonly used points — *hegu* (LI 4), *yifeng* (SJ 17) and *zusanli* (ST 36). Supplementary points — *quchi* (LI 11), *xingjian* (LV 2), *zhaohai* (KI 6) and *dazhui* (DU 14).

Manipulation: Select either physiological saline or vitamin B1 (50 mg/ml). Commonly used points taken as the main points, which may be replaced by supplementary points if no satisfactory result is achieved. Two or three points are employed at each session, lateral to the head or face, and lateral or bilateral to the four limbs. 0.30–1.0 ml of liquor is injected into each point, depending on the thickness of the local muscles. Take a No. 5 pinhead for dentistry in injection, and push in the liquor on the arrival of *qi*. The treatment is applied once daily, or twice daily for severe cases.

Rush-burning moxibustion (rush-fire cauterization)

Selection of points — Jiaosun (SJ 20).

Manipulation: Brush aside the hair on *jiaosun* (SJ 20), with the skin exposed. Dip the rush, about 2 cm long, into vegetable oil, ignite the oiled rush, and put it on the acupoint. When the burning rush touches the skin, a "pa" sound should be heard and the fire extinguished. The local skin then becomes reddish but it needs no treatment. Usually one burn is employed for each point, and another burn may be applied the next day if no satisfactory result is achieved.

Remarks

Among the three therapies introduced above, body acupuncture is the most commonly used one. A combination of filiform needling and pricking needling, it has been applied to 999 cases, with a total effective rate of 90%–100%. Acupoint injection has been applied to 173 patients, all of whom recovered except for 19 cases (discontinued). It generally works after 1–3 times. Rush-burning moxibustion comes from folk, is easy to perform, and has been applied to 316 cases with a recovery rate of 90.1%. The three therapies have their own features and are all available.

It should be pointed out that acupuncture and moxibustion can rapidly relieve the symptoms of acute tonsillitis, but since the pharyngeal bacterial culture may be positive, its mechanism of action is believed to lie in motivating and regulating the disease resistance of the body itself by means of meridians, nerves and body fluids so as to cure the disease.

QUESTIONS

(1) Restate in detail the acupuncture manipulation in treatment of chronic sinusitis.
(2) What characteristics does acupuncture and moxibustion have in treatment of allergic rhinitis?
(3) What characteristics does body acupuncture have in treatment of acute tonsillitis? How to manipulate it?

ACUTE TOOTHACHE

Overview

Toothache is a common symptom due to saprodontia, pulpitis, apical periodontitis or pericoronitis. In acute cases, the pain is severe and unendurable. Acute pulpitis manifests as pain at short intervals which is aggravated at night, and the sufferer cannot locate the affected tooth; acute apical periodontitis as rest pain, and the affected tooth can be clearly pointed out; acute pericoronitis as obvious gum swelling and redness. In TCM it is called *ya tong* (toothache) or *chi tong* (odontia), which was mentioned in the ancient silken book *Channels*. A great number of reports have been published about the treatment with acupuncture and moxibustion in modern times, and analysis shows that it is highly effective for acute apical periodontitis, with the longest time of pain relief, followed by acute pericoronitis and acute pulpitis. At present, the average effective rate is about 80%.

Treatment

Body acupuncture

Selection of points: Commonly used points — two groups, namely (1) *chongyang* (ST 42) (on the dome of the instep of the foot, posterior to the second and third metatarsal bones, inside the long extensor muscle of the toes) and *jiache* (ST 6); (2) *hegu* (LI 4) and *xiaguan* (ST 7). Supplementary points — *taiyang* (EX-HN5), *kunlun* (BL 60) and *neiting* (ST 44).

Manipulation: Commonly used points are taken as the main points, with the first group for upper tooth pain and the second for lower tooth pain; supplementary points are added if that fails to stop the pain. *Jiache* (ST 6) and *xiaguan* (ST 7) are given respectively perpendicular needling and deep needling, making the sensation radiate to the tooth root. *Taiyang* (Ex-HN5) is punctured at an angle of 45° toward the tooth root by slowly twirling and rotating the needle to a depth of 1.5–1.8 *cun*; *hegu* (LI 4), *neiting* (ST 44) and *chongyang* (ST 42) are punctured, tips upward, with the detecting technique by lifting and thrusting, trying to radiate the sensation to the affected area. *Kunlun* (BL 60) is inserted into with the tip obliquely toward the anterior border of the medial malleolus, to a depth of 0.3–0.5 *cun*. On the arrival of *qi*, all the points are given manipulation by twirling and rotating combined with lifting and thrusting the needles for 2–3 min, at an angle of 150°–180°, with the frequency of twirling and rotating at 100–140 cpm, the amplitude of lifting and thrusting at 0.5 cm, and the intensity tolerable to the patient. The needles are retained in each point for 20–40 min, during which they are manipulated once every 5–10 min. The treatment is performed once or twice a day.

Ear acupuncture

Selection of points: Commonly used points — tragic apex and cheek. Supplementary points — *shenmen* (HT 7) and mouth.

Manipulation: Generally one or two commonly used points are employed, and supplementary points are added according to symptoms. First, the sensitive spot is located and punctured with a 5-*fen*-long No. 28 filiform needle by repeatedly twirling and rotating with strong stimulation, with the needle retained for 30 min, during which stimulation is applied two or three times, 1–2 min each time, once or twice each day. If recurrent attacks occur, needle embedding with a thumbtack needle may be applied to ear points on one side, which requires rigid sterilization.

Remarks

There are many therapies for toothache with acupuncture and moxibustion, but only the two most frequently used ones in clinics have been introduced here. Body acupuncture has been applied to 794 cases, with an effective rate ranging from 57.9% to 100%. Ear acupuncture is easy and convenient to perform, and has been applied to 214 cases, with an average effective rate of 93.5%. During the treatment, it is of great importance to induce the needling sensation, which is achieved by directing the needle tips to the affected area, and close detection through lifting and thrusting. Once an upward sensation occurs, twirl and rotate the needle in combination with gentle lifting and thrusting, for the purpose of inducing transmission of the sensation.

RECURRENT APHTHOUS ULCER

Overview

A recurrent aphthous ulcer (RAU), also called an aphthous ulcer, is an ulcerative lesion commonly affecting the mucous membrane of the oral cavity. It is clinically manifested by a lesion in the superficial mucous membrane, and recurrent attacks, with characteristics such as being red (ulcer border), yellow (accidental membrane) or curved (ulcer invagination), and pain (scorching heat and pain). An RAU is similar to *kou chuang* (oral sore), *kou gan* (oral erosion) and *kou yang* (oral ulcer) in TCM. Treatment with acupuncture and moxibustion appears many times in the literature of acupuncture and moxibustion from the Song Dynasty.

Modern treatment was reported in 1958, and since then great development has been achieved, with an effective rate of 80%–90%.

Treatment

Body acupuncture

Selection of points: Commonly used points — *chengjiang* (RN 24), *dicang* (ST 4) and *ashi* points (local ulcer side). Supplementary points — *hegu* (LI 4), *quchi* (LI 11), *zusanli* (ST 36), *Sanyinjiao* (SP 6). *jinjin* (EX-HN12) and *yuye* (EX-HN13) added for aphtha on the tongue, and *yingxiang* (LI 20) for aphtha on the lips or cheeks.

Manipulation: Commonly used points are employed at each session, and supplementary points are added according to symptoms. *Ashi, Jinjin* (EX-HN12) and *yuye* (EX-HN13) are given pricking needling after rinsing the mouth. A No. 28 filiform needle is inserted into the *ashi* point once for small ulcers, and 2–4 times for ulcers larger than 0.3 cm in diameter; *jinjin* (EX-HN12) and *yuye* (EX-HN13) are punctured with three-edged needles for bloodletting. The rest of the points are given manipulations on the arrival of *qi* by lifting and thrusting combined with twirling and rotating, with the needles retained for 15–20 min. Treatment is performed once daily or every other day, at 10 sessions as a course. Generally, two courses are needed, and other therapies are available if that fails to induce satisfactory results.

Ear acupuncture

Selection of points: Commonly used points — mouth, tongue (second area of the earlobe), lung and *shenmen* (HT 7). Supplementary points — sympathetic, liver, heart, spleen, kidney and adrenal gland.

Manipulation: Two or three commonly used points are employed at each session, and supplementary points are selected according to syndrome differentiation by tongue inspection, heart and lung for ulcers on the apex linguae, and liver and gallbladder for ulcers on the lateral borders of the tongue. Sensitive spots having been detected, rapid insertion is applied, twirling and rotating the needle several times for the arrival of *qi*, with the needles retained for 30 min, during which manipulate them once every 10 min. Needle embedding or pill pressing is also available (*Vaccaria segetalis* seeds or magnetic beads). Bilateral points are selected for acupuncture, and lateral points for needle embedding or pill pressing, with the former applied once daily at 6 sessions as a course, and the latter twice a week at 12 sessions. The next course begins after an interval of 3–7 days.

Acupoint laser irradiation

Selection of points: Cavum concha.

Manipulation: The cavum concha is the superficial anatomic site of the auricle, including points such as heart, lung and mouth. The He–Ne laser apparatus is used for scattered irradiation, 1 m between the orifice opening and the point area, 1.5 cm in facula diameter, output current 20 mW, wavelength 632.8 nm, for 5 min on one ear. The treatment is applied once daily, for 5 days as a course, at an interval of 3 days between courses.

Remarks

An RAU is one of the refractory diseases in the stomatological department, and the three therapies of acupoint stimulation are all commonly used in the clinic. Body acupuncture has been applied to 184 cases, with 97 recovered (the ulcer surface was healed and no recurrence occurred in two more months), and the total effective rate was 82.1%. Ear acupuncture and acupoint laser irradiation have a similar curative effect, but protective efficacy has not been achieved. Other therapies are available, like acupoint injection, pricking for blood with a lance needle and application to *yongquan* (KI 1), which are omitted here.

TEMPOROMANDIBULAR JOINT DISORDER

Overview

Temporomandibular joint disorder (TMJD or TMD), or TMJ syndrome, is one of the frequently occurring diseases in the stomatological department. It is clinically manifested by a clicking or popping sound and pain when the patient opens or closes the mouth, an excessively large or small opening degree, bias or retorting of opening, joint twisting and locking, accompanied by tinnitus, dizziness and headache. It usually has a long course of disease, and relapses easily, commonly attacking people aged 20–40. TMJD belongs to the category of *bi zheng* (arthralgia syndrome) in TCM, similar to *kou jin bu kai* (lockjaw). The treatment with acupuncture and moxibustion was recorded in *Zhen Jiu Jia Yi Jing* (*The Systematic Classic of Acupuncture and Moxibustion*). Modern reports began in the mid-1950s, and increasingly more clinical articles have been published since the 1980s. At present, an average recovery rate of 90% has been achieved, with a similar curative effect for different therapies.

Treatment

Body acupuncture

Selection of points: Commonly used points — *xiaguan* (ST 7), *jiaozhong* [middle point on the connecting line between *xiaguan* (ST 7) and *jiache* (ST 6)] and *tinggong* (SI 19). Supplementary points — *tongli* (HT 5), *taiyang* (EX-HN 5), *zusanli* (ST 36) and *hegu* (LI 4).

Manipulation: Commonly used points are taken as the main points, and supplementary points as adjuvant, with three or four points employed at each session. With the patient in the decubitus or sitting position, apply perpendicular needling with sligHT twirling, rotating, lifting and thrusting till the arrival of *qi*, and then manipulate the needle with medium or strong stimulation for 1–2 min for a stronger sensation. The needle is retained for 30 min, during which manipulate it once every 5–10 min. Do massage on the obvious tenderness 1–3 min after the withdrawal of the needle. The treatment is applied once daily, at 10 sessions as a course, at an interval of 5 days between courses.

Ear acupuncture

Selection of points: Commonly used points — apex of the antitragus. Supplementary points — cheeks, liver and gallbladder.

Manipulation: Commonly used points are taken as the main points, and supplementary points are added according to symptoms. The sensitive spot detected, a 5-*fen*-long No. 30 filiform needle is inserted perpendicularly with an obvious sensation of pain, the more the better. If there is no pain, lift the needle *in situ*, moving it a little, until the tenderness spot is found. Generally, points on the affected side are selected, but bilateral points are selected for acupuncture for bilateral diseases. Pressing with *Vaccaria segetalis* seeds is also available to the degree that the patient complains of pain; otherwise, press upward, downward, forward and backward till the tenderness is detected. The pressing times should be 15–20 min. The needles are retained for 20 min. Ear acupuncture is applied once every other day, pressing once every two days.

Acupuncture with intradermal needling

Selection of points: *Ashi* point (the tenderness spot on the face, often lateral to the condyle).

Manipulation: A 5-mm-long No. 34 thumbtack intradermal needle is inserted into the point after sterilization of the local area, and fixed with adhesive plaster, and pressing is done to induce an obvious sensation of soreness and distension. The patient is asked to press once or twice every day, two embeddings a week, at three sessions as a course, at an interval of five days between courses.

Remarks

There are a variety of treatment approaches to TMJD with point stimulation, including electroacupuncture, medicinal cupping, acupoint laser irradiation, ear acupuncture and needle embedding, in addition to traditional acupuncture and moxibustion. Even for the same stimulation, there are two or more treatment schedules. The three methods introduced here are representative of different acupuncture and moxibustion. Among them, body acupuncture is superior in curative effect, and has been applied to 133 patients with 125 recovered (94%), and the total effective rate was 100%. Ear acupuncture is easy to perform, and has been applied to 123 patients with 56 recovered (45.5%), and the effective rate was 86.7%. It was found that combination of two approaches can enhance the recovery rate. Consequently, it is advisable to combine with intradermal needling or ear acupuncture when body acupuncture is applied.

QUESTIONS

(1) Describe briefly the two commonly used therapies in treatment of acute toothache with acupuncture and moxibustion.

(2) Describe how to select points and manipulate needling in treatment of an RAU.

(3) What approaches of point stimulation are there in treatment of TMJD?

CHAPTER 29

Acupuncture and Moxibustion
for Dermatological and Other Diseases

NEURODERMATITIS

Overview

Neurodermatitis is a frequent chronic skin condition characterized by itching and lichenification, usually on the neck, the extensor aspect of the elbow joints, poples, thighs and lumbosacral, mostly in the local area but sometimes widespread. It often occurs in young people and adults. The exact cause remains unknown but is obviously related to nerves or psychological factors.

Reports about acupuncture treatment in modern times began in the mid-1950s, and many cases proved it to be effective. In the 1960s, tapping needling with dermal needles became popular because of its convenience and rapid effectiveness. Traditional therapies found that medicinal moxibustion by pellet fire was also effective, according to *Ben Cao Gang Mu Shi Yi* (*Supplement to "The Grand Compendium of Materia Medica"*), by Zhao Xue-min in the Qing Dynasty. In the late 1970s, the treatment with acupuncture and moxibustion underwent great development, and various therapies were applied to the disease and produced affirmative effect, including scalp acupuncture, embedding, electroacupuncture, acupoint injection and bloodletting. With the increase in clinical practice, there is a tendency toward comprehensive application of multiple stimulations, with tapping needling as the main method. Articles and experiences collected by the writer show that acupuncture and moxibustion should mainly be applied to localized neurodermatitis with an average effective rate of more than 85%; among them, there are some recurrences.

Treatment

Acupuncture with skin needling

Selection of points: Commonly used points — bilateral to vertebration, *ashi* point (skin lesion area and tenderness spot or something positive in a trabs shape. Supplementary points — *quchi* (LI 11), *neiguan* (PC 6), *tai-yuan* (LU 9) and *hegu* (LI 4) are added for dermatitis on the face, neck and head; *neiguan* (PC 6), *quchi* (LI 11), *feishu* (BL 13) and *xinshu* (BL 15) for dermatitis on the upper limbs; *xuehai* (SP 10), *zusanli* (ST 36) and *shenshu* (BL 23) for dermatitis on the lower limbs; *pishu* (BL 20), *weishu* (BL 21), *guanyuan* (RN 4) and *sanyinjiao* (SP 6) for dermatitis on the perineum and the abdomen.

Manipulation: Commonly used points are taken as the main points, and supplementary points are added according to symptoms. First, *ashi* is given tapping needling with forceful tapping till there is a little bleeding, followed by tapping the area bilateral to vertebration with mild or medium strength making the local skin reddish. Tap the area of the supplementary point till it becomes reddish. Generally, 3–5 times of tapping are required. On the lesion area, tap around with mild stimulation, followed by repeatedly tapping on the lesion area, with the length of the tapping time depending on the area of the lesion, 4–6 min if the area is 10 cm in diameter; on the area bilateral to vertebration, tap from inside to outside, top to bottom. After that, fumigating moxibustion may be applied to the lesion with moxa sticks till the skin becomes reddish. The treatment is performed once daily or once every other day, at 15 sessions as a course, at an interval of 3–7 days between courses.

Moxibustion

Selection of points: Commonly used points — *ashi* point (skin lesion area) (the same as below).

Manipulation: Direct moxibustion is applied. A moxa cone, made of pure moxa wool, is put near the *ashi* point for moxibustion, 1.5 cm between the moxibustion spots, with garlic juice smeared on previously for more viscosity. When the cone burns out, clear away the ash and keep it clean with saline, covered with dressings. If the patient fears pain, put the cone out before it burns out with a tongue spatula and pat the patient gently around the moxibustion spot. One cone is needed, twice a week, and change to another spot until complete recovery. If water blisters occur without suppuration, paracentesis for drainage may be applied and gentian violet is smeared on it. If suppuration occurs, ointment for eliminating inflammation is applied so that no cicatrix will be left after recovery.

Surrounding needling

Selection of points: Commonly used point — *ashi* point. Supplementary points — *hegu* (LI 4), *quchi* (LI 11), *zusanli* (ST 36), *xuehai* (SP 10) and *sanyinjiao* (SP 6).

Manipulation: Commonly used points and two or three supplementary points are employed at each session. A 1.5-*cun*-long No. 28 filiform needle is inserted from the *ashi* point toward the center along the skin, to a depth of 0.5–1 *cun*. Ten to thirty insertions are applied, depending on the area of the skin lesion, with the tips all directed to the center of the lesion, without retention; or only four needles around are left, connected to the electroacupuncture apparatus with a frequency (500–600 cpm), a continuous wave and an intensity tolerable to the patient, for 15–20 min. The treatment is performed once daily or once every other day at 10 sessions as a course, at an interval of 3 days between courses. Supplementary points are given uniform reinforcing–reducing manipulation, with the needles retained for 15–20 min.

Electro-acupuncture

Selection of points: Commonly used points — *dazhui* (DU 14) and *lingtai* (DU 10). Supplementary points — *quchi* (LI 11) is added for affected skin on the head, neck and upper limbs; *weizhong* (BL 40) for affected skin on the trunk and lower limbs; *quchi* (LI 11) and *weizhong* (BL 40) are alternately used for dermatitis affecting the whole body.

Manipulation: Commonly used points are taken as the main points, and supplementary points are selected according to different areas of the skin lesion. The patient is in the prone position. On the arrival of *qi*, the electroacupuncture apparatus is connected, the cathode conductor to commonly used points and the anode conductor to supplementary points, with a frequency (more than 400 cpm) and an intensity tolerable to the patient, and the needles are retained for 20 min. The treatment is applied once daily, at 10 sessions as a course. The next course begins after a week's rest. Generally, two or three courses are needed, during which no other therapy is applied.

Remarks

All the four therapies are commonly used in the clinic. Tapping with a dermal needle is applicable to cases with a large lesion area, and is the first choice for neurodermatitis. Generally, tapping therapy is enough, but fumigating moxibustion is applied in addition for cases with a long course of disease or intractable symptoms. Moxibustion is mainly for localized neurodermatitis and is effective in cases with a small lesion area and less onset parts, but less effective for neurodermatitis of the scattering type. It is nonscarring moxibustion — the cone is not too big, it is done no more than twice, and it is better not to have blisters. Surrounding needling is for cases with a large lesion area, not in bends of the elbow or the poples. Tapping with a dermal needle may be used in combination for the purpose of enhancing the curative effect for cases with intractable symptoms and severe itching. Electroacupuncture is for cases with a generalized skin lesion, and tapping with a dermal needle may be applied to the local skin for enhancement of the curative effect.

VITILIGO

Overview

Vitiligo is a skin disorder of acquired localized depigmentation, clinically manifested by localized depigmentation patches with clear margins, hair whitening in the lesion area, no rational symptoms, and burning itching when there is exposure to the sun. Called *bai bo feng* (vitiligo) in TCM, it is easy to diagnose, but hard to cure because of its unknown causes. Acupuncture for vitiligo was portrayed in *Bei Ji Qian Jin Yao Fang* (*Important Formulas Worth a Thousand Gold Pieces for Emergencies*) and *Qian Jin Yi Fang* (*Supplement to "Important Formulas Worth a Thousand Gold Pieces"*) in the Tang Dynasty. Modern documents did not appear until the 1980s, not only in China, where many clinical papers were published, but also in Sri Lanka, where a practitioner cured a patient with acupuncture and moxibustion. Nowadays, acupoint stimulation therapies are widely used, including acupuncture, moxibustion, tapping needling with a dermal needle, ear acupuncture, otopoint pressing, catgut embedding at acupoints, acupuncture combined with electromagnetic waves, and bee needles. The characteristics of acupuncture therapy for vitiligo are: (1) emphasis on combination of multiple stimulations to improve the curative effect; (2) a high effective rate of about 90% but a lower recovery rate of 4%–7% with long-term effectiveness requiring further observation; (3) a long course of treatment, with 2–6 months needed for white patches changing to pink and to normal, and it is necessary for patients to keep to treatment; (4) applicability to vitiligo in the early stage.

Treatment

Otopoint pill pressing

Selection of points: Commonly used points — lung, endocrine, adrenal gland and *shenmen* (HT 7). Supplementary points — *ashi* point, diaphragm, subcortex, central rim and sympathetic. The *ashi* point is located in the vitiligo area.

Manipulation: Three or four commonly used points and one or two supplementary points are employed at each session. The treatment begins with needle embedding. Find the sensitive spot, and insert a thumbtack needle into it, fixing it with an adhesive plaster. Change to another one after 3–5 days of retention, at 5 sessions as a course. The second course involves otopoint pressing with *Vaccaria segetalis* seeds or magnetic beads (380 G) on a square adhesive plaster measuring 0.7 cm × 0.7 cm; press it several times a day to reinforce the stimulation. For cases of deficiency cold, gentle manipulation is performed; for cases of sthenic heat, force manipulation. Change to another plaster in a week. The treatment is applied to one ear at each session, the two ears alternately, during which mild tapping needling is given on the depigmented patches with the plum blossom needle, combined with moxibustion with moxa sticks till the local skin becomes reddish, in order to reinforce the curative effect.

Drug moxibustion

Selection of points: Commonly used point — *ashi* point.

Manipulation: Sterilize *ashi* with 75% alcohol, applying a thin layer of golden cream, and then employ revolving moxibustion with moxa sticks for 30 min until the affected skin becomes pink. District moxibustion should be applied to cases with a generalized pattern. Lastly, wipe clean the affected area. The treatment is performed once daily, at 12 sessions as a course. Take Huanyuandan (recovery pill) in addition, one pill each time for patients older than 15, three times a day; for those younger than 15, one pill each time, twice a day.

Fire needling

Selection of points: Commonly used point — *ashi point*. Supplementary points — *neiguan* (PC 6), *gongsun* (SP 4), *zusanli* (ST 36) and *taichong* (LR 3).

Manipulation: Commonly used points are employed at each session, and two supplementary points may be added according to symptoms. The former are given fire needling, which starts with routine sterilization of the local area and injection of 1% lidocaine for local anesthesia. A No. 26 fire needle with the tip burnt red is inserted into the lesion area by pricking needling, one pricking after one burning, one after another, until the whole lesion area is full of needling spots. Supplementary points are punctured with filiform needles using uniform reinforcing–reducing manipulation on the arrival of *qi*, with the needles retained for 20 min. After the treatment, *ashi* is bound up with antiseptic gauze for 7–10 days, until it crusts over and ablates, and this is followed by another treatment. Generally, one course consists of 10 sessions. Treatment does not stop until the white patches disappear completely and the skin color returns to normal.

Remarks

There are many treatment options available for vitiligo, but only three which are easy to perform in clinic have been introduced here. Ear acupuncture is used in more cases, with a higher effective rate but a lower recovery rate, and is applicable to cases with a small lesion area in the early stage. Drug moxibustion is also convenient and is advised to be combined with the otopoint pressing method. Fire needling has a higher recovery rate but requires experienced practitioners. During treatment with fire needling, the needle tip must be burnt red, and the pricking must be rapid and not too deep. It is also applicable to cases with a small lesion area in the early stage. At the beginning, bleeding points may not be seen and local capillaries start to fill; the pigment is to increase after two or three times of treatment. Bleeding points occurring with the manipulation of pricking signifies that recovery is approaching. During the treatment, hot food and seafood should be avoided.

QUESTIONS

(1) Which method is preferable in treatment of neurodermatitis with acupuncture and moxibustion? Describe the manipulation in detail.

(2) What should be noted in treatment of vitiligo with fire needling?

URTICARIA

Overview

Urticaria is a kind of skin rash notable for pale-red, raised, itchy weals which may come and go rapidly, and is associated with fever, nausea, vomiting and abdominal pain in some cases. It is often acute and recurrent, as well as chronic, lasting years or even dozens of years. In TCM it is called *yin zhen* (urticant eruptions), and its treatment with acupuncture and moxibustion was recorded in *Qian Jin Yi Fang (Supplement to "Important Formulas Worth a Thousand Gold Pieces")* in the Tang Dynasty. Modern reports appeared in the early 1950s. Methods of point stimulation practiced during early times tend to be diversified instead of being acupuncture only, and the effective rate ranges from 75% to 95% in different places.

Treatments

Body acupuncture

Selection of points: Commonly used points — quchi (LI 11), *xuehai* (SP 10), *sanyinjiao* (SP 6) and *dachangshu* (BL 25). Supplementary points — *houxi* (SI 3), *weizhong* (BL 40), *chize* (LU 5), and *dazhui* (DU 14) penetrating to *zhiyang* (DU 9).

Manipulation: Two or three commonly used points and one supplementary point are employed at each session, and penetration may be added for cases with recurrent attacks. On the arrival of *qi*, reducing manipulation is applied by lifting and thrusting or twirling and rotating with strong stimulation for 1–2 min, with the needles retained for 20 min, during which manipulate the needle two or three times. Filiform needles 4–5 *cun* long are inserted into *dazhui* (DU 14) and *zhiyang* (DU 9) penetrating to the middle of the two points, with a retention of 1–2 h. *Houxi* (SI 3), *weizhong* (BL 40) and *chize* (LU 5) are pricked for bloodletting with three-edged needles, once daily or once every other day.

Cupping

Selection of points: Shenque (RN 8).

Manipulation: With the patient in the supine position, cup on *shenque* (RN 8) with flash-fire cupping or with a vacuum aspiration cup for 3–5 min. Repeat the cupping several times, until the local skin becomes reddish or ecchymosis apppears. The treatment is applied once daily.

Ear acupuncture

Selection of points: Commonly used points — lung, *fengxi*, and adrenal gland. Supplementary points — heart, *shenmen* (HT 7), endocrine and liver.

Manipulation: Generally, commonly used points are employed, and supplementary points are added if there is no obvious effect. The sensitive spot found, keep twirling and rotating with strong stimulation until the auricle becomes reddish and hot, with a retention of 30 min, on one ear at each session, with the two ears used alternately. The treatment is applied two or three times a day for extreme itching, and once for ordinary cases.

Remarks

Body acupuncture is the most common method in clinics. It is applicable to acute or chronic urticaria, and especially effective for acute cases. It was applied to 387 cases, with an effective rate of 76.9%–96.5%. While penetrating *dazhui* (DU 14) and *zhiyang* (DU 9), be sure to manipulate the needle subcutaneously to a depth of 4 *cun*, respectively. Cupping has been popular in recent years and is mainly applicable to acute urticaria at the first onset, while for recurrent or chronic cases it should be combined with body acupuncture. Ear acupuncture is also effective, but it is advisable to combine it with body acupuncture.

SHINGLES (HERPES ZOSTER)

Overview

Shingles is an acute inflammatory skin disease involving skin and nerves. It is clinically manifested by rapid onset, burning heat in the affected area, and first-irregular lamellar erythema which soon forms gregarious bean-sized papulae or blisters on a red base, often in a stripe. The skin between stripes is normal. The skin lesion is limited to one side of the body, and is commonly seen in intercostal nerve distributions on the torso, and also in trigeminal nerve distribustions on the face, usually accompanied by neuralgia, or even fever in severe cases. It is called *chan yao huo dan* (serpiginous belt eruption) in TCM but there were no records about acupuncture treatment in ancient literature. In the early 1950s reports about treatment of shingles with acupuncture and moxibustion were published. Practice of more than 50 years supports the view that acupuncture and moxibustion is able to control extreme neuralgia, and to help dry the blisters and remove the erythema. The average effective rate is about 95% now.

Treatment

Body acupuncture

Selection of points: Commonly used points — *ashi* point (around the skin lesion, 0.5–1 *cun* to the shingles), *jiaji* (EX-B2), *zhigou* (TE 6) and *yanglingquan* (GB 34). Supplementary points — *quchi* (LI 11), *hegu* (LI 4) and *waiguan* (SJ 5) added for the focus below the waist; *sanyinjiao* (SP 6), *taichong* (LR 3) and *xuehai* (SP 10) for the focus above the waist.

Manipulation: Commonly used points are employed at each session, and one or two supplementary points are added if no obvious effect achieved. *Ashi* is punctured with 1–2-*cun*-long filiform needles at an angle of 25° obliquely toward the shingles (4–8 needles are needed), slightly lifting, thrusting, twirling and rotating until the arrival of *qi*. *Jiaji* (EX-B2), usually the point on the nerve segment corresponding to the skin lesion, is obliquely punctured deep, slightly toward the vertebral column, transmitting the sensation along the nerve distribution paths. The rest of the points are given reducing manipulation on the arrival of *qi* by lifting, thrusting, twirling and rotating. The needles are retained in each point for 20–30 min, during which manipulate them once every 5–10 min.

Acupoint laser irradiation

Selection of points: Commonly used points — two groups, namely (1) *ashi point* (focus area); (2) focus above the waist: *hegu* (LI 4) and *quchi* (LI 11); below the waist: *yanglingquan* (GB 34) and *xiaxi* (GB 43) (on the lateral side of the instep of the foot, between the fourth and fifth toes, at the junction of the red and white skin, proximal to the margin of the web). Supplementary points — *zhigou* (TE 6) and *taichong* (LR 3).

Manipulation: A H–Ne laser apparatus is employed with wavelength 632.8 nm and output current 28 mm, 2–3 mW at the exit. The first group of points is for cases with a larger skin lesion area, more blisters, more infection and mild pain. Laser defocusing irradiation is applied with a distance of 40–60 mm and a density of 0.5–1 mW/cm², for 5–10 min in each area. The second group of points is for cases with pain as the main symptom, a localized skin lesion, and only red papules or rashes that have crusted over. For extreme pain, supplementary points may be added for irradiation for 5 min, respectively. If the lesion area is large and the pain is obvious, the two groups should be combined. The treatment is applied once daily, at 10 sessions as a course.

Remarks

There are many treatment therapies for shingles. Body acupuncture is traditional and preferable in treatment, and has been applied to 495 cases, with an effective rate of 96%. The modern therapy of acupoint laser irradiation has been applied to 311 cases, the total effective rate reaching 94.2% after 5 treatments. Other therapies are still available, like ear acupuncture, acupoint injection, dermal acupuncture, moxibustion and fire needling. The main characteristics of acupuncture are relieving pain and taking about one week for blisters to dry and crust over, with the development of skin lesions.

QUESTIONS

(1) Which method of point stimulation is preferable in treatment of recurrent urticaria? How to manipulate it?
(2) What are the characteristics of point selection and manipulation in treatment of shingles?

ACNE

Overview

Acne, or acne vulgaris, is a chronic inflammatory disorder of hair follicles and sebaceous glands, occurring most commonly in young men and women, often on the face with comedones, papules, abscess nodes, and cysts. In TCM it is called *jiu ci* (acne), *fei feng fen ci* (anemopulmonary acne) and *mian chuang* (facial sore), but no records about acupuncture therapy can be found in ancient literature. Modern reports began in the 1960s. In recent years, with the pursuit of beauty by people, a great number of clinical articles have been published and the average effective rate is 95% or so.

Treatment

Acupuncture and moxibustion

Selection of points: Commonly used points — two groups, namely (1) *quchi* (LI 11) and *hegu* (LI 4), and (2) *houxi* (SI 3) and *laogong* (PC 8). Supplementary points — *dazhui* (DU 14), *zusanli* (ST 36), *yingxiang* (LI 20), *xiaguan* (ST 7) and *jiache* (ST 6).

Manipulation: One group is employed at each session, the two groups alternately, and two or three supplementary points are selected according to symptoms. On the arrival of *qi*, *quchi* (LI 11) and *hegu* (LI 4) are punctured by lifting and thrusting with medium stimulation, with a retention of 30 min. *Houxi* (SI 3) is punctured with a 2-*cun*-long filiform needle penetrating to *laogong* (PC 8), with the needle retained for 20 min, followed by drops of blood being pressed out after the needle is withdrawn. Supplementary points are given medium stimulation, and then connected to an electroacupuncture apparatus with an interrupted wave and an intensity tolerable to the patient, for 20–30 min. After withdrawal of the needles, the face and *zusanli* (ST 36) are given revolving moxibustion for 10–15 min, till the local skin becomes reddish. The treatment is applied once daily or once every other day, at seven sessions as a course, at an interval of five days between courses. Penetrating needling is applied to *houxi* (SI 3) and *laogong* (PC 8) once a week.

Ear acupuncture

Selection of points: Commonly used points — sympathetic, hot spot (the antihelix zone on the same line as the medial border of the upper crus of the antihelix), endocrine, subcortex and central rim. Supplementary points — adrenal gland and *shenmen* (HT 7).

Manipulation: Two or three commonly used points are employed at each session, with all points selected alternately; if the effect is not satisfactory, supplementary points may be added. Rapid pricking needling is applied with sterilized three-edged needles to a depth of 0.1 cm, without penetrating cartilages, and 1–3 drops of blood are pressed out. One ear is employed each time, once every other day, at 10 sessions as a course.

Pricking and cupping

Selection of points: Commonly used points — *dazhui* (DU 14), and *zhi-yang* (DU 9). Supplementary points — groove on the back of the auricle, hot spot, and stomach.

Manipulation: Commonly used points are given tapping needling with three-edged needles or dermal needles several times before cupping for 20 min. Supplementary points are pricked for drops of blood pressed out, one or two points at each session. The treatment is applied once every other day, at 10 sessions as a course, at an interval of 5–7 days between courses.

Remarks

There are many treatment approaches to acne with point stimulation, but here only the common ones in the clinic have been introduced. The first is a comprehensive method of acupoint stimulation which has been proven to have a high effective rate and a high recovery rate, but the complicated manipulation requires more clinical experience to obtain high effectiveness. Ear acupuncture is the most commonly used approach with more reformed methods, among which bloodletting on otopoints is reported to have been applied to more than 1000 cases with an average effective rate of 95%, and a recovery rate of over 80%, but rigid sterilization is imperative, in order to avoid infection. Pricking for blood with cupping is easy and convenient to perform, and has been applied to 354 cases, with a total effective rate of 99.4% but a lower recovery rate.

ALOPECIA AREATA

Overview

Alopecia areata is a localized area of nonscarring hair loss. It often affects the young with one or more coin-sized, round, smooth, bare patches without any rational symptoms. In TCM it belongs to the category of *you feng* (alopecia), commonly called *gui ti tou*. There were rare records about the acupuncture treatment for *you feng* in ancient literature, while modern reports appeared in 1958. Since the 1960s, dermal acupuncture has been applied to treatment of alopecia areata, and thousands of cases in 40 years have confirmed the effectiveness of acupuncture therapy with an effective rate of about 85%.

Treatment

Acupuncture with skin needling

Selection of points: Commonly used points — *ashi* point (alopecia area), positive reaction spot (bilateral to the spinal column, or positive soft reactors in trabs, nodes or bubbles if touched, or a positive reaction spot with soreness and numbness when pressed) and *fengchi* (GB 20). Supplementary points — *taiyuan* (LU 9), *neiguan* (PC 6), neck, sacrum, and lower back.

Manipulation: *Ashi* and *fengchi* (GB 20) are employed at each session, and supplementary points selected from the lumbosacral region. A positive spot is the main area for tapping needling. A seven-star needle is inserted into the baldness area densely and evenly, first tapping in bostrychoid from the border of the baldness to the center, then from the nonbaldness to the center of the baldness. *Fengchi* (GB 20) is densely punctured by tapping an area 0.5–1 cm in diameter from about 20 times at the beginning to 40–50 times, until the skin becomes red or there is a little bleeding. Other points are punctured in the same way as *fengchi* (GB 20). Points on the back are punctured by tapping both sides of the vertebrae and the center of the spinal column from the nape to the sacrococcygeal region several times, with positive spots as the main area for tapping. In order to enhance the curative effect, a ginger slice may be used to rub on the baldness with a slight burning sensation in the local area. Treatment with dermal acupuncture is applied once daily or once every other day, at 15 sessions as a course, at an interval of 5–7 days between courses.

Body acupuncture

Selection of points: Commonly used points — *baihui* (DU 20), *ashi* point (alopecia area), *shengfaxue* [the middle of the line between fengchi (GB 20) and *fengfu* (DU 16), *fanglaoxue* 1 *cun* posterior to *Baihui* (DU 20)] and *jiannaoxue* [5 *fen* below *fengchi* (GB 20)]. Supplementary points — *yiming* (EX-HN14), taiyang (EX-HN5), *fengchi* (GB 20), *Waiguan* (SJ 5) and *tianjing* (SJ 10).

Manipulation: Two or three commonly used points are employed at each session, and *ashi* is vital; others, alternately. Supplementary points may be added if there is no obvious effect. *Ashi* is punctured horizontally with a No. 30 filiform needle, 1–1.5 *cun* long, from peripheric to the center of the baldness; *fanglaoxue* is punctured with the tip obliquely forward, and the handle parallel to the scalp, to 1 *fen* along the skin; *jiannaoxue* is punctured with the tip obliquely downward to 2 *fen*, avoiding too-deep or too-shallow puncture. *Fengchi* (GB 20) is punctured, obliquely downward to a depth of 1.0–1.5 *cun*, till the arrival of *qi*. The other points are punctured, and the needles are retained for 15–20 min. The treatment is applied once daily, at 10 sessions as a course.

Remarks

Of the two methods introduced above, dermal acupuncture is more common and more confirmed in effectiveness. Over 1000 cases have shown its effective rate to be 87%–97%. Points in body acupuncture are newly discovered and are highly effective with correct point selection and manipulation. Besides, laser irradiation on the focal area is effective for a single alopecia areata. Acupoint injection into the baldness area and pricking for blood on *weizhong* (BL 40) are also available.

MELANOSIS

Overview

Melanosis, also known as chloasma hepaticum, is a patchy brown or dark brown skin discoloration that usually occurs on the face and the forehead, and is particularly common in pregnant women. In TCM it is called *mian chen* ("dusty complexion") and no records about acupuncture treatment were found in ancient literature, or even in modern times until recent years. The most important therapy is ear acupuncture, but body acupuncture and point injection are also available, with better effectiveness. At present, the average effective rate is over 85%.

Treatment

Ear acupuncture

Selection of points: Commonly used points — Heat spot, *jiezhongxue* (above the posterior surface of the ear, the outside lower part of the ear apex when the ear is folded forward) and subcortex. Supplementary points — endocrine, spleen, and stomach.

Manipulation: Commonly used points are taken as the main points, and supplementary points are added according to symptoms. The patient is sitting upright. Following rigid sterilization, take a three-edged needle to pierce the epidermis to 0.1 cm, with blood coming out. Three cotton balls are dipped in 75% alcohol and squeezed to clean the blood. Cover the pore with a sterilized dry cotton ball to avoid infection, one point at each session. Pricking for blood is applied once every other day, with the points taken alternately, at 15 sessions as a course, at an interval of 7–10 days between courses. While cleaning off the bloodstains, slightly move the external helix zone to avoid bleeding obstruction by pressing forcefully. Ask the patient to keep the cotton ball on the pore for 24 h, avoiding dampening. If the pricking pore is hard to heal, avoid bloodletting in this area.

Ear (body) acupuncture

Selection of points: Commonly used points — kidney, liver, spleen and endocrine. Supplementary points — *yangbai* (GB 14) added for chloasma on the forehead, *jiache* (ST 6) and *sibai* (ST 2) for the cheeks, *yintang* (EX-HN3) and *yingxiang* (LI 20) for the bridge of the nose, and *dicang* (ST 4) and *chengjiang* (RN 24) for the areas around the nose and lips.

Manipulation: Commonly used points are employed at each session. Acupuncture with 5-*fen*-long No. 28 filiform needles is combined with pressing *Vaccaria segetalis* seeds. Insert the needle into the sensitive spot of the otopoint on one side, not too deep, till a sensation of distending pain arises; press on the other side, once daily or once every two days, with the two ears employed alternately. Supplementary points are selected according to pigmentation parts. One-*cun*-long No. 30 filiform needles are horizontally inserted from points to pigmentation parts with mild stimulation on the arrival of *qi*, by slightly twirling and rotating. The needles of ear and body acupuncture are all retained for 30 min, during which manipulate them two or three times. Electroacupuncture is also available with a continuous wave and a frequency of 90–120 cmp for the same time. The needles on the otopoints are withdrawn before a little blood is let out. Body acupuncture is applied once every other day or every three days, at the same time as ear acupuncture, at 15 sessions as a course, at an interval of 5–7 days between courses.

Remarks

Both of the therapies introduced above are effective in treatment of melanosis. Ear acupuncture for bloodletting is applied to more cases and more confirmed, and was applied to 283 cases, with 165 recovered (the pigmentation patches faded completely and the skin color returned to normal), a total effective rate of 85% and good long-term effectiveness. Otopoint pricking is applicable to cases with a course of 1–6 years and ages from 17 to 22. In addition, ear and body acupuncture are effective not only in melanosis but also in menopathy.

QUESTIONS

(1) How many treatment approaches are there to acne with acupuncture and moxibustion? What are they?

(2) Restate the two methods of point stimulation for alopecia areata.

(3) What are the differences and similarities in point selection and manipulation in treatment of melanosis and acne?

CHAPTER 30

Acupuncture and Moxibustion
for Healthcare

SMOKING CESSATION

Overview

Tobacco smoking is a bad habit. According to scientific research, tobacco contains about 100 poisonous compounds like nicotine, tar and benzopyrene, which are related to coronary artery disease, hypertensive disease, chronic bronchitis, and emphysema, and are able to increase the incidence of many malignant tumors. Quitting smoking by acupuncture and moxibustion is not found in ancient literature, but is a development of modern healthcare with acupuncture and moxibustion, which was first suggested by a foreign practitioner in the 1950s. Since the early 1980s, more and more clinical reports have been published in China. Tens of thousands of cases have proven its effectiveness with a total effective rate of 70%–90%, although different methods of point stimulation are applied, and the effect varies for different criteria due to different smoking amounts per day and smoking lengths.

Treatment

Ear acupuncture

Selection of points: Commonly used points — mouth, lung and *shenmen* (HT 7). Supplementary points — subcortex, endocrine and adrenal gland.

Manipulation: Generally, commonly used points are employed at each session, and one or two supplementary points may be added if no satisfactory result is achieved. Sensitive spots having been detected on both ears, No. 28–30 filiform needles are inserted rapidly into the points till a sensation of distending pain arises, twirling and rotating rapidly and slightly for half a minute at a frequency of 120 cpm till the auricle becomes hot and red, with the needles retained for 15–20 min. The treatment is applied once every other day, at 10 sessions as a course. The next course begins after a 3-day interval.

Body acupuncture

Selection of points: Commonly used points — *tianweixue* between *lieque* (LU 7) and *yangxi* (LI 5), a soft spot one thumb away from the border of the radius cervcial papilla, a depression spot with obvious tenderness]. Supplementary points — *hegu* (LI 4) and *zusanli* (ST 36).

Manipulation: Commonly used points are first employed, and if the therapeutic effect is not satisfactory, supplementary points are replaced or added. *Tianweixue* on both sides having been selected, the smoker keeps the dorsum of the hand upward to locate the tenderness spot, which is perpendicularly punctured with a 1-*cun*-long No. 28 filiform to a depth of 3 mm. In doing so, the smoker makes a deep aspiration before holding the breath till the finish of the insertion. Twirl and rotate the needle to induce a sensation of soreness and distension, with a retention of 15 min. The smoker should finally feel heaviness of the hands. Either of the supplementary points on both sides is employed at each session, and punctured with the No. 28 filiform needles till the arrival of *qi*, repeating rapid lifting and slight thrusting of the needles combined with twirling at high frequency for 1–2 min to strengthen the sensation. Then connect to the electroacupuncture apparatus with a continuous wave and an intensity tolerable to the patient for 15 min. Withdraw the needles, and insert a grainlike intradermal needle into the point along the skin to 1 cm, the needle body and the running course of the meridian being vertical to each other in a cross that is fixed with adhesive plaster, with the needles retained for one day, during which the smoker is asked to press the embedding points three or four times a day, for 2–3 min each time, with the two supplementary points taken alternately. The treatment is applied once daily, at five sessions as a course. Another type of acupuncture will be performed after an interval of 3–5 days if that fails to help the smoker quit smoking completely.

Remarks

There are many treatment approaches to smoking cessation, but only two have been introduced here. The first proves by rigid contrast and observation that cases of both active and passive smoking cessation will experience the different smell of cigarettes after ear acupuncture. In a followup lasting 3–8 months, 71% of active quitters stayed abstinent, which shows that ear acupuncture has long-term as well as short-term effectiveness, while only 39% of passive quitters stayed abstinent. Ear acupuncture is therefore preferable in quitting smoking. *Tianweixue*, discovered by an American named Olms, is a point for smoking cessation, and has been proven to be highly effective by physicians and acupuncturists. Fewer supplementary points are employed with complicated manipulation, mainly applicable to smokers with great nicotine addiction, long-term smoking and no response to other methods.

It has been found that acupuncture has both short-term and long-term effectiveness in active smoking quitters with shorter-term and less smoking per day, while being less effective in passive quitters with long-time smoking, and nicotine addiction. Many ex-smokers say that they feel the tobacco changing to hot, fierce or tasteless, and out of sorts in the throat.

DRUG REHABILITATION

Overview

Drug abuse, a global problem today, not only presents risks to human health, but also brings a series of difficult social problems, and has attracted widespread international attention. How to control drug abuse, i.e. drug treatment, has become one of the urgent problems to be solved in the world. For long-term drug users, stopping the supply of drugs will lead to a series of intolerable withdrawal symptoms, such as restlessness, insomnia, abdominal pain, chest tightness, limb pain, sneezing and yawning, tears, or even collapse, loss of consciousness, or a life-threatening state.

Acupuncture for drug rehabilitation was discovered by chance by a surgeon named H. L. Wen in Hong Kong, when performing an anesthesia operation on a drug user. Now, acupuncture for drug rehabilitation has been studied and developed in many countries. Foreign practitioners prefer ear acupuncture, while domestic acupuncturists tend to choose body acupuncture, or electroacupuncture, or combined with ear acupuncture, and also bloodletting, fire needling and point electric stimulation, with points of the head as the main points and points of the limbs as adjuvant. According to statistics from 21 records of foreign countries involving more than 2500 drug users, the average withdrawal rate is about 46%, and 10% in one-year followup. It is higher in China, but the precise therapeutic effect needs further investigation as there are insufficient cases in practice and the mechanism remains unknown. Generally speaking, acupuncture for drug rehabilitation has been accepted to be safe, effective, convenient and inexpensive, with fewer side effects and less pain. Not only is its therapeutic effect lower than that of other therapies, but also it has been found to be able to temporarily or continuously change addictive behaviors. When other therapies are inefficacious, it is a method worth promoting.

Acupuncture for drug rehabilitation, like other drug treatments, has a serious problem of relapse that tends to decline with time. Chinese acupuncture practitioners have made some progress but it is still very difficult to solve the problem.

Treatment

Electric ear acupuncture

Selection of points: Commonly used points — lung. Supplementary points — sympathetic, *shenmen* (HT 7), liver, lung and kidney.

Manipulation: Commonly used points are employed, and supplementary points are added or replaced according to symptoms. Commonly used points of bilateral auricles of the ear are punctured with 5-*fen*-long filiform needles to induce *qi*, and connected to the electroacupuncture apparatus with a continuous wave, a frequency (300–1000 cpm) and an intensity tolerable to the patient, for 30–60 min. Lateral supplementary points are punctured with filiform needles till there is a sensation of distending pain, with the needles retained for 1 h. The treatment is applied once or twice a day, for eight days as a course. Commonly used points may also be inserted into two or three times in the first three days, and once daily in the following five days.

Body acupuncture (I)

Selection of points: Commonly used points — *neiguan* (PC 6), *shuigou* (DU 26), and *suliao* (DU 25). Supplementary points — *quchi* (LI 11), *hegu* (LI 4), *yinlingquan* (SP 9), *shenmen* (HT 7) and *zusanli* (ST 36); *baihui* (DU 20) and *yintang* (EX-HN3) added for insomnia; *yongquan* (KI 1) for obnubilation; *laogong* (PC 8) for irritation.

Manipulation: Commonly used points are employed at each session, and supplementary points are added according to symptoms. Acupuncture is performed at a fixed time every morning. *Neiguan* (PC 6) is inserted into perpendicularly to a depth of 1 *cun*, lifting, thrusting, twirling and rotating the needle on the arrival of *qi* for 1 min. Then *shuigou* (DU 26) is punctured to a depth of 0.5 *cun* with sparrow-pecking needling, until tears drop or are in the eyes; *suliao* (DU 25) is punctured perpendicularly to a depth of 0.3 *cun*, until there is obvious distending pain; and *dazhui* (DU 14) is punctured obliquely downward to a depth of 1.2 *cun* to make the sensation radiate downward. Supplementary points are punctured to induce *qi*, twirling and rotating the needles with a large amplitude for 2–5 min, with the intensity tolerable to the patient. The needles are all retained for 20 min, during which manipulate them in the same way once or twice. The treatment is applied once or twice a day, for 10 days as a course.

Electroacupuncture

Selection of points: Commonly used points — two groups, namely (1) *zusanli* (ST 36), *sanyinjiao* (SP 6) and tenderness spot (most centralized between T5 and T7; secondly around L2 and T3); (2) *baihui* (DU 20), *yintang* (EX-HN3), *neiguan* (PC 6) and *shenshu* (BL 23). Supplementary points — *laogong* (PC 8), *hegu* (LI 4), *shuigou* (DU 26), *suliao* (DU 25) and *shenmen* (HT 7).

Manipulation: Commonly used points are employed, one group a day, the two groups alternately. Tenderness spot, *zusanli* (ST 36) and *sanyinjiao* (SP 6) are connected to a G6805-2 electroacupuncture apparatus with a frequency of 3–5 Hz, a sparse wave at 2–200 cps, and stimulating the intensity to the maximum tolerance value of the patient. The treatment is applied two or three times a day, for 30 min each time, for 10 days as a course.

Body acupuncture (II)

Selection of points: Commonly used points — *sishencong* (EX-HN1), *neiguan* (PC 6), *hegu* (LI 4), *zusanli* (ST 36), and *sanyinjiao* (SP 6). Supplementary points — *shuigou* (DU 26), *laogong* (PC 8) and *zhiyang* (DU 9).

Manipulation: Sishencong (EX-HN1) is given uniform reinforcing–reducing manipulation, *neiguan* (PC 6) and *hegu* (LI 4) are given reducing manipulation by forcefully lifting and slightly thrusting three times, and *zusanli* (ST 36) is given reinforcing manipulation by forcefully thrusting and slightly lifting three times. On the arrival of *qi*, the needles are retained for 30 min, during which they are regulated once every 5 min. The treatment is applied twice a day in the first three days (one at 9–11 in the morning and the other at 3–5 in the afternoon, and another added at 9–11 in the night for severe cases), and once daily in the following seven days (at 3–5 in the afternoon). For severe cases, puncture *shuigou* (DU 26) and *laogong* (PC 8), or apply pricking and cupping to *zhiyang* (SP 6).

Remarks

Among the four methods for drug rehabilitation introduced here, the first three are applicable to rapid rehabilitation and the last to prevention of relapse. Electric ear acupuncture is more commonly used at home and abroad, with a higher withdrawal rate, but the long-term effectiveness is not ideal. Body acupuncture is more often applied to drug users with mild symptoms, and needs combination with appropriate assisting measures for drug users with intense manifestations. Electroacupuncture is highly effective for emotional disturbance, skeletal and muscle pain, and insomnia. Body acupuncture (II) is mainly for preventing relapse, and should be employed as soon as possible after detoxification; it generally works in one course. It is advisable to treat drug addiction in coordination with Chinese or Western medication for antirelapse.

QUESTIONS

(1) What method do you prefer in quitting smoking with acupuncture?
(2) What are the characteristics of the four acupuncture methods for drug rehabilitation?

ATHLETIC SYNDROME

Overview

Athletic syndrome refers to a series of symptoms before or during a competition (such as an examination or a game), like palpitations, shortness of breath, dry mouth, dizziness, irritability, loss of appetite, nausea, vomiting, diarrhea or constipation, abdominal pain, menstrual disorders, blurred vision, trembling hands, intellectual deterioration, rigidity of thinking, increased blood pressure, psychopathy, syncope, or even sudden death. Psychotherapy or taking sedative drugs before competitions or examinations leads to results that are unsatisfactory. In recent years, some acupuncture practitioners have been exploring the use of acupuncture for preventing athletic syndrome, especially exam room syndrome, and have achieved satisfactory results, and to some extent can improve the performances of the candidates.

Prevention Methods

Ear acupuncture

Selection of points: Commonly used points — heart, *shenmen* (HT 7), subcortex and spleen. Supplementary points — sympathetic, liver, stomach, large intestine, central rim and adrenal gland.

Manipulation: Commonly used points are taken as the main points, and according to some accompanying symptoms, supplementary points may be added, such as liver for irritability, stomach for nausea and vomiting, large intestine for constipation or diarrhea, and central rim for intellectual deterioration. *Huangjingzi (Fructus Viticis Negundo)* is used for application; *Vaccaria segetalis* seeds or magnetic beads are also available. The individual for prevention is asked to press the points 3–5 times a day, for 10–20 min each time. He or she is to press again, for 20 min, before retiring.

Body acupuncture

Selection of points: *Baihui* (DU 20).

Manipulation: A No. 30 filiform needle is inserted horizontally to a depth of 1.2 *cun*, with reinforcing manipulation on the arrival of *qi*, by lifting and thrusting or twirling and rotating with mild stimulation. Generally, acupuncture is applied the night before the examination or competition, and withdraw the needles in the morning before getting up, with the needles retained for 8 h. If the examination or competition is held in the afternoon, retain the needles before noon for about 2 h.

Remarks

Both methods are mainly to prevent exam room syndrome. Compared with medication, *tui na* or other therapies, acupuncture is more convenient and less expensive, with no time or condition limits, and no negative influence on the studies and reviews. As for the prevention results, ear pressing has been applied to 213 cases, which began prevention six days before the examination, and were followed up every night during the examination till it finished. A total effective rate of 92.8% has been achieved. Body acupuncture has been applied to 532 cases. The needles were retained for 8 h the night before the examination. Most of the participants had improved sleep, and also a steady mental state during the examination. Compared with the control group, each person improved the score for each subject by 3.4; in particular, reinforcing manipulation produced a much higher score. For those who are apparently nervous, the needles may be retained during the examination, but most of the participants will fail to improve their scores. Apply acupuncture before noon for an examination in the afternoon; this will result in clear-headedness and a score 2.75 higher for each course subject.

CHRONIC FATIGUE SYNDROME

Overview

Chronic fatigue syndrome, officially named by the Centers for Disease Control (CDC) of the U.S. in 1988, refers specifically to unexplained significant systemic fatigue in healthy subjects who fail to lead a normal social life for six months or more. It is characterized by long-term, chronic and recurrent fatigue, often associated with headache, dizziness, palpitations, shortness of breath, fewer words, insomnia and dreaminess, mild fever, depression, lack of concentration, joint and muscle pain and weakness, and other symptoms. In recent years, the number of patients with chronic fatigue syndrome have been increasing. Since it happens to healthy people, the exact cause remains unknown and the treatment therefore is at the passive and primary stage.

Acupuncture has a more significant role in eliminating fatigue. Back in the 1950s, foreign practitioners tried gold and silver needle acupuncture at different points to eliminate muscle fatigue caused by excessive stress. Later on, some acupuncturists and physiologists in China established relevant indicators and made a more in-depth study of it. For example, the application of the ergograph showing index finger contraction and fatigue curves found that puncturing of *zusanli* (ST 36) combined with reinforcing manipulation is able to significantly promote recovery from fatigue. Compared to acupuncture practitioners of the last century, modern acupuncture practioners place more emphasis on prevention and treatment of chronic fatigue syndrome. It is worth mentioning that in recent years many approaches to the syndrome, including body acupuncture, electroacupuncture, cupping and magnetic circular needling, have obtained more satisfactory results.

Treatment

Otopoint pill pressing

Selection of points: Commonly used points — kidney, spleen and subcortex. Supplementary points — pancreas and gallbladder and *shenmen* (HT 7).

Manipulation: Otopoint application is performed using commonly used points as the main points, and pancreas and gallbladder are added for poor appetite, and *shenmen* (HT 7) for poor sleep. Apply *Vaccaria segetalis* seeds or magnetic beads to bilateral points. Press once respectively in the morning, at noon and in the evening, for 2–3 min each time, until the auricle of the ear becomes hot and red. It is not necessary to press magnetic beads. Remove them before retiring, and use another plaster the next morning. Apply once daily during the intense work.

Body acupuncture

Selection of points: Commonly used points — *baihui* (DU 20), *neiguan* (PC 6) and *zusanli* (ST 36). Supplementary points — *liangmen* (ST 21), *tianshu* (ST 25), *yinbai* (SP 1), *shenmai* (BL 62) and *houxi* (SI 3).

Manipulation: Commonly used points are employed at each session, and supplementary points added according to symptoms. 1.0–1.5-*cun*-long needles are taken according to different constitutions and acupoint locations. On the arrival of *qi*, uniform reinforcing–reducing manipulation is applied, with a retention of 20 min, during which there is no manipulation at all. The treatment is given once every 3 days, with 2 days' rest on weekends, for 12 weeks as a course.

Acupoint injection

Selection of points: Zusanli (ST 36).

Manipulation: Bilateral points are employed. The patient is in the sitting or supine position. Both *zusanli* points (ST 36), after routine sterilization, are perpendicularly punctured to a depth of 4 cm, lifting and thrusting appropriately till there is a sensation of soreness and distension, followed by astragalus injection, 2 ml at each point, once every other day, at 10 sessions as a course. The next course begins after a 5-day interval.

Electroacupuncture coupled with cupping

Selection of points: Commonly used points — *baihui* (DU 20), *danzhong* (RN 17), *zhongwan* (RN 20), *guanyuan* (RN 4), *neiguan* (PC 6) and *zusanli* (St 36). Supplementary points — points of *du* and bladder channels (level of *DU* 14–*DU* 3).

Manipulation: Four or five commonly used points are employed for acupuncture at each session. The patient, in the supine position, is treated with a 1.5-*cun*-long No. 30 filiform needle with rapid insertion, slowly lifting, thrusting, twirling and rotating to induce *qi*. Uniform reinforcing–reducing manipulation is applied with medium stimulation, for 0.5 min at each point. Connect to the electroacupuncture apparatus with a continuous wave, a low frequency (60–80 cpm) and mild stimulation tolerable to the patient, with the needles retained for 30 min.

Supplementary points are given cupping. The patient is in the prone position, with the back naked, and a pillow under the chest to relax the shoulders and the neck. The cupping glass with a thick and smooth mouth, 3.5 cm in diameter, is smeared with a thin layer of lubricant on the mouth and the area for moving cupping. Hold the bottom of the glass with both hands and push it horizontally or obliquely a little up and down five or more times, until the skin becomes reddish, dark-red, or there are scarlatina spots, and the patient feels hot in the back. The treatment is applied twice a week, at six sessions as course. The next course begins after a 5-day interval.

Remarks

The four methods for prevention of chronic fatigue syndrome vary in application according to their own characteristics. Otopoint pressing is for preventing or eliminating general physiological fatigue. Observations show that this method plays a role in eliminating fatigue of athletes by heavy stress training, as well as fatigue of tourists and brain-workers. Body acupuncture is mainly for chronic fatigue syndrome. In this method, the commonly used points may be applicable to prevention. The sufferer should be informed in advance that it needs a three-month treatment, which will not stop until clinical recovery has been achieved. Acupoint injection is applicable to chronic fatigue syndrome in the early stage or with mild symptoms. It will also take about three months. Electroacupuncture and cupping is applied to cases with severe symptoms and a long course of disease. Wipe the local skin clean with *Gossypium* absorbents after moving cupping. And be sure to keep the body warm and avoid bathing on the day of treatment.

QUESTIONS

(1) Have you thought of combining the two methods of point stimulation in prevention and treatment of athletic syndrome?
(2) What are the acupuncture approaches to chronic fatigue syndrome and general fatigue?

SUBHEALTH

Overview

Subhealth refers to an unhealthy state between health and disease, also known as the third state, gray state, somatopsychic disturbance state, latent clinical state or preclinical state. It is a new medical concept raised in the 1990s, and is in fact a reflection of a conceptual shift from the focus on disease to the human being. According to a survey, 60% of the Chinese population are in a subhealth condition, and only 5.6% are really ill. The occupations related to subhealth show mental stress, overload of intellectual work, and interpersonal tension. Unhealthy lifestyles include smoking, irregular work and rest, improper diet and lack of exercise. The following are the events in sequence easily leading to subhealth conditions: sudden injury or natural disasters, family overburden, loss of a spouse, love lost, etc. It is worth noting that subhealth is rather prevalent among white-collar workers, undergraduates, teachers in primary or middle schools and administrators of enterprises.

The main symptoms of the subhealth condition are loss of memory and concentration, a great deal of anxiety about the health, insomnia, dreaminess, agitation, irritability, emotional lability, fatigue, sensation of weakness and depression, oppression of the chest, shortness of breath, hyperhidrosis and muscle pain. It occurs in males and females with similar symptoms, but different features at different ages; for example, forgetfulness, fatigue and defective ejaculation tend to increase with aging, while teenagers usually have symptoms like inattention, low spirits, dreaminess and emotional lability. In addition, with the widespread use of computers and televisions, long-time fixing of the eyes on the electronic screen will definitely lead to dryness and irritation of the eyes, blurred vision and asthenopia.

It is generally believed that healthy people must attach importance to daily care and exercises, and diseases should be treated early, while a subhealth focus on regulation, i.e. regulating the slight disequilibrium of the body, is the principal method for correcting the subhealth condition. Besides adjusting unhealthy lifestyles and eating health foods (including medicated dietary therapy of TCM), acupuncture and moxibustion is one of the preferred methods, and has attracted increasing attention from the public, especially electroacupuncture and moxibustion.

Treatment

Electroacupuncture

Selection of points: Commonly used points — *baihui* (DU 20) and *yintang* (EX-HN3). Supplementary points — *shenmen* (HT 7), *sanyinjiao* (SP 6) and *neiguan* (PC 6).

Manipulation: Commonly used points are employed at each session, and supplementary points are added according to symptoms. *Baihui* (DU 20) is punctured with the tip backward, and *yintang* (EX-HN3) downward, horizontally to 0.8 *cun*. Uniform reinforcing–reducing manipulation is applied till the arrival of *qi* (a sensation of distension and heaviness), before connecting both handles to the G6805 electroacupuncture apparatus with a continuous wave, a frequency (6–8 Hz) and an output tolerable to the patient. Two of the supplementary points are selected alternately, and are perpendicularly punctured before uniform reinforcing–reducing manipulation is applied, with the needles retained for 30 min. Nasal oxygen may be used in combination if possible. The treatment is applied once every other day, at 15 sessions as a course. Generally, one or two courses are needed in treatment.

Moxibustion

Selection of points: Commonly used points — *dazhui* (DU 14), *mingmen* (DU 4) and *shenque* (RN 8). Supplementary points — *zusanli* (ST 36) and *guanyuan* (RN 4).

Manipulation: Generally, commonly used points are employed at each session, and supplementary points are added for weak constitutions. With the patient in the prone position, apply mild–warm moxibustion to points of the back with moxa sticks, to *dazhui* (DU 14) and *mingmen* (DU 4) at the same time, for 15 min each time, until local skin becomes reddish. Then the patient changes to the supine position and is given salt-separated moxibustion with moxa sticks to *shenque* (RN 8) for 15–20 min. Supplementary points are treated the same way with *dazhui* (DU 14). The treatment is applied once every other day or twice a week.

Remarks

Electroacupuncture is preferable and effective for regulation, since it needs fewer acupoints, only commonly used points selected, the patient can fall asleep during the treatment, and the retention may be extended according to the sleeping time. Moxibustion requires sufficient time till the patient feels unusually relaxed after treatment. Be sure to avoid scalding due to moxa fire dropping.

ELIMINATING DEPRESSION

Overview

Depressive neurosis is a kind of mental disorder characterized by a lasting low mood and prolonged pathogenesis. In recent years, with economic development, acceleration of the rhythm of work and life, lifestyle changes, and increasing pressures from society, mental disorder has played an important part in affecting human health, and the incidence of the illness tends to increase every year, interfering with daily life and the ability to work. The main symptoms are a low mood, low affective activity and giving up of interests, accompanied by slow reaction, insomnia, weight reduction, decreased activeness, lack of interest in life, early awakening, anorexia, poor appetite and hyposexuality, but no illusions or delusions. Depressive disorder is different from organic mental disorder or schizophrenia. It is sorted out to mild depression in the world, and in TCM it belongs to the category of *yu zheng* (melancholia).

In addition, poststroke depression is one of the complications after cerebrovascular accidents. It has been reported that the incidence is about 25%–60%, while the rate of missed diagnosis is 75%. The main symptoms are a low mood, thought slowness, and reduction in speech and movement.

Acupuncture treatment for depression began in the mid-1980s, and more related reports have appeared in recent years. Much experience has also been accumulated. Electroacupuncture is the most commonly used method, and scalp needling and moxibustion are also available.

Treatment

Electroacupuncture

Selection of points: Commonly used points — *baihui* (DU 20) and *yintang* (EX-HN3). Supplementary points — *yamen* (DU 15) and *tiantu* (RN 22) added for melancholy and taciturnity; *taixi* (KI 3) and *neiguan* (PC 6) for insomnia and amnesia; *sanyinjiao* (SP 6) and *taichong* (LR 3) for anxiety and irritation; *shaoshang* (LU 11) and *shixuan* (EX-UE11) for sluggishness and inactiveness.

Manipulation: Generally, commonly used points are employed, and supplementary points are added for cases with severe symptoms. Sterilize the local skin and the filiform needles, which are inserted into *baihui* (DU 20) obliquely forward to 5–8 *fen*, and into *yintang* (EX-HN3) obliquely upward to 5–8 *fen*, combined with a 701-IIA electric needling therapeutic device with a frequency of 80–90 cpm, or a G6805 electroacupuncture apparatus with an irregular wave, voltage 6 V, frequency 6–8 Hz, and output current to a limit where muscle contracts slightly and which the patient can tolerate. Supplementary points are given uniform reinforcing–reducing manipulation without electroacupuncture. Usually, the treatment is applied once daily, for 45–60 min each time, six times a week except for Sundays, for six weeks as a course. Effective cases may be given a second course according to the patient's condition, to enhance or strengthen the curative effect.

Body acupuncture

Selection of points: Commonly used points — *zhisanzhen, shouzhizhen*, and *siguanxue*. Location of *zhisanzhen*: three points — one is the junction of the anterior hairline and the midline of the head, and the other two are 3 *cun* bilateral to the first point. *Shouzhizhen* consisting of *neiguan* (PC 6), *shenmen* (HT 7) and *laogong* (PC 8). *Siguanxue* consisting of *hegu* (LI 4) and *taichong* (LR 3). Supplementary points — *shenmen* (HT 7), *sanyinjiao* (SP 6), *taixi* (KI 3), *daling* (PC 7) and *yinbai* (SP 1).

Manipulation: Either group is employed at each session, and the two groups alternately or together. Two or three supplementary points may be added according to symptoms. *Zhisanzhen* points are inserted into horizontally with 1.5-*cun*-long No. 28 filiform needles to 1.5 *cun* with strong stimulation, with the needles retained for 1–2 h; *shouzhizhen* points are given routine manipulation till the arrival of *qi*, with the needles retained for 30 min, during which manipulate them once every 5–10 min; *siguanxue* points are punctured with filiform needles, followed by inducing *qi* on the arrival of *qi*, i.e. slow lifting and slow thrusting. Breathe deeply through the nose six times and repeat that after 1 min of rest, until withdrawal of the needles. The needles are retained for 30 min during which manipulate them once every 10 min. Routine acupuncture is applied to supplementary points, with a retention of 30 min. The treatment is performed twice a week, for eight weeks on end.

Remarks

Depressive neurosis is one of the affective disorders, and so requires persuasion of spirit and emotion to help in the treatment; music, physical exercises, mesmerism and suggestion therapies are also available for achieving self-relaxation, a cheerful mood and regulation of *qi* activity, and the strengthening of acupuncture helps patients recover earlier. Electroacupuncture is applied not only to treatment of depressive neurosis (mild depression), but also to medium and severe depression. In doing so, electric pulse stimulation should not be too strong or last for a long period. Body acupuncture is mainly applicable to depressive neurosis, as well as poststroke depression.

DELAYING SENILITY

Overview

Delaying senility and promoting longevity is the common ideal of humankind. There is no final answer as to how long a human being can live on earth, but according to scientists it should be at least 120 years. Therefore, preventing senilism and delaying aging has become one of the important issues facing modern preventive medicine.

It is believed in TCM that premature aging is related to deficiency of kidney essence, decline of vital gate fire, and yang *qi* deficiency, which leads to *qi* deficiency and blood insufficiency, and yin and yang disequilibrium promotes some senile syndromes, like luxated teeth, loss of hair, blurred vision and deafness. Acupuncture therapy works to assist kidney yang, generate *qi* and blood, dredge the channels, and balance yin and yang, and therefore has been an important method for healthcare, delaying aging and lengthening human life. Since premature aging is the result of various physiological, psychological and social factors, acupuncture for delaying aging is to prevent or cure diseases leading to premature aging or consequences like stroke or coronary heart disease, which have been introduced in previous chapters; on the other hand, acupuncture stimulation of different acupoints is applied to enhance the disease resistance of the body, regulate human physiological function, maintain health and lengthen human life.

Treatment

Ginger moxibustion

Selection of points: Zusanli (ST 36).

Manipulation: Bilateral points are employed. Locate them exactly and mark them with gentian violet. Put a slice of fresh ginger 1.5 cm in diameter and 2–3 mm in thickness on the points, respectively. Moxa cones 1 cm in diameter and 350 mg in weight are ignited and put on the ginger slices, during which try to avoid burning the skin. When the patient complains of burning heat, pat the skin around the point or lift a little the ginger. Each point requires seven cones. The moxibustion is applied once daily, six times on end, at an interval of one day. A course of treatment lasts three months.

Mild-warming moxibustion

Selection of points: Shenque (RN 8), and *zusanli* (ST 36).

Manipulation: Shenque (RN 8) and *zusanli* (ST 36) on both sides are employed at each session for mild-warming moxibustion with moxa sticks for 10 min at each point, until the local skin becomes reddish. The treatment is applied once every other day, for two months as a course.

Acupuncture and moxibustion

Selection of points: Commonly used point — *zusanli* (ST 36). Supplementary points — *qihai* (RN 6) and *guanyuan* (RN 4).

Manipulation: One commonly used point and one supplementary point are employed at each session for acupuncture and moxibustion once daily or once every other day, in which *zusanli* (ST 36) (bilateral) is punctured with 1.5-*cun*-long No. 30 filiform needles by rapid insertion with mild stimulation, and slow–rapid reinforcing–reducing manipulation is applied by slow thrusting and rapid lifting for 1 min. For a weak constitution, sparrow-pecking moxibustion is applied with moxa sticks in addition to acupuncture. *Guanyuan* (RN 4) and *qihai* (RN 6) are alternately given revolving moxibustion with moxa sticks for 3–5 min, until the local skin becomes reddish. The treatment is applied once daily or once every other day, at 15–30 sessions as a course, at an interval of 15 days between courses.

Body acupuncture

Selection of points: Commonly used points — *jiankang-changshou-xue*. Supplementary points — *baihui* (DU 20), *qihai* (RN 6), *guanyuan* (RN 4), *zusanli* (ST 36), *sanyinjiao* (SP 6), *dazhui* (DU 14), *pishu* (BL 20) and *shenshu* (BL 23). Location of *jiankang-changshou-xue*: upper top of the philtrum groove under the nose.

Manipulation: Commonly used point is employed at each session, and three or four supplementary points are added according to symptoms, with the points selected alternately. The commonly used point is punctured with a 1-*cun*-long No. 28 filiform needle obliquely toward the nasal septum, twirling and rotating swiftly to induce a sensation of soreness and distension. Other points are given routine acupuncture with 1.5-*cun*-long No. 28 filiform needles till the arrival of *qi*, lifting, thrusting, twirling and rotating slightly. The needles are retained in each point for 15–20 min. The treatment is applied once every other day, 20 times as a course, but twice a week from the second course, then reducing to once a week for half a year.

Drug-cake-separated moxibustion

Selection of points: Commonly used points — *danzhong* (RN 17), *zhongwan* (RN 20), *shenque* (RN 8), *guanyuan* (RN 4) and *zusanli* (ST 36). Supplementary points — *dazhui* (DU 14), *shenshu* (BL 23) and *pishu* (BL 20).

Manipulation: The drug cake is made of Huangqi (*Radix Astragali*), Danggui (*Radix Angelicae Sinensis*), Buguzhi (*Fructus Psoraleae*), Yinyanghuo (*Herba Epimedii*), Dahuang (*Radix et Rhizoma Rhei*) and Danshen (*Radix et Rhizoma Salviae Miltiorrhizae*), which are ground to powder, sieved by a 120-mesh sieve, and mixed evenly in 80% alcohol, to make cakes 3 cm in diameter and 0.8 cm in thickness with a drug cake mold. The cup-shaped moxa cone is made of moxa wool weighing about 1.2 g.

Manipulation: Commonly used points are employed, or alternately used with supplementary points, three points on both sides at each session, three cones for each point, once every other day for 24 times as a course.

Remarks

Moxibustion is the most important therapy for delaying senility, so here three moxibustion methods and one combined method with acupuncture and moxibustion have been introduced. Ginger moxibustion is usually applicable to the healthy elderly regardless of age, who are advised to take moxibustion for two or three courses. Mild-warming moxibustion, also applicable to the healthy elderly, is for postponing the decline of recent memory, improve the senile balance ability, improve the cardiac function, and delay visual accommodation function and skeletal muscle aging. Drug-cake-separated moxibustion is applicable to cases with yang deficiency syndrome and is able to improve symptoms like soreness and weakness of the waist and knees, aversion to cold and extremity cold, fatigue, frequent nocturia, forgetfulness and insomnia. Acupuncture and moxibustion is mainly applied to patients who fail to respond to moxibustion alone. In the early stage, it is performed for one course and from the second course the treatment should be applied once a week. Acupuncture is effective for delaying aging, but is not suitable for the old who are weak or fear pain because of the strong sensation induced by acupuncture.

QUESTIONS

(1) What are the respective characteristics of electroacupuncture and moxibustion in preventing subhealth conditions?
(2) What are the characteristics of point selection in eliminating depression?
(3) Describe the characteristics of the three moxibustion therapies in delaying senility.

Index